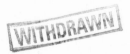

Microbial Diseases
of Fish

Special Publications of the Society for General Microbiology

Publications Officer: Colin Ratledge, 62 London Road, Reading, UK.

1. Coryneform Bacteria,
      eds. I. J. Bousfield and A. G. Callely

2. Adhesion of Microorganisms to Surfaces,
      eds. D. C. Ellwood, J. Melling and P. Rutter

3. Microbial Polysaccharides and Polysaccharases,
      eds. R. C. W. Berkeley, G. W. Gooday and D. C. Ellwood

4. The Aerobic Endospore-forming Bacteria:
   Classification and Identification,
      eds. R. C. W. Berkeley and M. Goodfellow

5. Mixed Culture Fermentations,
      eds. M. E. Bushell and J. H. Slater

6. Bioactive Microbial Products: Search and Discovery,
      eds. J. D. Bu'Lock, L. J. Nisbet and D. J. Winstanley

7. Sediment Microbiology,
      eds. D. B. Nedwell and C. M. Brown

8. Sourcebook of Experiments for the Teaching of Microbiology,
      eds. S. B. Primrose and A. C. Wardlaw

9. Microbial Diseases of Fish,
      ed. R. J. Roberts

This book is based on a Symposium of the Pathogenicity Group of the S.G.M. held at Edinburgh, 17th September 1981.

Microbial Diseases of Fish

Edited by

R. J. Roberts

University of Stirling,
Scotland, UK

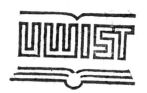

1982
Published for the
Society for General Microbiology
by
ACADEMIC PRESS
A Subsidiary of Harcourt Brace Jovanovich, Publishers
London   New York
Paris   San Diego   San Francisco   São Paulo
Sydney   Tokyo   Toronto

ACADEMIC PRESS INC. (LONDON) LTD.
24/28 Oval Road
London NW1

United States Edition published by
ACADEMIC PRESS INC.
111 Fifth Avenue
New York, New York 10003

British Library Cataloguing in Publication Data
Microbial diseases of fish. — (Special publications
   of the Society for General Microbiology; 9)
   1. Fishes — Diseases — Congresses
   2. Fishes — Microbiology — Congresses
   I. Roberts, R.J.   II. Series
   597.2   SH171

   ISBN 0-12-589660-3

   LCCCN 82-72335

Phototypeset by Dobbie Typesetting Service, Plymouth, Devon, England
Printed by Thomson Litho, East Kilbride, Scotland

Contributors

C. AGIUS   *Institute of Aquaculture, University of Stirling, Stirling FK9 4LA, U.K.*

D. J. ALDERMAN   *Ministry of Agriculture, Fisheries and Food, Directorate of Fisheries Research, Fish Diseases Laboratory, Weymouth, Dorset DT4 8UB, U.K.*

A. E. ELLIS   *Department of Agriculture and Fisheries for Scotland, Marine Laboratory, P.O. Box 101, Victoria Road, Aberdeen AB9 8DB, U.K.*

MARY F. GRACE   *Department of Zoology, University of Hull, Hull HU6 7RX, U.K. (Present address: Institute of Aquaculture, University of Stirling, Stirling FK9 4LA, U.K.)*

B. J. HILL   *Ministry of Agriculture, Fisheries and Food, Directorate of Fisheries Research, Fish Diseases Laboratory, The Nothe, Weymouth, Dorset DT4 8UB, U.K.*

MICHAEL T. HORNE   *The University of Stirling, Stirling, U.K.*

MARGARET J. MANNING   *Department of Zoology, University of Hull, Hull HU6 7RX, U.K. (Present address: Department of Biological Sciences, Plymouth Polytechnic, Drake Circus, Plymouth, Devon PL4 8AA, U.K.)*

A. H. McVICAR   *Department of Agriculture and Fisheries for Scotland, Marine Laboratory, P.O. Box 101, Victoria Road, Torry, Aberdeen AB9 8DB, U.K.*

C. MICHEL   *Laboratoire d'Icthyopathologie, I.N.R.A., Route de Thiverval, 78850 Thiverval-Grignon, France.*

A. L. S. MUNRO   *Department of Agriculture and Fisheries for Scotland, Marine Laboratory, P.O. Box 101, Victoria Road, Aberdeen AB9 8DB, U.K.*

A. D. PICKERING   *Freshwater Biological Association, Windermere Laboratory, The Ferry House, Far Sawrey, Nr. Ambleside, Cumbria LA22 0UP, U.K.*

CHRISTOPHER J. SECOMBES   *Department of Zoology, University of Hull, Hull HU6 7RX, U.K. (Present address: Department of Zoology, University of Aberdeen, Aberdeen AB9 1AS, U.K.)*

P. D. WARD   *Wellcome Research Laboratories, Langley Court, Beckenham, Kent, U.K.*

L. G. WILLOUGHBY   *Freshwater Biological Association, Windermere Laboratory, The Ferry House, Far Sawrey, Nr. Ambleside, Cumbria LA22 0LP, U.K.*

KENNETH E. WOLF   *United States Department of the Interior, Fish and Wildlife Service, National Fish Health Research Laboratory, Box 700, Kearneysville, West Virginia 25430, U.S.A.*

Editor's Foreword

The study of fish microbial diseases has recently been greatly accelerated by the rapid growth of both marine and freshwater fish culture, since the importance of epizootics, and equally of low grade chronic infections, in affecting the profitability of an enterprise, has justified considerable expansion of microbial research facilities in Universities, Government Institutions and in commercial companies.

The range of microorganisms involved is very wide and for the newcomer to the field there are many interesting and novel aspects of the subject such as the irridovirus, lymphocystis virus, which stimulates fibroblasts to hypertrophy to a size where they can be clearly seen with the naked eye, and *Ichthyophonus*, the subject of a major review in this volume, over which there is still considerable dispute as to whether it is in fact a fungus or a protozoan. However, the principles of the subject and the techniques used are all modifications of the standard techniques of medical and veterinary microbiology, and thus there is likely to be much of interest to the general microbiologist in the proceedings of this the thirty-second symposium of the Society for General Microbiology.

It is thoroughly appropriate that this symposium, which in many ways marks a coming of age of the subject, should have been held in the University of Edinburgh, for it was here that possibly the most significant of all fish bacteriological studies was carried out, the extensive study on furunculosis by Professor Mackie and his colleagues. This work which formed the basis of the famous Furunculosis Report to the British Government, is rightly recognized as a major milestone in fish pathology.

Another aspect of the symposium equally appropriate, was the presence, as keynote speaker, of Dr. Ken Wolf, from Leetown, U.S.A. Dr. Wolf isolated the first fish virus, IPN virus, in 1959 and he has been largely responsible for most of the subsequent development of both poikilotherm tissue culture and virology.

The role of the Society for General Microbiology in setting up this most agreeable symposium is greatly appreciated by all fish microbiologists and it is hoped that these proceedings will act as both a guide to the subject and a stimulus to the further development of this fascinating aspect of microbiology.

February 1982   Ronald J Roberts

Contents

1

Differences Between the Immune Mechanisms of Fish and Higher Vertebrates

A. E. ELLIS

DAFS Marine Laboratory
Victoria Road, Aberdeen, Scotland, U.K.

Introduction

During the past decade a considerable interest in the immune mechanisms of bony fish (teleosts) has been generated. Initially this interest followed the rapid expansion of fish farming and the need to control disease in fish farms. It was soon discovered, however, that fish provided a valuable experimental animal for study by comparative immunologists, where work has contributed significantly to an understanding of immune mechanisms in general, especially in the field of ontogeny and development of immune mechanisms and in the field of T lymphocyte antigen-receptors. Some work has been done with fish other than teleosts such as the Agnatha, Chondrichthyes, Holocephali and Dipnoa. Immune mechanisms differ between all these groups and a comparison of such could form a topic unto itself. However, this review will be restricted mainly to the immune mechanisms in teleosts and a comparison of them with higher vertebrates.

In contrasting the fish system with the higher vertebrates (principally the mammal) I hope not merely to indicate that the immune system of the fish is more primitive than that of the mammal, though this is indeed the case in that it is less complex, but to interpret the function of the immune system of the fish in regard to the needs of the fish. In such a way we may gain greater insight into how the system works and possibly discover important ways of manipulating conditions conducive to the optimum development of immunity in fish.

An important aspect of such an approach is the ontogenetic development of the immune system and this is dealt with in greater detail in the chapter by Dr Manning and her colleagues. Other aspects will be presented here. Some of the topics such as the work on T-like lymphocyte antigen-receptors may prove important in understanding issues of significance to general

1

immunology. I am sure that work on the fishes, the most primitive of vertebrates, will continue to be of value in this regard. Other topics are addressed mainly to the field of fish immunology where the mechanisms are quite different from those of the mammal and peculiar to the fish. Such areas, of importance to those of us concerned with fish diseases, are in urgent need of further research and I hope to highlight some of these, such as antigen-processing, factors affecting antibody production, inter-relationships between specific and non-specific immune mechanisms, inflammation and hypersensitivity responses, in order to stimulate such studies.

Stem Cells

In adult anurans and all other higher vertebrates, haemopoietic stem cells, capable of reconstituting all lymphoid organs, are found in the bone marrow (Cooper et al., 1980). Fish do not possess bone marrow. However, haemopoietic bone marrow-like microenvironments are well developed in the kidney and spleen of the teleosts and, in the Chondrichthyes (sharks and rays), in a variety of other organs such as the oesophageal wall (Leydig's organ), the liver and the gonads (Ellis, 1977a; Zapata, 1979, 1980; Fänge, 1981).

There is no available experimental data concerning the source of stem cells in fish but in teleosts the kidney would appear important on onto-genetic and histological criteria. Haemopoiesis is first seen in the kidney, early in ontogeny, though erythrocytes and macrophages are present before differentiation of the kidney so the yolk sac is probably the earliest organ of limited haemopoiesis (Ellis, 1977b; Grace et al., 1980). Lymphocytes do not appear until the thymus has become lymphoid. In the Salmonidae this is a few days before hatching (Ellis, 1977b; Grace et al., 1980) whereas in the plaice (*Pleuronectes platessa*) this does not occur until the time of metamorphosis (Lele, 1933).

How is the fish kidney possibly analogous to higher vertebrate bone marrow in fulfilling the needs of haemopoietic stem cell differentiation? Two requirements for stem cell differentiation may be of importance in this regard. These are the great radio sensitivity of stem cells and their requirement as free cells loosely aggregated, for a low pressure and slow-moving blood supply, i.e. sinuses.

The vertebrate kidney arose as a filtration–excretory organ which would inevitably also filter antigenic material from the circulating fluids. It would seem advantageous if the cells responsive to antigens (lymphocytes and phagocytes) gathered in this filter bed. A microenvironment suitable for the differentiation of progenitors of these cells would suitably be supplied by development of a low pressure renal-portal system like that found in the teleost kidney (Randall, 1970). In respect to the radiation-sensitivity of stem cells, the aquatic environment provides a good shield to environmental radiation (Cooper *et al.*, 1980) but the large amounts of melanin present in the fish kidney (see below) and its anatomical situation under the vertebral column may also assist in radiation shielding.

Structure and Function of the Kidney

The kidney of fish differentiates ontogenetically in two phases. The first to develop is the pronephros, or head kidney, which loses its excretory function as the opisthonephros develops. The latter forms the bulk of the adult organ and contains the excretory tubules. Both parts of the kidney contain a generalized haemopoietic tissue, rich in lymphoid cells and granulocytes (Ellis, 1976), which resembles bone marrow in many respects (Zapata, 1979). However, unlike bone marrow, the kidney haemopoietic tissue contains many antibody producing cells and phagocytes (Rijkers *et al.*, 1980) and following antigenic stimulation many pyroninophilic cells appear, often in large clusters (Secombes *et al.*, 1982). Thus, the kidney tissue performs functions which are associated with both mammalian bone marrow and lymph nodes.

Pigment-containing cells are commonly found in the kidney of fish. Most of this pigment is melanin but variable amounts of lipofuscin and haemosiderin are also present (Ellis, 1977a; Agius, 1979). In the Salmonidae, the pigment-containing cells are scattered randomly throughout the tissue while in other teleosts they are frequently aggregated into so-called melano-macrophage centres (Agius, 1980). Most of the pigment-bearing cells appear to be macrophages and Roberts (1975) designated them melano-macrophages. More recently, George and Wolke (in preparation) have identified some of the pigment-bearing cells as melanocytes.

Also present within the melano-macrophage aggregates are lymphocytes and antibody-containing cells. Small circulating lymphocytes have been reported to 'home' onto the melano-macrophage aggregates where they are metabolically active in RNA synthesis (Ellis and de Sousa, 1974). The function of these pigmented cells is unknown but they will be discussed in more detail in the sections dealing with the spleen and inflammatory responses below.

Structure and Function of the Spleen

The spleen is the last organ to become lymphoid during ontogeny in teleosts and develops a lymphoid population about the time of first feeding (Ellis, 1977b; van Loon et al., 1980; Grace et al., 1980). An arterial supply divides into narrow-lumened capillaries which ramify throughout the organ. These capillaries (ellipsoids) possess a thick wall composed of reticulin fibres and macrophages (Ellis et al., 1976). The ellipsoid capillaries open into red pulp sinuses which drain into the splenic venous system. Reticulin fibres extend from the ellipsoid sheath through the splenic white pulp which is rarely well developed in the teleosts. Also enmeshed in these reticulin fibres are melano-macrophage centres which are believed to originate in the ellipsoid walls (Ferguson, 1976; Secombes et al., 1982). The presence, arrangement and content of pigment cells in the spleen are similar to that already described for the kidney except that the iron content is more characteristic of pigment cells in the spleen (Agius, 1979).

The spleen also contains many antibody-producing cells (Rijkers et al., 1980) and, following antigenic stimulation, clusters of pyroninophilic cells appear in the ellipsoid walls. Observations suggest that these clusters may develop into melano-macrophage aggregates (Secombes et al., 1982).

The ellipsoid walls are important in phagocytosis and antigen-trapping. Colloidal carbon particles are rapidly phagocytosed by the ellipsoid macrophages which, when replete, migrate into existing melano-macrophage aggregates or form neo-aggregates (Ellis et al., 1976). Soluble protein antigens such as bovine serum albumin (BSA) and human gamma-globulin (HGG) appear to be trapped as immune complexes on the reticulin fibres of the ellipsoid walls where they are retained for prolonged periods (Ellis, 1980; Secombes and Manning, 1980; Secombes et al., 1980). This trapping of antigen on reticulin fibres should be confirmed by ultrastructural studies but if found to be true this phenomenon would be very different from the trapping of antigen on dendritic cells in higher vertebrates (Baldwin and Cohen, 1980; van Rooijen, 1980). The functional significance of antigen-trapping in mammals is thought to be involved with the development of immune-memory (Klaus et al., 1980) but its functional significance in fish awaits investigation.

Structure and Function of the Thymus

The thymus of teleosts is, in most species, an extremely superficial, paired organ being located immediately below the epithelium in the dorsoposterior part of the branchial cavity. It is the first organ to become lymphoid and in *Salmo salar* it arises, prior to hatching, as three separate buds dorsal to the first three gill arches as collections of lymphoid cells in the pharyngeal epithelium external to the basement membrane. Subsequently, the thymus buds grow and coalesce into a single organ on either side of the fish and by the third day prior to hatching the mass of the organ is located over the third gill arch and is contained within a thin connective tissue capsule (Ellis, 1977b). In some species such as the plaice, lymphoid differentiation does not occur until metamorphosis of the larvae (Lele, 1933). Here is an interesting example of a vertebrate which, in its early free-living stages, does not possess a lymphoid system. Furthermore, Grace *et al.* (1980), in an ultrastructural study of the rainbow trout (*Salmo gairdneri*) thymus, have found that the external surface of the organ is covered only by a single layer of epithelium which has no apparent specialization. This very superficial location of the thymus and its late development in some species of fish suggests the thymus may not be well protected from antigenic material and poses interesting questions as to the functional importance of excluding foreign material from the thymus with regard to the possibility of inducing tolerance.

With regard to these developmental differences between the thymus of fish and mammals, is there any evidence that the thymus of fish is a primary lymphoid organ? The thymus is composed principally of mitotically active and differentiating lymphocytes with small numbers of macrophages and epithelioid cells. There is little differentiation into cortex and medulla, and antibody producing cells are not present (Bogner and Ellis, 1977). Foreign material such as colloidal carbon or bovine serum albumin (BSA) injected parenterally cannot be detected in the thymus (Ellis *et al.*, 1976; Ellis, 1980) and circulating lymphocytes do not migrate through the thymus (Ellis and de Sousa, 1974). Although experimental evidence of the kind that neonatal thymectomy has afforded in higher vertebrates is lacking for fish, thymectomy performed in two-month-old rainbow trout was found to lead to a prolongation of allograft rejection (Grace, 1981). Involution of the fish thymus with age is well documented. In the rainbow trout this occurs at about the onset of maturity but in the plaice it appears to be a more prolonged process (Lele, 1933). Thus, the thymus of fish has many features of a primary, non-executive lymphoid organ as in mammals. However, as far as this may be true for antibody producing cells, the results of Ruben *et al.* (1977) deserve further study. These workers found that in goldfish injected intraperitoneally (i.p.) with sheep erythrocytes (Srbc) in low dose amounts, antigen-binding cells (ABC), though not antibody-secreting cells, appeared in the thymus and the numbers peaked earlier (day 4) in the thymus than in the kidney or spleen (days 6–10). This kind of responsiveness to antigens is not found in the mammalian thymus. As low-dose carrier priming was also most conducive to stimulating T helper function in the goldfish, the authors suggested these ABC in the thymus may be T helper cells (see also below) which differentiated intra-thymically in the fish rather than extra-thymically, as in the mammal. The implication that antigen can exert positive immunological effects in the thymus of fish raises many questions concerning the applicability to the fish of the concept that the thymus in mammals is closed to foreign antigens and where antigen-responsive lymphocyte clones which may arise in the thymus from somatic mutation are deleted (Jerne, 1980).

Other evidence suggests that the thymocytes of fish may not be comprised only of T-like cells but that B-like cells may also be present. The question of T and B cells in fish will now be considered.

Lymphocyte Subpopulations in Fish — The Question of T and B Cells

Three main lines of enquiry have been undertaken to investigate the existence of T and B-like lymphocytes in fish. These are the presence of membrane-bound immunoglobulins (mIg), responsiveness to mitogens and the carrier-hapten effect to detect helper cells. All of these give rise to arguments for the existence of lymphocyte subpopulations similar to T and B cells by analogy with higher vertebrates. The necessary experiments to prove this directly (thymic ablation in the embryo and reconstitution with labelled syngeneic cells) have not been done. Though such is the case, present data are strongly suggestive of the existence of T-like and B-like populations in fish.

The Presence of Membrane-bound Immunoglobulin (mIg)

Fish appear to be unique amongst vertebrates in that in adults, lymphocytes from all organs (thymus, kidney, spleen and blood) possess mIg detectable by immunofluorescent (IF) techniques (Ellis and Parkhouse, 1975; Emmrich et al., 1975; Etlinger et al., 1976; Clem et al., 1977; Warr et al., 1977; Warr and Marchalonis, 1980). This observation is different from that obtained in adults of all higher vertebrates where only the B lymphocytes are positive for mIg by IF and similar techniques (Warr, 1980). This raises several important issues including the existence of T and B-like cells in fish and also the question of the mechanism of immune recognition by T cells in general, which is still a point of contention amongst mammalian immunologists. However, a word must first be said concerning the validity of the observation in fish.

It has been shown that anti-Ig antisera can react with the carbohydrate moiety of the IgM molecule and this may cross-react with non-IgM carbohydrate groups in the lymphocyte membrane. Yamaga *et al.* (1978) described a cross-reaction of rabbit antisera to rainbow trout IgM with L-fucose and these authors cautioned that the immunofluorescent reaction with trout thymocytes could be due to this cross-reactivity and not to the presence of mIgM. Albeit, immunochemical data have confirmed the presence of mIg on thymocytes of fish using radioimmunoassay and extraction procedures (Warr and Marchalonis, 1980; Fiebig *et al.*, 1980) which have also provided evidence of lymphocyte subpopulations in fish. The mIgM of fish kidney lymphocytes occurs in a monomeric form as two heavy and two light (2H2L) chains and also as an HL subunit. In contrast, the thymocyte mIgM lacks the L chain. Instead, the molecule is thought to consist of two H chains covalently linked. These may dimerize non-covalently as a 4H unit (Fiebig *et al.*, 1980). While these immunochemical data appear convincing, recent work with monoclonal antibodies to catfish Ig reveal that no more than 35% of catfish lymphocytes possess mIg by immunofluorescence studies (L. W. Clem, personal communication). Further work is in progress to solve this controversy but if it is proved that thymocytes (or T cells) do possess mIg what are the implications?

Does the mIg on fish lymphocytes act as an antigen receptor? No conclusive evidence exists to confirm this but anti-IgM antisera inhibit antigen-binding by lymphocytes from all anatomical sites in fish (Ruben *et al.*, 1977; Azzolina, 1978; DeLuca *et al.*, 1978). Also, use of double-fluorescent label techniques have demonstrated that anti-IgM antibody (in non-inhibiting concentration), and antigen co-distribute on the membrane surface (DeLuca *et al.*, 1978; Warr and Marchalonis, 1980). These data do not prove that the antigen-receptor and mIgM are the same but they do suggest that at least they are in very close proximity to each other.

If it is accepted that all vertebrates possess an adaptive immune system based on immunoglobulins, it would seem unlikely that antigen-specific recognition molecules other than immunoglobulins would have arisen. Hence the observations that all fish lymphocytes possess mIg and that a functional dichotomy into T and B-like cells already exists in fish (Ruben and Edwards, 1980) strongly suggest that Ig plays a universal role in immune recognition in vertebrates. The reason why Ig has not been readily detected in T cells in mammals may be failure of the anti-Ig antisera to recognize determinants in relatively evolutionarily conserved regions (such as the variable region) of Ig molecules of closely related species. Using the principle of phylogenetic distance whereby species of different classes rather than genera might be expected to recognize such determinants, Warr *et al.* (1980) have been able to demonstrate the presence of mIg in the thymocytes of rodents using an anti-Ig antiserum prepared in chickens. There is now growing evidence that antibodies directed to isotype determinants of Ig do not react with mammalian T cells while, on the other hand, antibodies to the combining-site region determinants of Ig can react with T cell-associated molecules (Warr *et al.*, 1980). This may reflect the orientation of the Ig molecule in the lymphocyte membrane. Whether the apparent ease of detection of mIg on fish thymocytes is a reflection of a greater exposure of the molecule in fish than in higher vertebrates or of the principle of phylo-genetic distance, or both, or a complete artifact is yet to be determined.

Lymphocyte Responses to Mitogens

The proliferation responses of different lymphocyte populations to different mitogens have proved very useful in distinguishing T and B lymphocytes in mammals. Similar work with fish lymphocytes so far remains inconclusive and, while evidence for lymphocyte subpopulations in fish has been forthcoming, some interesting differences in the distribution of these populations between certain fish species and mammals appears to exist.

Etlinger *et al.* (1976) studied the responses of rainbow trout lymphocytes from different anatomical sites to a variety of mitogens. It was found that the species origin of the serum supplement to the culture medium was important. Lipopolysaccharide (LPS) and purified protein derivative (PPD), both mammalian B cell mitogens, caused proliferative responses in lymphocytes from spleen and blood when the culture medium contained rainbow trout serum (RTS), whereas only peripheral blood lymphocytes (PBL) responded in medium supplemented with foetal bovine serum (FBS). Anterior kidney cells responded only to LPS and only when the medium was supplemented with RTS. Thymocytes did not respond to LPS or PPD in either serum supplement. Concanavalin A (Con A) stimulated lymphocytes from all the lymphoid organs in medium supplemented with RTS and, with the exception of cells from the anterior kidney, also stimulated cells from each tissue in medium supplemented with FBS. These findings, that the patterns of mitogenic responses of cells from different tissues were significantly different, suggested that lymphocyte heterogeneity existed in rainbow trout and that they had a unique tissue distribution.

The above results are similar to those expected by analogy with mammalian responses, for a T and B cell dichotomy. However, Cuchens and Clem (1977) were unable to find a similar distributional dichotomy in the blue gill *Lepomis macrochirus*, in that the thymocytes, as well as lymphocytes from other organs, were stimulated by both T cell mitogens (phytohaemagglutinin (PHA) and Con A) and also by the B cell mitogen LPS. Nevertheless, further evidence was reported which suggested that the cells responding to the different mitogens belonged to distinct populations. In all tissues, there was a differential effect of temperature on the mitogenic responses. At low temperature (22°C) the mitogenic effect of PHA and Con A was either markedly decreased (in the case of the thymocytes) or completely abolished (in the case of the anterior kidney) in comparison with stimulation at 32°C. Conversely, the mitogenic response to LPS was either unaffected (in the case of anterior kidney) or enhanced (in the case of the thymus) by lowering the temperature of incubation from 32° to 22°C. Also, on examination of the anterior kidney cells, it was shown that the cells responding to PHA and Con A contained surface antigens in common with blue gill brain and did not form spontaneous rosettes with rabbit erythrocytes while the converse was the case for the cells which responded to LPS.

This pattern of mitogenic responses and brain-antigen distribution coupled with observations that mixed lymphocyte responses were obtained at 32°C but not at 22°C strongly suggests that the PHA/Con A responsive cell population represents the fish equivalent of T cells. The other population may be B cell equivalents. These results raise two significant points. Firstly, the greater temperature dependency of the putative T cell response as compared with the B cell response, which will be discussed further below, and secondly, the finding that the thymus apparently contains both putative T and B cells. This contrasts with the work of Etlinger et al. (1976) on the rainbow trout and may reflect a species difference but further work on the fish thymus cell populations, especially functional studies, are needed before definitive statements can be made concerning lymphocyte populations in the periphery or in the thymus of fish. One such approach has so far been carried out and the significance of this will now be discussed.

Helper Cell Function — The Carrier/Hapten Effect

It is now well established in mammals that a population of T cells performs a helper function in the antigen stimulation of B cells to produce antibody to most antigens (T-dependent antigens). The carrier effect is generally accepted as a means of detecting cells that do not produce antibody (the carrier-reactive T cell) but which act as helper cells in the induction of antibody production by the hapten-reactive B cell. The demonstration of a carrier effect requires that an antibody response to a hapten conjugated to a carrier antigen should be elicited only in animals pre-immunized with the same carrier. Using a variety of antigens, such carrier effects have been demonstrated in the winter flounder *Pseudopleuronectes americanus* (Stolen and Makala, 1976) and in the goldfish *Carassius auratus* (Warr et al., 1977; Ruben et al., 1977). These studies have also helped to throw light on the phenomenon of antigen-reactive cells in the fish thymus already referred to and also the effects of temperature and antigen dose on the induction of helper cell function in fish (see below).

Immunoglobulins of Fish: Structure and Function

Immunoglobulins (Ig) are found in most of the tissue fluids in fish (plasma, lymph, skin and gut mucus and bile). In the blood, they comprise about 40–50% of the total serum proteins which in the brown trout, *S. trutta*, range from 4.5–10.8g 100ml^{-1} (Ingram and Alexander, 1977). In immunoelectrophoresis, the immunoglobulins are found in the gamma and beta regions (Ingram and Alexander, 1980).

The blood vascular system of fish is evidently quite permeable to serum Ig. Mackie and Wardle (1971) demonstrated that in polyacrylamide-gel electrophoresis, the protein content of the serum and that of lymph from the neural lymphatic duct of the plaice *Pleuronectes platessa*, was qualitatively identical and the lymph contained as high as 80% of the protein concentration of the blood plasma (Wardle, 1971). This situation contrasts with the mammalian condition where tissue (afferent) lymph, under normal circumstances, contains very little Ig.

Little work has been done on the half-life of serum antibody in fish. From kinetic studies of antibody titres in the carp, Avtalion *et al.* (1976) calculated the half-life as 12.5 days. However, Voss *et al.* (1980), in radiolabel studies of purified Ig in the coho salmon (*Oncorhynchus kisutch*), found a much lower half-life (about 49 hours at 12°C) though the use of similar techniques in the sheepshead (*Archosargus probatocephalus*) has given half-lives of 16 days for both high molecular weight (HMW) and low molecular weight (LMW) Ig (Lobb and Clem, 1981a).

A striking feature of the fish Ig is the presence of only one class. In terms of heavy chain mass, interchain disulphide bonding, amino acid and carbohydrate content and solution conformation, the fish Ig resembles mammalian IgM (Litman, 1975). The teleost IgM is mainly a HMW molecule composed of 4 subunits of 8 heavy (H) and 8 light (L) chains. It has a sedimentation coefficient of about 16S and approximate molecular weight of 700,000. Some species, for example the plaice (Fletcher and Grant, 1969) and the margate (Clem and McLean, 1975), also possess a 7S monomeric form of IgM, while other species, such as salmonids and carp, only possess the tetrameric form (Shelton and Smith, 1970; Litman, 1975). Chondrichthyean fish also possess only IgM but in a pentameric and monomeric form. Dipnoans (lungfish) are the only group of fish to possess a second Ig class which is a 7S monomer, though controversy exists with regard to the goldfish where a LMW Ig has been reported to be induced by prolonged immunization (Uhr *et al.*, 1962) and to be antigenetically and electrophoretically distinct from the HMW polymer (Trump and Hildemann, 1970). With this exception, all studies have shown the absence of a shift from HMW to LMW Ig in fish during an immune response.

The functional specialization of the different Ig classes in mammals is a property of the structure of the heavy chains which determine the class. Evidence exists for structural heterogeneity of IgM in fish (Lobb and Clem, 1981a) and this raises the question as to the functional repertoire of fish IgM. Exhaustive studies in this field have not yet been done but some data can be mentioned.

Fish antibody, in the presence of normal serum as a complement source, is capable of lysing target cells (Nonaka *et al.*, 1981) and this forms the basis of the plaque antibody assay (Rijkers *et al.*, 1980). Thus, fish Ig is capable of complement activation though few investigations to date have addressed the question of IgM subclasses in respect to complement fixation. A possibility exists that this may be the case. Yamaguchi *et al.* (1980) found seasonal variation in the agglutinating and cytolytic activities of rainbow trout antiserum, even when environmental conditions were maintained constant. While the two assay techniques gave titres which followed similar kinetics when fish were immunized in summer, in winter-immunized fish the cytolytic titres were lower than agglutinating titres. One possible explanation of this is that the agglutinating and cytolytic activity of the trout antibody may be performed by different IgM subclasses.

While agglutinating activity is readily demonstrated by fish, antibody precipitating activity is not. Hodgins *et al.* (1967) found rainbow trout possessed only HMW IgM and could detect passive haemagglutinating antibodies to BSA early in the response but precipitating activity was not detected until much later. Clem and McLean (1975) found that the 16S IgM of the margate (*Haemulon album*) possessed high agglutinating activity to BSA. Similar concentration of the 7S IgM, as measured by antigen-binding capacity in the Farr test, possessed very little agglutinating activity. In the grouper (*Epinephalus tauvina*), the HMW Ig possessed efficient pre-cipitating activity while the LMW Ig did not. It is thus apparent that teleost fish may possess functional subclasses of IgM with differing activities (complement fixing, agglutinating and precipitating) and seasonally variable proportional titres. This should be borne in mind when the type of antibody assay is chosen.

An important function of antibody in mammals is its opsonic activity. This is based on the steric change in conformation of the Fc portion of the antibody molecule on binding antigen and the subsequent binding of the immune-complex by Fc receptors on the surface of phagocytes enabling the complexes to be phagocytosed more readily. Recent studies by Wrathmell and Parrish (1980a) have been unable to find evidence of an opsonic role for fish antibody or the presence of Fc receptors on fish phagocytic cells. These observations have not been confirmed in recent work by Sakai (personal communication) who found opsonizing activity associated with complement and antibody in salmonids. It is possible the conflicting results are due to species differences.

Little work has been done on the IgM found in fish secretions (mucus and bile). Fletcher and Grant (1969) reported that the mucus IgM of plaice was similar to serum IgM. Recently, Lobb and Clem (1981b, c) have reported IgM in the mucus and bile of the sheepshead (*Archosargus probato-cephalus*) a marine teleost. They demonstrated that this IgM was not derived by exudation from the serum Ig pool. Although it was antigenically identical to the serum Ig, several structural differences were noted between the Ig from all these sites. For instance, serum Ig was composed of tetrameric and monomeric forms, while that in the mucus and bile was dimeric. As antibody production can be stimulated systematically or locally, depending on the method of antigen administration (Fletcher and White, 1973), a better understanding of the nature, function and induction of the secretory and systemic IgM may have significant bearing on deciding the most appropriate techniques for use in vaccination programmes.

Finally, the possible existence of a histamine-releasing function for fish IgM is worthy of mention. In mammals, IgE is responsible for mediating the antigen-induced release of histamine from mast cells, an activity which is important in inflammation and allergic responses. IgE has not been identified in fish but criteria for immune anaphylaxis have been reported in the goldfish where behavioural and physiological changes were induced by antigen-specific sensitization which could be transferred to normal fish by injecting serum from a sensitized individual (Goven *et al.*, 1980). Little is understood of the mechanisms of hypersensitivity responses in fish (Ellis, 1981a) but the evidence that antigen-specific systemic sensitization with lethal consequences can occur in fish deserves further study, not least because of the implications for vaccination procedures.

In summary, the fish appears phylogenetically primitive in possessing only a single class of Ig in comparison to at least two and up to five distinct classes in higher vertebrates. It is possible that the evolution of multiple Ig classes, particularly low molecular weight forms, arose to meet the demands for a more efficient vascular system connected with air-breathing and terrestrial locomotion. A higher blood pressure would require tighter junctions between vascular endothelial cells in order to prevent the exudation of plasma fluids and proteins. This would result in the inability of Ig macromolecules to escape into the tissue spaces and would favour low molecular weight Ig forms. The fish is not presented with these problems and its metabolic needs can be met by a vascular system of low hydrostatic pressure and endothelial fenestrations allowing the escape of Ig macro-molecules. In order to maintain the body's integrity, the ectothermal epithelium requires tight intercellular junctions and in this regard it may be significant that the secretory IgM of teleosts is dimeric. Structural hetero-geneity of the IgM in fish is rapidly becoming recognized and much of the functional specialization of the Ig classes in higher vertebrates may be performed by IgM subclasses in the fish.

Factors Affecting the Immune Response in Fish

Temperature

Amongst the best studied and most significant factors affecting the immune response (both humoral and cell mediated) in fish is temperature. Generally speaking, the higher the temperature in the physiologically tolerated range, the faster the onset of the response and the higher its magnitude. At low temperatures there is either a prolongation of the induction period with low antibody titres being reached or a complete absence of a response. The critical temperature for development of an immune response in fish appears to be related to the natural environmental temperatures experienced by a particular species. Hence, the warm water carp may not respond when held at temperatures below 15°C (Avtalion *et al.*, 1976) while in temperate and cold-water species, such as salmonids, the immune response is not inhibited until temperatures reach as low as 4°C (Fryer *et al.*, 1976).

Only certain phases of the antibody response are temperature dependent. Avtalion *et al.* (1976) found that in carp immunized with BSA, normal secondary responses could be elicited at low temperatures so long as primary stimulation was carried out at high temperature. Furthermore, these authors demonstrated that the temperature-dependent phase of the primary response occurred during antibody induction in the first few days after immunization. Thereafter, antibody production was normal and independent of temperature.

Other workers have failed to confirm the all or none effect of temperature. Rijkers *et al.* (1980) reported successful antibody production to sheep red blood cells (Srbc) in the carp at temperatures between 8 and 28°C. However, the ability of the fish to respond in a typical secondary manner was absent when the fish were maintained below 18°C throughout.

Some evidence exists that acclimatization to low temperatures can occur. In this respect, Azzolina (1978) found that goldfish acclimated to 4°C or 22°C and immunized with polymerized flagellar antigens (POL) produced similar numbers of antibody-forming cells. The time course of antibody production was also identical in the two groups but the peak serum antibody titre was lower in the 4°C acclimated group. This was interpreted as reflecting a lower anabolic activity of plasma cells at low temperatures and a more efficient retention of immune capacity to bacterial antigens.

The nature of the antigen may indeed be important (see also below). Cuchens and Clem (1977) reported that responsiveness to T cell mitogens (PHA and Con A) and also mixed leucocyte responses (MLR) in the bluegill were inhibited by low temperatures. Recently, Abruzzini *et al.* (1981) reported results from studies on lymphocyte membrane fluidity and Con A responsiveness in the pinfish (*Lagodon rhomboides*). The lymphocyte membrane fluidity was reduced by lowering the ambient temperature but adaptive changes, probably mediated by changes in the degree of saturation of the membrane lipids, were found to occur with recovery of fluidity in about 12 days. Pinfish lymphocyte responses to Con A were found to be temperature dependent but acclimation of the fish for 2 weeks to the lower temperature regime, allowed the lymphocytes to recover the magnitude of the response although it was still somewhat delayed. No information concerning the temperature adaptation of B cell mitogen responses could be obtained with the experiments on the pinfish but the temperature dependency of T-like cell responsiveness and the lack of it for LPS responsiveness in the blue gill lymphocytes (Cuchens and Clem, 1977) suggests that the homoeoviscous adaptation of T-like cells may be slower, or at least more critical for their responsiveness, than for B-like cells. Thus, responses to T-dependent antigens, like BSA and Srbc may be expected to be affected to a greater degree than T-independent antigens like POL.

In a series of elegant experiments using immunogenically altered forms of BSA, Avtalion *et al.* (1980) have obtained data which are consistent with an interpretation based on the existence of helper and suppressor cells (T cell function) in carp with the induction of helper cell function being preferentially suppressed at low temperatures.

There is much interest in the mechanism of the effect of temperature on the immune response in fish and while there is still much to understand, the data so far can be summarized as follows. The first temperature-dependent phase is thought to involve interaction between T and B-like cells. It has been suggested that the mechanism involves a block of T helper function or an increase in "T suppressor" activity. The subsequent multiplication and differentiation of activated antibody producing cells (B-like cells) is thought to be temperature independent with a final temperature-dependent phase involving the level of antibody production by plasma cells.

The importance of temperature acclimation to the responsiveness of fish lymphocytes has not been a major consideration to workers in either the field of basic or applied research. This should be considered, since by simply raising the temperature at certain times of year when vaccinating fish, an efficient antibody response with long-term memory formation could be achieved where otherwise there would be none. The implications for disease outbreaks may be pronounced. Exposure to antigen at low temperature (winter) may lead to suppression of immunity. This may account for the prevalence of disease outbreaks on fish farms in spring.

Effect of Dose and Route of Administration of Antigen

The magnitude of the primary and secondary response has been reported to be dose and route dependent. Rijkers *et al.* (1980) showed that the priming route, antigen dose and timing of the secondary stimulation were important in determining the magnitude of the primary and secondary antibody response in carp. When the fish were primed intravenously (i.v.), the magnitude of the primary and secondary response to Srbc increased with antigen dose. However, after intramuscular (i.m.) priming, a high dose resulted in a high primary response but poor secondary response. Low-dose priming i.m. resulted in a low primary response but a high secondary response when the booster was given not less than 6 months after primary stimulation. The highest secondary response attained at all times of secondary stimulation (1–10 months) was obtained by primary immunization with an intermediate dose administered i.m.

The high secondary response resulting from low-dose priming may be due to the more effective stimulation of T helper function by low doses of antigen (Trizio and Cudkowicz, 1978). In this regard, Ruben *et al.* (1977) found that low-dose carrier-priming in the goldfish induced the highest carrier effect (T helper function) and the highest numbers of ABC in the thymus.

The route of primary immunization with certain antigens may have drastic consequences in certain species. For example, if carp are given a primary injection of soluble BSA intracardially, antigen-specific tolerance may be induced (Serero and Avtalion, 1978). This was not found to occur if the antigen was injected outwith the vascular system (see also Nature of the Antigen).

Nature of the Antigen

Not all antigens are effective immunogens in fish, particularly soluble protein antigens. Hodgins *et al.* (1967) found that BSA was poorly immunogenic in rainbow trout and bovine gamma globulin elicited no response. However, keyhole limpet haemocyanin was found to be highly immunogenic in this species.

In the carp, Avtalion *et al.* (1980) found that BSA in complete Freund's adjuvant (CFA) was immunogenic but soluble BSA in saline was not, unless the fish had first been primed with BSA in CFA or with acetylated BSA in CFA which is itself non-immunogenic. Furthermore, injection of soluble BSA given intracardially, but not i.p., induced specific tolerance to secondary challenge with BSA in CFA. Tolerance induction was not only route dependent but also dose and temperature dependent. Species variation was also found by these authors, since *Tilapia* spp. were found to be capable of responding to soluble BSA under all variations of dose, route and temperature without induction of tolerance.

Other types of antigens, including viral, bacterial and erythrocyte antigens, appear to be effective immunogens in most teleosts studied.

Seasonal Effects on Antibody Production in Fish

Evidence suggests that many poikilotherms possess endogenous rhythms and even when environmental conditions of light and temperature are kept constant, non-maturing animals still exhibit a seasonally correlated variability of the antibody response (Hussein *et al.*, 1978). Under constant conditions of light and temperature, immature rainbow trout produce lower titres of agglutinating and cytolytic antibodies to *Aeromonas salmonicida* cells when immunized prior to winter as compared with immunization prior to spring (Yamaguchi *et al.*, 1980). The mechanisms of these endogenous rhythms are not understood but they are of obvious significance for vaccination programmes.

The Effect of Social Interactions and Pheromones on Antibody Production in Fish

Several instances of pheromone-induced physiological changes in fish have been reported. One report exists of the immune suppressive effects of a "crowding pheromone" produced by blue gourami (*Trichogaster trichopterus*) when held at high population density (Perlmutter *et al.*, 1973). The suppression of antibody production to IPN virus was removed if the water in which the fish were held was extracted with methylchloroform. The mechanism of this immune suppression is not known but it may be linked to stress. Modulation of immune responses in fish by stress has been reviewed by Ellis (1981c).

Complement in Fish

This very important defence system is known to exist in fish but little is understood concerning its biochemical components, mechanisms of activation and functional significance. Nonaka *et al.* (1981) have demonstrated the ability of trout IgM to fix trout complement and activate its lytic properties. Instances of inter-species incompatibility between complement and antibody is known even amongst mammals (Gigli and Austen, 1971). Similarly, fish antibody–antigen complexes do not activate mammalian complement and data suggest that for antibody-activation of complement the two components must be derived from fairly closely related species (Chiller *et al.*, 1969; Smith *et al.*, 1967; Sakai, 1981a).

The work of Nonaka *et al.* (1981) has shown the complement system in rainbow trout to have many characteristics in common with mammalian complement. For instance, the requirement of Ca^{2+} and Mg^{2+} ions and the presence, on fragments of lysed target cells, of multi-component macro-molecular proteins that had many physicochemical properties in common with the membrane-attack complexes of the complement system of mammals. Furthermore, prior incubation of trout serum with LPS, zymosan or inulin depleted the lytic activity of complement and also, rabbit erythrocytes were lysed by the complement system in the absence of antibody. This suggests that an alternative pathway of complement activation, which was shown to require only Mg^{2+} ions, exists in the trout and is similar to that of mammals.

Some minor differences between trout and mammalian complement were reported (Nonaka *et al.*, 1981). The optimum temperature for trout complement activity was 25°C (that of mammalian complement is 37°C). Also, the protein component of trout complement, which corresponded electrophoretically with mammalian C9 component, was present in much higher proportional concentration than in the mammal. Fish complement is more heat labile than that of mammals. Also, the optimum temperature for 20 minutes to inactivate complement of fish sera differs between species, e.g. 44°C for rainbow trout (*Salmo gairdneri*), 45°C for coho salmon (*Oncorhynchus kisutch*) and goldfish (*Carassius auratus*) and 47°C for tilapia (*Sarotherodon nilotica*) (Sakai, 1981b).

There is more detailed information available of the complement system in sharks. Although the antibody-mediated lytic activity of nurse shark (*Ginglymostoma cirratum*) serum is similar to mammalian, there are major differences in the physicochemical characteristics. Jensen and Festa (1980) purified the components of the nurse shark complement and found only six components of which only three showed compatibility with three of the nine components of mammalian complement. No labile intermediate complexes were found in the nurse shark system and no evidence for an alternative pathway of activation of complement was obtained. In mammals, the labile components of complement, particularly C3a and C5a are potent mediators of many events which occur in inflammatory responses such as chemotaxis of leucocytes and release of histamine from mast cells. The nature and function of these cells in fish and the nature of the inflammatory responses will now be discussed.

Phagocytic Cells and Inflammation in Fish

Macrophages

These cells are present in many tissue sites in fish especially in the mesenteries as free cells and in the splenic ellipsoids, the kidney and, at least in some species like the plaice, in the atrium of the heart, as reticulo-endothelial cells (Ellis *et al.*, 1976). *In vivo* and *in vitro* studies have demonstrated these cells to be highly phagocytic for inert and antigenic material (Ellis *et al.*, 1976; McKinney *et al.*, 1977). In histochemical staining and ultrastructure, they closely resemble mammalian macrophages but little is known about other functional aspects, such as factors affecting their phagocytic responsiveness or their interaction with other host defence mechanisms and no data exists on chemotactic responses of fish leucocytes. The macrophage migration inhibition test has been used with positive results so presumably lymphokines like MIF may exert physiological influences on macrophages in fish. An important difference between macrophages of certain fish species and those of mammals is the apparent lack of Fc and C3 receptors on fish macrophages and the lack of opsonic activity of fish antibody and complement (Wrathmell and Parrish, 1980a, b). These results suggest that the mechanisms of phagocytosis and intra-cellular killing, both of which are significantly enhanced by antibody-complement complexes in mammals, may be different in some fish species but more work is necessary before reliable statements can be made. Indeed, recent work has demonstrated opsonization of bacteria by homologous antibody and complement in phagocytic responses of rainbow trout peritoneal exudate cells (Sakai, unpublished data).

Neutrophils in Fish

Fish neutrophils have very similar morphology and histochemical staining properties to mammalian neutrophils (Ellis, 1976, 1981b; Ferguson, 1976) and they are frequently seen in inflammatory lesions (Roberts, 1978). However, there is very little evidence that neutrophils in fish are actively phagocytic and where these cells have been identified on histochemical or ultrastructural grounds they have been reported to have no phagocytic properties (Ellis *et al.*, 1976; McKinney *et al.*, 1977) or to be only weakly phagocytic (Young and Chapman, 1978). The precise role of neutrophils in fish therefore remains poorly defined.

The findings that fish neutrophils possess most of the enzymes found in mammalian neutrophils and their obvious presence in many inflammatory lesions suggests they play an active role in defence mechanisms. Ellis (1981b) has suggested that the fish neutrophil may carry out a bactericidal role extracellularly rather than intracellularly. Assuming that these cells utilize similar bactericidal mechanisms to those that occur intracellularly in mammals, this would have significant consequences for host tissue damage during inflammation. In mammals, phagocytosing neutrophils generate O_2^-, H_2O_2 and $OH^\bullet$ in the phagosomes and also over their surface. These substances are highly damaging to the neutrophil membrane and also to adjacent cells and fibres. It is considered that superoxide dismutase (SOD) and peroxidases control these toxic ions and free radicals intracellularly but these enzymes are not present in high concentration in extracellular fluids (Huber, 1980). The escape of these free radicals from activated neutrophils causes early death of the phagocytosing neutrophil and accounts for much of the host tissue damage which occurs during inflammatory reactions. Consider what the case may be if fish neutrophils generate O_2^-, and $OH^\bullet$ extracellularly. The resultant tissue damage would be considerable. In fact, this is frequently the case in inflammatory responses in fish, with extensive tissue liquefaction and ulceration of the integument. The fish may require powerful and diverse means of modulating such a response and the involvement of melanin may be one (see below). This postulated self-tissue destructive power of neutrophils in fish may not be as drastic as it sounds. Fish probably have better tissue-regenerating powers than mammals with injured epidermal cells responding within hours and cells such as myofibrils retain their ability to divide throughout life (see Ellis, 1981b). If fish neutrophils exert their effect extracellularly it may not be surprising that they lack Fc and C3 receptors. More information on the role of the fish neutrophil in inflammation is required before we can gain an understanding of the inflammatory reactions and disease processes of fish.

Pigment-Containing Macrophages and Melanocytes

In the lymphoid tissues of most teleosts, and also in many inflammatory lesions, are to be found cells containing dark-coloured pigment. This is mainly melanin but ceroid and sometimes haemosiderin are also present (Ellis, 1977a; Agius, 1980). The function of this melanin within these tissues is obscure. On the basis of the stable free-radical properties of melanin and its ability to quench free-radical reactions, Ellis (1981b) has postulated that the visceral melanin may provide a means of protection from free-radical damage, similar to its function in protection from radiation-induced free-radicals in the skin. In the case of lymphoid tissue, melanin may protect against free-radicals produced by phagocytic cells, particularly neutrophils. The lipids of fish tissues are mainly composed of polyunsaturated fatty acids, probably as an adaptation to low temperatures (Cossins, 1977). Polyunsaturated fats are very prone to oxidation by free-radical reactions with the production of ceroid substances (Miquel *et al.*, 1977). It is likely that fish neutrophils may generate free-radicals extra-cellularly (as described above) causing host tissue damage and oxidation of tissue lipids to ceroid substances. It is possible that macrophages which contain melanosomes and which are phagocytosing tissue debris rich in free-radicals may be protected against damage to themselves. The function of melanocytes in phagocyte-rich tissues may be to furnish the macrophages with melanosomes in an analogous way to the supply of melanosomes to malpighian cells by melanocytes in the epidermis of mammals (George and Wolke, in preparation).

It would seem that the possible protective role of melanin against lytic enzyme systems in general is worthy of investigation. Tyramine, a substrate for melanin production (Edelstein, 1971) is known to be a scavenger of superoxide ions (Huber, 1980). Many organisms, including micro-organisms, produce melanin and the ability to do so appears to confer resistance to lytic action of potential parasites (Bloomfield and Alexander, 1967) or conversely to host defences (Zambon *et al.*, 1981). In higher organisms, melanin may play a widespread role in protection against invasion of the tissue by certain parasitic organisms and also defence against the potentially self-harmful mechanisms induced during activation of the host's own defence systems. The interaction of peroxide and free-radical generating systems with peroxidase and melanin pigment may provide useful investigations for understanding host–parasite relationships in respect to their mutual attack mechanisms.

Hypersensitivity Responses in Fish

This controversial topic has recently been reviewed by Ellis (1981a). Much more work is needed to establish the nature of hypersensitivity responses in fish. Mast cells, high tissue histamine levels and IgE appear to be difficult to demonstrate in or are absent from fish. However, antigen-specific lethal anaphylactic responses have been reported in some species (Dreyer and King, 1948; Goven *et al.*, 1980) but not in others (Clem and Leslie, 1969; Harris, 1973). Immediate hypersensitivity skin reactions have been reported in several flatfish species induced by C-polysaccharide substances (Baldo and Fletcher, 1975). The mechanism of these responses is not known, but the last authors suggested that slow reacting substance of anaphylaxis (SRS-A), rather than histamine, may be the mediator in flatfish.

Physiological responses of fish to exogenous histamine is very variable and there may be significant species differences in their sensitivity to this substance. Some workers have dismissed the potential role for histamine in fish (Reite, 1972) but Ellis (in preparation) has found that histamine levels of the rainbow trout intestine markedly decrease after i.p. injection of furunculosis toxin, suggesting this depot is mobilizable and may contribute to disease processes in fish.

The responsive cell in hypersensitivity responses in fish is not definitively known. Typical mammalian-like mast cells are not present in fish. In the Cyprinidae and their close relatives, a PAS-positive granular leucocyte (PAS-GL) has been suggested to be the analogue of the mammalian mast cell (Barber and Westermann, 1978). In flatfish and the Salmonidae, the eosinophilic granular cell (EGC) has been suggested to be the responsive cell. Baldo and Fletcher (1975) have reported localized degranulation of this cell in plaice undergoing skin hypersensitivity responses, and Ellis (in preparation) found a degranulation of the EGCs in the stratum compactum of the intestine of rainbow trout, coincidental with a decrease in the histamine content of this tissue, after i.p. injection of the furunculosis toxin.

The report of Goven et al. (1980) that a large proportion of catfish died after sensitization and challenge, may be highly significant. If immune hypersensitivity responses are widespread in fish, an understanding of the mechanisms involved would have important bearing on designing vaccination procedures and greatly aid our understanding of pathophysiological processes in fish.

Summary and Conclusions

Many aspects of immune mechanisms in fish are similar to those of the mammal but significant differences also exist. An understanding of these differences is important from the comparative immunological view point and also to fish pathologists interested in the disease processes in fish and the prospects of using vaccination methods to control disease.

Many differences also exist in the defence mechanisms between fish species. This is not surprising since there are over 20,000 recent species of fish. The most recent group, and the one of major commercial importance, are the teleosts which first appeared in the late Devonian Age, 300 million years ago. They are also the most numerous with some 16,000 species (compared with the 4,500 species of mammals). Fish, including the Agnatha, Chondrichthyes and Osteichthyes represent a diverse group, extending over a wide variety of habitats and, in time, over widely divergent evolutionary pathways. The constraints of an aquatic environment enforce similarities of morphology and physiology between the groups but these similarities are superficial and one must be aware of the danger of assuming conformity in physiology because of general structural resemblances. In view of this, it may be difficult to make generalizations, even amongst the teleosts, and extension of observations from one species to another should be done with caution.

Nevertheless, it is evident that fish possess all of the characteristics of adaptive immunity, both humoral and cell-mediated. There is much evidence to believe that lymphocyte subpopulations, with functional dichotomy, have evolved at the level of the fishes but it is still not clear if these subpopulations arise in discrete organs equivalent to the thymus and bone-marrow of mammals.

Some features of the immune system of fish are quite different from that of the mammal and a greater understanding of these could have considerable importance to immunological theory and greatly aid effective immunization of fish. Present data suggest that in some species of teleosts, both B-like and T-like cells exist in the thymus. Though antibody-producing cells are absent from the thymus, low-dose antigen stimulation results in the proliferation of antigen-binding cells in the thymus which are suggested to have T-helper function. The ontogeny and structure of the thymus in fish also suggests that under certain circumstances, antigen may gain access to the thymus. Such observations raise important questions about mechanisms of tolerance induction by deletion of "forbidden" clones in the thymus.

The apparent presence of Ig on the membranes of all lymphocytes in fish provides further evidence that the antigen-receptor of T cells is in fact Ig. This is still a controversial subject in immunology in general and comparative studies on lower vertebrates have contributed a great deal to the debate about the antigen-recognition mechanisms of T cells. However, all our knowledge relating to putative T and B cells in fish comes from arguments by analogy with higher vertebrates and the necessary experiments of thymic ablation and reconstitution by identifiable cell populations have not been done in fish owing to the lack of syngeneic strains. Once the latter become available, important issues for fish and mammalian immunology may be solved.

Other aspects discussed in this paper, while having importance to comparative immunologists, are of particular relevance to our understanding of fish immune mechanisms in relationship to disease control and diagnosis. These include the antigen-trapping mechanisms on reticulin fibres rather than dendritic cells in the splenic ellipsoids and associated structures such as the melano-macrophage centres. The function of phagocytic cells in fish is still little understood. Macrophages are avidly phagocytic but little is known of their relationship to the specific immune response or complement system. Further work concerning neutrophil function would be fruitful in understanding the nature of many disease processes in fish. Little evidence exists of the phagocytic nature of these cells and it has been suggested here that they may exert bactericidal effects extracellularly with important consequences to our understanding of inflammatory events and their control in fish.

Many features such as the effect of temperature, antigen dose and route of immunization upon the production of antibody and development of immune memory are being studied with important results. Manipulation of temperature, consideration of season and timing of booster injections are all important for developing appropriate vaccination programmes and may prove important in understanding some of the adaptational aspects of fish host–parasite interrelationships.

A recognition of structural heterogeneity in the single (IgM) class of fish antibody is emerging but little is yet understood about their properties and functions. Thus, subclasses of IgM may exist in fish and we know nothing of the functional implications of this. A secretory IgM has been identified in fish mucus and bile and further work on its functional properties and mechanisms of elicitation combined with disease-protection studies may prove highly significant for development of vaccines.

Finally, the nature of hypersensitivity responses in fish has been discussed and is an area worthy of further study from the viewpoints of understanding the phylogenetic origin of hypersensitivity responses, mechanisms of inflammation in fish and the consequences for vaccination techniques.

References

Abruzzini, A. F., Ingram, L. O. and Clem, L. W. (1981). Temperature mediated processes in teleost immunity: Homeoviscous adaptation in teleost lymphocytes. *Proceedings of the Society of Experimental Biology and Medicine*, in press.

Agius, C. (1979). The role of melano-macrophage centres in iron storage in normal and diseased fish. *Journal of Fish Diseases* 2, 337–343.

Agius, C. (1980). Phylogenetic development of melano-macrophage centres in fish. *Journal of Zoology* 191, 11–32.

Avtalion, R. R., Weiss, E. and Moalem, T. (1976). Regulatory effects of temperature upon immunity in Ectothermic Vertebrates. *In* "Comparative Immunology" (Ed. J. J. Marchalonis), pp.227–238. Blackwell . Scientific Publication, Oxford.

Avtalion, R. R., Wishkovsky, A. and Katz, D. (1980). Regulatory effect of temperature on specific suppression and enhancement of the humoral response in fish. *In* "Immunological Memory" (Ed. by M. J. Manning), pp.113–121. Elsevier/North Holland, Amsterdam.

Azzolina, L. S. (1978). Antigen recognition and immune response in goldfish *Carassius auratus* at different temperatures. *Developmental and Comparative Immunology* **2**, 77–86.

Baldo, B. A. and Fletcher, T. C . (1975). Phylogenetic aspects of hypersensitivity reactions in flatfish. *In* "Immunologic Phylogeny" (Eds. W. H. Hildemann and A. A. Benedict), pp.365–372. Plenum Press, London.

Baldwin, W. M. and Cohen, M. (1980). A primitive dendritic splenocyte in *Xenopus laevis* with morphological similarities to Reed-Sternberg cells. *In* "Aspects of Developmental and Comparative Immunology I" (Ed. J. B. Solomon), pp.179–182. Pergamon Press, Oxford.

Barber, D. L. and Mills Westermann, J. E. (1978). Observations on development and morphological effects of histamine liberator 48/80 on PAS-positive granular leukocytes and heterophils of *Catostomus commersoni*. *Journal of Fish Biology* **13**, 563–574.

Bloomfield, B. J. and Alexander, M. (1967). Melanins and resistance of fungus to lysis. *Journal of Bacteriology* **93**, 1276–1280.

Bogner, K. H. and Ellis, A. E. (1977). Properties and functions of lymphocytes and lymphoid tissues in teleost fish. *Beitrage zür Histopathologie der Fische* **4**, 59–72.

Chiller, J. M., Hodgins, H. O. and Weiser, R. S. (1969). Antibody response in rainbow trout (*Salmo gairdneri*). II. Studies on the kinetic development of antibody-producing cells and on complement and natural hemolysin. *Journal of Immunology* **102**, 1202–1207.

Clem, L. W. and Leslie, G. A. (1969). Phylogeny of immunoglobulin structure and function. *In* "Immunology and Development" (Ed. M. Adinolfi), pp.62–88. Lavenham Press, England.

Clem, L. W. and McLean, W. E. (1975). Phylogeny of immunoglobulin structure and function. VII. Monomeric and tetrameric immunoglobulins of the margate, a marine teleost fish. *Immunology* **29**, 791–799.

Clem, L. W., McLean, W. E., Shankey, V. T. and Cuchens, M. A. (1977). Phylogeny of lymphocyte heterogeneity. I. Membrane immunoglobulins of teleost lymphocytes. *Developmental and Comparative Immunology* **1**, 105–118.

Cooper, E. L., Klempau, A. E., Ramirez, J. A. and Zapata, A. G. (1980). Source of stem cells in evolution. *In* "Development and Differentiation of vertebrate lymphocytes" (Ed. J. D. Horton), pp.3–14. Elsevier/North Holland Biomedical, Amsterdam.

Cossins, A. R. (1977). Adaptation of biological membranes to temperature. The effects of temperature acclimation of goldfish upon the viscosity of synaptosomal membranes. *Biochimica Biophysica Acta* **470**, 395–411.

Cuchens, M. A. and Clem, L. W. (1977). Phylogeny of lymphocyte heterogeneity II. Differential effects of temperature on fish T-like and B-like cells. *Cellular Immunology* **34**, 219–230.

DeLuca, D., Warr, G. W. and Marchalonis, J. J. (1978). Phylogenetic origins of immune recognition: lymphocyte surface immunoglobulins and antigen binding in the genus *Carassius* (Teleostii). *European Journal of Immunology* **8**, 525–530.

Dreyer, N. B. and King, J. W. (1948). Anaphylaxis in fish. *Journal of Immunology* **60**, 277–282.

Edelstein, L. M. (1971). Melanin: A unique biopolymer. *In* "Pathobiology Annual" Vol. 1 (Ed. H. L. Ioachim), pp.309–324. Appleton-Century-Crofts, New York.

Ellis, A. E. (1976). Leucocytes and related cells in the plaice (*Pleuronectes platessa*). *Journal of Fish Biology* **8**, 143–156.

Ellis, A. E. (1977a). The leucocytes of fish: A review. *Journal of Fish Biology* **11**, 453–491.

Ellis, A. E. (1977b). Ontogeny of the immune response in *Salmo salar*. Histogenesis of the lymphoid organs and appearance of membrane immunoglobulin and mixed leucocyte reactivity. *In* "Developmental Immunobiology" (Eds. J. B. Solomon and J. D. Horton), pp.225–231. Elsevier/North Holland Biomedical Press, Amsterdam.

Ellis, A. E. (1980). Antigen-trapping in the spleen and kidney of the plaice *Pleuronectes platessa* L. *Journal of Fish Diseases* **3**, 413–426.

Ellis, A. E. (1981a). Histamine, mast cells and hypersensitivity responses in fish. *Developmental and Comparative Immunology* **6**, Suppl. 1. (in press).

Ellis, A. E. (1981b). Non-specific defence mechanisms in fish and their role in disease processes. *In* "Developments in Biological Standardization", Vol. 49, Symposium on Fish Biologics: Serodiagnostics and Vaccines (Eds. D. P. Anderson and W. Hennessen), pp.337–352. S. Karger, Basel, Switzerland.

Ellis, A. E. (1981c). Stress and modulation of the immune response in fish. *In* "Stress and Fish" (Ed. A. D. Pickering), pp.147–169. Academic Press, London.

Ellis, A. E. (in preparation). Eosinophilic granular cells (EGC) and histamine responses to *Aeromonas salmonicida* toxins in rainbow trout.

Ellis, A. E. and de Sousa, M. A. B. (1974). Phylogeny of the lymphoid system I. A study of the fate of circulating lymphocytes in plaice. *European Journal of Immunology* **4**, 338–343.

Ellis, A. E. and Parkhouse, R. M. E. (1975). Surface immunoglobulin on the lymphocytes of the skate, *Raja naevus*. *European Journal of Immunology* **5**, 726–728.

Ellis, A. E., Munro, A. L. S. and Roberts, R. J. (1976). Defense mechanisms in fish I. A study of the phagocytic system and the fate of intraperitoneally injected particulate material in the plaice (*Pleuronectes platessa*). *Journal of Fish Biology* **8**, 67–78.

Emmrich, F., Richter, R. F. and Ambrosius, H. (1975). Immunoglobulin determinants on the surface of lymphoid cells in carp. *European Journal of Immunology* **5**, 76–78.

Etlinger, H. M., Hodgins, H. O. and Chiller, J. M. (1976). Evolution of the lymphoid system I. Evidence for lymphocyte heterogeneity in rainbow trout revealed by the organ distribution of mitogenic responses. *Journal of Immunology* **116**, 1547–1553.

Fänge, R. (1981). Aspects of lymphomyeloid tissue of fish. *In* "Developmental and Comparative Immunology, Vol. 6, Suppl. 1. Pergamon Press, Oxford (in press).

Ferguson, H. W. (1976). The relationship between ellipsoids and melano-macrophage centres in the spleen of turbot (*Scophthalmus maximus*). *Journal of Comparative Pathology* **86**, 377–380.

Fiebig, H., Scherbaum, I. and Ambrosius, H. (1980). Evolutionary origin of the T lymphocyte receptor I. Immunochemical investigation of immunoglobulin-like cell surface protein of carp thymocytes. *Molecular Immunology* **17**, 971–984.

Fletcher, T. C. and Grant, P. T. (1969). Immunoglobulins in the serum and mucus of the plaice (*Pleuronectes platessa*). *Biochemical Journal* **115**, 65.

Fletcher, T. C. and White, A. (1973). Antibody production in the plaice after oral and parenteral immunization with *Vibrio anguillarum* antigens. *Aquaculture* **1**, 417–428.

Fryer, J. L., Pilcher, K. S., Sanders, J. E., Rohovec, J. S., Zinn, J. L., Groberg, W. J. and McCoy, R. H. (1976). Temperature, infectious diseases, and the immune response in salmonid fish. United States Department of Commerce. *National Technical Information Service*, PB-253 191 72pp.

George, C. J. and Wolke, R. (in preparation). Morphology of pigmented cell aggregates (Mictic corpuscles) in the viscera of the Teleostei.

Gigli, I. and Austen, R. F. (1971). Phylogeny and function of the complement system. *Annual Review of Microbiology* **25**, 309–330.

Goven, B. A., Dawe, D. L. and Gratzek, J. B. (1980). *In vivo* and *in vitro* anaphylactic type reactions in fish. *Developmental and Comparative Immunology* **4**, 55–64.

Grace, M. F. (1981). The functional histogenesis of the immune system in rainbow trout (*Salmo gairdneri*). PhD Thesis, Hull University, England.

Grace, M. F., Botham, J. W. and Manning, M. J. (1980). Ontogeny of lymphoid organ function in fish. *In* "Aspects of Developmental and Comparative Immunology I" (Ed. J. B. Solomon), pp.467–468. Pergamon Press, Oxford and New York.

Harris, J. E. (1973). The apparent inability of cyprinid fish to produce skin-sensitizing antibody. *Journal of Fish Biology* **5**, 535–540.

Hodgins, H. O., Weiser, R. S. and Ridgeway, J. J. (1967). The nature of antibodies and the immune response in rainbow trout. *Journal of Immunology* **99**, 534–544.

Huber, W. (1980). Future trends in free radical studies. *In* "Inflammation: Mechanisms and Treatment" (Eds. D. A. Willoughby and J. P. Giroud), pp.27–42. MTP Press, Lancaster.

Hussein, M. E., Badir, N., Elridi, R. and Akef, M. (1979). Lymphoid tissues of the snake *Spalerosophis diadema*, in the different seasons. *Developmental and Comparative Immunology* **3**, 77–88.

Ingram, G. A. and Alexander, J. B. (1977). Serum protein changes in brown trout (*Salmo trutta* L.) after single injections of soluble and cellular antigens. *Journal of Fish Biology* **11**, 283–292.

Ingram, G. A. and Alexander, J. B. (1980). The immune response of brown trout *Salmo trutta* to lipopolysaccharide. *Journal of Fish Biology* **16**, 181–197.

Jensen, J. A. and Festa, E. (1980). The 6-component complement system of the nurse shark (*Ginglymostoma cirratum*). *In* "Aspects of Developmental and Comparative Immunology I." (Ed. J. B. Solomon), pp.485–486. Pergamon Press, Oxford.

Jerne, N. K. (1980). The somatic generation of immune recognition. *Developmental and Comparative Immunology* **4**, 189.

Klaus, G. G. B., Humphrey, J. H., Kunkl, A. and Dongworth, D. W. (1980). The follicular dendritic cell: Its role in antigen presentation in the generation of immunological memory. *Immunological Reviews* **53**, 3–28.

Lele, S. H. (1933). On the phasical history of the thymus gland in plaice of various ages with note on the involution of the organ, including also notes on the other ductless glands in this species. *Journal of University of Bombay* **1**, 37–53.

Litman, G. W. (1975). Physical properties of immunoglobulins of lower species: A comparison with immunoglobulins of mammals. *In* "Comparative Immunology" (Ed. J. J. Marchalonis), pp.239–275. Blackwell, Oxford.

Lobb, C. J. and Clem, L. W. (1981a). The metabolic relationships of the immunoglobulins in fish serum, cutaneous mucus and bile. *Journal of Immunology* **127**, 1525–1529.

Lobb, C. J. and Clem, L. W. (1981b). Phylogeny of immunoglobulin structure and function XI. Secretory immunoglobulins in the cutaneous mucus of the sheepshead, *Archosargus probatocephalus*. *Developmental and Comparative Immunology* **5**, 587–596.

Lobb, C. J. and Clem, L. W. (1981c). Phylogeny of immunoglobulin structure and function XII. Secretory immunoglobulins in the bile of the marine teleost *Archosargus probatocephalus*. *Molecular Immunology* **18**, 615–619.

Loon van, J. J. A., Oosterom van, R. and Muiswinkel, van, W. B. (1980). Development of the immune system in carp. *In* "Aspects of Developmental and Comparative Immunology I." (Ed. J. B. Solomon), pp.469–470. Pergamon Press, Oxford.

Mackie, I. M. and Wardle, C. S. (1971). Electrophoretic identification of lymph from muscle tissue of plaice (*Pleuronectes platessa* L.). *International Journal of Biochemistry* **2**. 409–413.

McKinney, E. C., Smith, S. B., Haines, H. G. and Sigel, M. M. (1977). Phagocytosis by fish cells. *Journal of the Reticuloendothial Society* **21**, 89–95.

Miquel, J., Oro, J., Bensch, K. G. and Johnson, J. E. (1977). Lipofuscin: Finestructural and biochemical studies. *In* "Free Radicals in Biology" Vol. III. (Ed. W. A. Pryor), pp.133–182. Academic Press, New York and London.

Nonaka, M., Yamaguchi, N., Natsuume-Sakai, S. and Takahashi, M. (1981). The complement system of rainbow trout (*Salmo gairdneri*) I. Identification of the serum lytic system homologous to mammalian complement. *Journal of Immunology* **126**, 1489–1494.

Perlmutter, A., Sarot, D. A., Yu, M., Filazzola, R. J. and Seeley, R. J. (1973). The effect of crowding on the immune response of the blue gourami, *Trichogaster trichopterus*, to infectious pancreatic necrosis (IPN) virus. *Life Sciences* **13**, 363–375.

Randall, D. J. (1970). The circulatory system. *In* "Fish Physiology" Vol. IV, (Eds. W. S. Hoar, and J. Randall), pp.133–172. Academic Press, New York and London.

Reite, O. B. (1972). Comparative Physiology of histamine. *Physiology Reviews* **52**, 778–819.

Rijkers, G. T., Frederix-Wolters, E. M. H. and Muiswinkel van, W. B. (1980). The immune system of cyprinid fish. Kinetics and temperature dependence of antibody-producing cells in carp (*Cyprinus carpio*). *Immunology* **41**, 91–97.

Roberts, R. J. (1975). Melanin-containing cells of teleost fish and their relation to disease. *In* "The Pathology of Fishes" (Eds. W. E. Ribelin and G. Migaki), pp.399–428. University of Wisconsin Press.

Roberts, R. J. (Ed.) (1978). Fish Pathology. Bailliere Tindall, London.

Rooijen van, N. (1980). Localisation of antigens and immune complexes in the spleen of mammals compared with lower vertebrates. *In* "Aspects of Developmental and Comparative Immunology I." (Ed. J. B. Solomon), pp.73–79. Pergamon Press, Oxford.

Ruben, L. N. and Edwards, B. F. (1980). Phylogeny of the emergence of T-B collaboration in humoral immunity. *In* "Contemporary aspects in Immunobiology", Vol. 9, (Eds. N. Cohen and J. J. Marchalonis), pp.55–89. Plenum Press, New York.

Ruben, L. N., Warr, G. W., Decker, J. M. and Marchalonis, J. J. (1977). Phylogenetic origins of immune recognition: Lymphoid heterogeneity and the hapten/carrier effect in the goldfish, *Carassius auratus*. *Cellular Immunology* **31**, 266–283.

Sakai, D. K. (1981a). Spontaneous and antibody-dependent hemolysis activities of fish sera and inapplicability of mammalian complements to the immune hemolysis reactions of fishes. *Bulletin of the Japanese Society of Scientific Fisheries* **47**, 979–991.

Sakai, D. K. (1981b). Heat inactivation of complements and immune hemolysis reaction in rainbow trout, masu salmon, coho salmon, goldfish and tilapia. *Bulletin of the Japanese Society of Scientific Fisheries* **47**, 565–571.

Secombes, C. J. and Manning, M. J. (1980). Comparative studies on the immune system of fishes and amphibians: antigen localization in the carp, *Cyprinus carpio* L. *Journal of Fish Diseases* **3**, 399–412.

Secombes, C. J., Manning, M. J. and Ellis, A. E. (1980). Antigen-trapping in the carp, *Cyprinus carpio*. *In* "Aspects of Developmental and Comparative Immunology I." (Ed. J. B. Solomon), pp.465–466. Pergamon Press, Oxford.

Secombes, C. J., Manning, M. J. and Ellis, A. E. (1982). The effects of primary and secondary immunization on the lymphoid tissues of the carp, *Cyprinus carpio* L. *Journal of Experimental Zoology* **220**, 277–287.

Serero, M. and Avtalion, R. R. (1978). Regulatory effect of temperature and antigen upon immunity in ectothermic vertebrates. III. Establishment of immunological suppression in fish. *Developmental and Comparative Immunology* **2**, 87–94.

Shelton, E. and Smith, M. (1970). The ultrastructure of carp (*Cyprinus carpio*) immunoglobulin: A tetrameric macroglobulin. *Journal of Molecular Biology* **54**, 615–617.

Smith, A. M., Potter, M. and Merchant, E. B. (1967). Antibody forming cells in the pronephros of the teleost *Lepomis macrochirus*. *Journal of Immunology* **99**, 876–882.

Stolen, J. S. and Makela, O. (1976). Cell collaboration in a marine fish: The effect of carrier preimmunisation on the anti-hapten response to NIP and NNP. *In* "Phylogeny of Thymus and Bone Marrow-Bursa Cells. (Ed. R. K. Wright and E. L. Cooper), pp.93–97. Elsevier/North Holland, Amsterdam.

Trizio, D. and Cudkowicz, G. (1978). The effect of selective T cell priming on anti-sheep and anti-hapten humoral responses. II. Separation by nylon-wool columns of the activated lymphocytes. *Journal of Immunology* **120**, 1028.

Trump, G. N. and Hildemann, W. H. (1970). Antibody responses of goldfish to bovine serum albumin. Primary and secondary responses. *Immunology* **19**, 621–627.

Uhr, J. W., Finkelstein, M. S. and Franklin, E. C. (1962). Antibody response to bacteriophage Phi X 174 in non-mammalian vertebrates. *Proceedings of the Society for Experimental Biology and Medicine* **111**, 13–15.

Voss, E. W., Groberg, W. J. and Fryer, J. L. (1980). Metabolism of coho salmon Ig. Catabolic rate of coho salmon tetrameric Ig in serum. *Molecular Immunology* **17**, 445–452.

Warr, G. W. (1980). Membrane immunoglobulins of vertebrate lymphocytes. *In* "Contemporary Topics in Immunobiology", Vol. 9. (Eds. J. J. Marchalonis and N. Cohen), pp.141–170. Plenum Press, New York.

Warr, G. W. and Marchalonis, J. J. (1980). Membrane immunoglobulins of teleost fish lymphocytes. *In* "Aspects of Developmental and Comparative Immunology I." (Ed. J. B. Solomon), pp.33–37. Pergamon Press, Oxford.

Warr, G. W., DeLuca, D., Decker, J. M., Marchalonis, J. J. and Ruben, L. N. (1977). Lymphoid heterogeneity in teleost fish: Studies on the genus *Carassius*. *In* "Developmental Immunology" (Eds. J. B. Solomon and J. D. Horton), pp.241–248. Elsevier/North Holland Biomedical Press, Amsterdam.

Warr, G. W., DeLuca, D. and Marchalonis, J. J. (1980). Phylogeny and ontogeny of antigen-specific T cell receptors. *In* "Development and Differentiation of Vertebrate Lymphocytes". (Ed. J. D. Horton), pp.99–110. Elsevier/North Holland, Amsterdam.

Wardle, C. S. (1971). New observations on the lymph system of the plaice, *Pleuronectes platessa* and other teleosts. *Journal of the Marine Biological Association, U.K.* **51**, 977–990.

Wrathmell, A. B. and Parish, N. M. (1980a). Cell surface receptors in the immune response in fish. *In* "Phylogeny of Immunological Memory" (Ed. M. J. Manning), pp.143–152. Elsevier/North Holland Biomedical Press, Amsterdam.

Wrathmell, A. B. and Parish, N. M. (1980b). Cell surface receptors and immune mechanisms in an elasmobranch fish *Scyliorhinus canicula*. *In* "Aspects of Development and Comparative Immunology I". (Ed. J. B. Solomon), pp.463–464. Pergamon Press, Oxford.

Yamaga, K. M., Kubo, R. T. and Etlinger, H. M. (1978). Studies on the question of conventional immunoglobulin on thymocytes from primitive vertebrates II. Delineation between Ig-specific and cross-reactive membrane components. *Journal of Immunology* **120**, 2074–2079.

Yamaguchi, N., Teshima, C., Kurashige, S., Saito, T. and Mitsuhashi, S. (1980). Seasonal modulation of antibody formation in rainbow trout (*Salmo gairdneri*). *In* "Aspects of Developmental and Comparative Immunology I" (Ed. J. B. Solomon), pp.483–484. Pergamon Press, Oxford.

Young, C. L. and Chapman, G. B. (1978). Ultrastructural aspects of the causative agent and renal histopathology of bacterial kidney disease in brook trout (*Salvelinus fontinalis*). *Journal of the Fisheries Research Board of Canada* **35**, 1234–1248.

Zambon, J. J., Reynolds, H. S. and Slots, J. (1981). Black-pigmented *Bacteroides* spp. in the human oral cavity. *Infection and Immunity* **32**, 198–203.

Zapata, A. (1979). Ultrastructural study of the teleost fish kidney. *Developmental and Comparative Immunology* **3**, 55–65.

Zapata, A. (1980). Ultrastructure of elasmobranch lymphoid tissue I. Thymus and spleen. *Developmental and Comparative Immunology* **4**, 459–472.

2

Developmental Aspects of
Immunity and Tolerance in Fish

MARGARET J. MANNING, MARY F. GRACE*
AND CHRISTOPHER J. SECOMBES[+]

*Department of Biological Sciences, Plymouth Polytechnic, Devon, U.K.
and Department of Zoology, University of Hull, Hull, U.K.*

Introduction

In fish which have free-living larvae, the maturation of the immune system takes place post-hatching when the animal is already being exposed to environmental antigens. The developmental stages are readily available for experimentation and young fry have been used in studies on the ontogeny of immunocompetence by Sailendri (1973) in the tilapia (*Sarotherodon mossambicus*), by Ellis (1977) in the salmon (*Salmo salar*), by Rijkers and van Muiswinkel (1977) in the rosy barb (*Barbus conchonius*), by van Loon *et al.* (1981) in the carp (*Cyprinus carpio*), and by Botham *et al.* (1980), Grace *et al.* (1981), Manning *et al.* (1981) and Secombes (1981) in the carp (*C. carpio*) and the rainbow trout (*Salmo gairdneri*). The present review brings together some of this information on the functional development of the immune system in fish and discusses the outcome of immunization during the first few months of life.

Histogenesis of the Lymphoid Organs

The thymus is the first lymphoid organ to develop in fish, as in other vertebrates. In the carp at $22 \pm 1°C$, the thymus first appears at 2 days post-hatching and becomes actively lymphopoietic by day 5. The kidney, which contains haemopoietic tissue at day 2, shows differentiating lymphoid cells

---

*Present address: Institute of Aquaculture, University of Stirling, FK9 4LA, U.K.
[+]Present address: Department of Zoology, University of Aberdeen, Aberdeen, AB9 1AS, U.K.

by day 6. The spleen first appears at day 5, but it develops more slowly than the kidney and remains predominantly erythroid for several months (Botham and Manning, 1981). Similar studies on rainbow trout at 14°C demonstrate the first appearance of the thymus at day 5 pre-hatching and the occurrence of lymphoid cells in the kidney at day 5 post-hatching, the spleen again remaining largely erythroid for the first few months of life (Grace and Manning, 1980). The same general picture has emerged from all ontogenetic studies carried out to date (Table 1), the thymus and the kidney being the most important lymphoid organs in the young fish.

Table 1. *Histogenesis of lymphoid organs in fish*

Species	Temperature (°C)	First appearance of lymphocytes in:			Reference
		Thymus	Kidney	Spleen	
Salmo gairdneri	14	3 days post-hatch	5 days post-hatch	6 days post-hatch; spleen still erythroid at day 28	Grace and Manning (1980)
Barbus conchonius	23	4 days post-hatch	4 days post-hatch	7 days post-hatch; spleen still erythroid at day 28	Grace (1981)
Cyprinus carpio	22	3 days post-hatch	6 days post-hatch	8 days post hatch; spleen still erythroid at day 28	Botham and Manning (1981)
Salmo salar	4–7	22 days pre-hatch	14 days pre-hatch	42 days post-hatch	Ellis (1977)
Sarotherodon mossambicus	Room temperature	6–8 days (late pre-larval)	13–16 days (mid post-larval)	30–80 days (juvenile)	Sailendri (1973)

The first occurrence of lymphocytes does not necessarily herald immunological maturity, however. In carp, although a few cells bearing surface immunoglobulin were found in suspensions taken from whole fish on day 7, such cells were not detected in the thymus or pronephros until day 14 (at 21°C), while cells with cytoplasmic immunoglobulin first appeared at day 21 in the pronephros (van Loon *et al.*, 1981). Similarly, in the salmon at 4–7°C, the presence of surface immunoglobulin on lymphocytes and the ability to give a proliferative response in mixed cell cultures did not occur until long after the lymphoid thymus and kidney had differentiated. Indeed, these two aspects of functional maturity occurred simultaneously and coincided with the onset of feeding at around day 45 (Ellis, 1977).

Humoral Antibody Responses

Antibody Production

Antibody production by young fish has been demonstrated in juvenile (1.2g) coho salmon (*Oncorhychus kisutch*) using *Aeromonas salmonicida* (Paterson and Fryer, 1974) and in rainbow trout fry 23 days after the commencement of feeding using *Aeromonas liquefaciens* (Khalifa and Post, 1976). Even younger rainbow trout can respond to DNP-KLH (dinitrophenol — keyhole limpet haemocyanin) when immunized at 1 month old and tested 3 months later (Dorson, 1974). This latter result agrees with the findings of Etlinger *et al.* (1979) who noted that juvenile rainbow trout react as intensively as adult fish to antigens that are thymus-independent in mammals, although their response to thymus-dependent antigens is only meagre.

Experiments designed to determine more precisely the age of maturation of humoral immunity in fish have been carried out on carp by van Loon *et al.* (1981) and in our own laboratory using carp and rainbow trout (Manning *et al.*, 1981; Secombes, 1981). Tables 2, 3 and 4 show some preliminary results obtained after immunizing young fish with a bacterial antigen (formalin killed *Aeromonas salmonicida*, 1×10^8 cells per g body weight) or with a soluble antigen HGG (human gamma globulin) or BSA (bovine serum albumin), 25 μg per g body weight administered either in saline or with an equal volume of FCA (Freund's complete adjuvant).

The young rainbow trout showed no response to either antigen when injected intramuscularly at day 1 post-hatching, day 7 post-hatching or day 14 post-hatching and tested 8 weeks later. A positive response against the bacterial antigen was, however, obtained following immunization on day 21 post-hatching, although antibody levels were not as high as those for 1 year old fish. On the other hand, the 21-day-old trout gave no response to HGG (Table 3).

When a second injection was given 8 weeks after the first, the young fish were again able to produce antibody against the bacterial antigen, although again the levels were lower than in the adult primary response. Furthermore, the responding groups included those given their first injection at 1 day old. Thus there is no evidence that early exposure to *Aeromonas salmonicida* is tolerogenic. This contrasts with the situation using soluble antigens (Table 3). Here young fish given HGG in their

Table 2. *Serum antibody (agglutination) titres against* Aeromonas salmonicida *in rainbow trout (*Salmo gairdneri*) kept at 14–17°C and immunized at an early stage of development*

	1 day	7 days	14 days	21 days	1 year[a]
	Age post-hatching when first injection given:				
Group A: tested 8 weeks after first antigen injection	0,0	0,0	0,0	3,3	5,7,7,7,7,8
Group B: tested 8 weeks after a second antigen injection given 8 weeks after the first	3,3	3,3	3,3	N.T.	N.T.

Group C: given injection of saline at age 1 day, and injected with antigen at week 8, then tested 8 weeks later: titres = 3,4.

[a] For 1 year old trout, each figure represents the −log 2 titre for one animal. For other groups, each figure represents the −log 2 titre for serum pooled from 10 animals.
N.T. = Not tested.
Antigen dose: 1×10^8 formalin-killed bacteria per g body weight.

primary immunization, followed by secondary challenge with the same antigen 8 weeks later, remained unresponsive, although normal fish and fish which had previously received BSA were able to give a fairly good antibody response to HGG by this age.

Our results with young trout agree with those of van Loon *et al.* (1981), who showed that carp aged 4 week are unable to mount a PFC (plaque forming cell) response to SRBC (sheep erythrocytes) at 21°C. Furthermore, when these fish were reimmunized 3 months later, they still failed to respond although animals which received their first injection of SRBC at 4 months of age showed normal anti-SRBC reactivity. Unfortunately, the specificity of this apparently tolerogenic effect has not been established since in our investigation (Table 3) none of the experimental groups showed any response to the "alternative" antigen, BSA. Moreover, in the anti-SRBC response of carp, the induced unresponsiveness may not be very long-lasting since by 5 or 13 months after the first injection a secondary challenge induced a normal "primary" reaction (W. B. van Muiswinkel, Wageningen, personal communication).

By the age of 8 weeks at 22°C, carp are able to respond to primary immunization using *Aeromonas salmonicida* or HGG in FCA almost as efficiently as adults. With the bacterial antigen, however, antibody levels

Table 3. *Serum antibody (passive haemagglutination) titres in rainbow trout (*Salmo gairdneri*) kept at 14–17°C and immunized with either human gamma globulin (HGG) or bovine serum albumin (BSA) at an early stage of development*

	Anti-HGG titres				
	Age post-hatching when antigen first given:				
Antigen initially injected	1 day	7 days	14 days	21 days	1 year[c]
Group A [a]					
HGG in saline	0,0	0,0	0,0	N.T.	N.T.
HGG in adjuvant	0,0	0,0	0,0	0,0	11,11,12,12,12,14
BSA in saline	0,0	0,0	0,0	N.T.	N.T.
BSA in adjuvant	0,0	0,0	0,0	N.T.	N.T.
Group B [b]					
HGG in saline	0	0	0	—	—
HGG in adjuvant	0	0	0	—	—
BSA in saline	2	3	2	—	—
BSA in adjuvant	4	6	6	—	—

An anti-BSA serum antibody response was lacking in all animals tested

[a]Group A were tested 8 weeks after first injection.
[b]Group B animals were reinjected 8 weeks after first injection with either HGG in adjuvant or BSA in adjuvant and tested 8 weeks after the second injection.
[c] For 1 year old trout each figure represents the $-\log 2$ titre for one animal. For other groups, each figure represents the $-\log 2$ titre for serum pooled from 10 animals.
N.T. = Not tested.
Antigen dose: 25 μg (g body weight)$^{-1}$.

following secondary challenge 8 weeks after the first injection did not increase to quite the high levels attained by older fish (Table 4), while with HGG in FCA, an analysis of the titres obtained after injecting fish of various ages and comparing those immunized above the age of 40 weeks with those receiving their primary injection at 8–40 weeks old indicated that in older fish antibody production commences somewhat earlier than in the younger animals (Secombes, 1981).

These studies suggest that full maturation of the antibody response is achieved during the first year of life, between months 2 to 10, but that (for certain antigens at least) non-responsiveness may be induced by premature immunization. Immunological tolerance is a phenomenon known to occur in fish as well as in mammals. It has already been demonstrated that, even in the adult (carp), a state of specific and long-lasting tolerance can be induced at low temperatures in fish previously injected with a high dose of soluble antigen (Serero and Avtalion, 1978; Avtalion *et al.*, 1980; Avtalion,

1981). The factors which might possibly lead to tolerance induction in young fish therefore require further investigation.

Table 4. *Serum antibody production at 22°C by young and 1-year-old carp,* Cyprinus carpio, *against* Aeromonas salmonicida *(agglutination titres) or HGG (human gamma globulin) in adjuvant (passive haemagglutination titres)*

	Age when first injection given:	
Time tested	8 weeks[a]	1 year
	Antibody titres against A. salmonicida	
4 weeks after 1st injection	6, 6	6, 6, 7, 7, 7, 8
4 weeks after 2nd injection		
given 8 weeks after the 1st	8, 9	11, 14, 14, 14, 15
	Antibody titres against HGG	
4 weeks after 1st injection	6, 7	11, 11, 12, 13, 14, 17
4 weeks after 2nd injection		
given 8 weeks after the 1st	>20, >20	>20, >20, >20, >20, >20

[a]For 8 weeks old fish, each figure represents the $-\log 2$ titre for pooled serum taken from 10 animals; for 1 year old fish, each figure represents the $-\log 2$ titre for one animal.

Histological Responses to Antigenic Stimulation

Carp aged 8 weeks respond to bacterial and soluble antigens in a manner essentially similar to that described for 6-month to 1-year-old fish by Secombes and Manning (1980, 1981). They show lymphoid cell proliferation and an increased number of pyroninophilic cells, especially in the pronephros and mesonephros during weeks 2 to 4 of the response. The trapping of soluble antigens, detected by immunofluorescence, was less efficient in the 8-week-old fish, however, particularly in the response of the spleen where the localization of immune complexes seen in the splenic ellipsoids of adult fish failed to occur. This indication that the spleen of 8-week-old fish is still somewhat immature is supported by the finding that melano-macrophage centre formation following antigenic stimulation occurs only to a limited extent in the young spleen.

Cell-Mediated Immunity

Histoincompatibility Reactions

Histoincompatibility reactions, manifested by the ability to reject allografts, provide an easy way to monitor the onset of cell-mediated immunity since it is possible to place grafts on delicate fish fry from an early stage of development. Such experiments indicate that the cellular component of the immune response matures rapidly in fish (Kallman and Gordon, 1957; Triplett and Barrymore, 1960; Sailendri, 1973; Botham *et al.*, 1980). Furthermore, this maturation can be correlated with critical stages in the histogenesis of the lymphoid organs in tilapia (Sailendri, 1973), carp (Botham and Manning, 1981) and rainbow trout (Grace, 1981; Manning *et al.*, 1981). Thus, in the trout, skin allograft reactivity relates to maturation of the thymus, the presence of small lymphocytes in the peripheral blood and the lymphocytic differentiation of the kidney.

In the carp, skin allografts in adults (Fig. 1) were found to have a mean survival time of 14 days at 22°C, with a lymphocytic invasion of the graft commencing at 2 to 4 days post-grafting and reaching a peak between 4 and 6 days. Fry of 16 days post-hatching were able to mount a cell-mediated response, although more slowly than adult fish. Lymphocytes were seen invading the graft by 4 to 8 days after grafting, but in much smaller

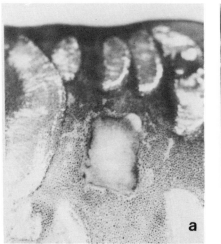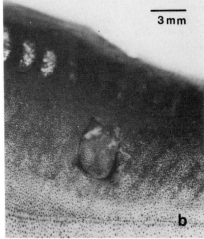

Fig. 1. Skin grafts on 1-year-old carp (22°C). (a) Allograft 12 days after grafting: note lack of pigment. (b) Autograft 11 days after grafting: note healthy appearance of the melanophores of the graft.

numbers than in adults. Thereafter, lymphocytic numbers increased rapidly with age of the host fish, possibly correlated with the large increase in lymphocytes in the pronephric and mesonephric kidneys, full adult reactivity being attained in 60-day-old fish. Young carp are capable not only of mounting an allograft response by day 16 post-hatching (albeit less efficiently than in adult fish) but also of developing a memory component in the response. Thus a skin graft applied to a carp at day 16 can induce an anamnestic (second-set) reaction at 1 month old to a graft taken from the same donor (Botham *et al.*, 1980; Botham and Manning, 1981).

In Vitro Correlates of Cell-Mediated Immunity

Specific inhibition of macrophage migration (Fig. 2) is an *in vitro* expression of delayed hypersensitivity which, in the mammal, is due to the liberation by specific antigen of a lymphokine factor, MIF (migration inhibition factor). Little is known about the relationship between lymphocytes and macrophages or the production of soluble non-immunoglobulin mediators of cellular immunity in fish, although the phenomenon of macrophage migration inhibition has been demonstrated both in elasmobranchs and in teleosts (McKinney *et al.*, 1976; O'Neill, 1978; Morrow, 1978; Jayaraman *et al.*, 1979).

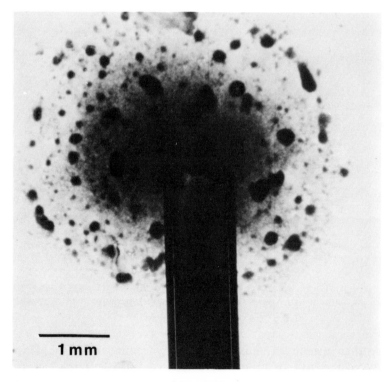

Fig. 2. Macrophage migration in carp, showing the normal fan which is produced when peripheral blood leucocytes are incubated for 24 hours at 26°C. Tests in which trays were everted and re-read 6 hours later indicate that the cell type which reaches the periphery of the fan is an adherent cell, probably a macrophage (see Secombes, 1981).

In mammals, MIF can readily be elicited non-specifically using T cell mitogens such as PHA (phytohaemagglutinin) and Con A (concanavalin A). These mitogens also inhibit macrophage migration in fish (P. D. Smith, personal communication). In our laboratory (Secombes, 1981), PHA at a concentration of 0.2 mg ml^{-1} and Con A at a concentration of 0.02 mg ml^{-1} elicited mean inhibition ratios respectively of 0.20 ± 0.05 and 0.37 ± 0.02 for blood leucocytes and 0.06 ± 0.09 and 0.20 ± 0.10 for pronephric cells when these were taken from normal carp weighing 30–40g. This migration inhibition could not be attributed solely to the cell agglutinating properties of the mitogen since in preliminary experiments using Con A (Table 5) it was found that the supernatant from a reaction could still effect macrophage migration inhibition after Con A had been removed by Sephadex G-200 gel filtration. There is therefore preliminary evidence for the occurrence of soluble lymphokine-like factors in mature fish. These play an important part in cell-mediated immunity but their presence has yet to be investigated in young fish fry.

Table 5. *MIF (Migration Inhibition Factor) in carp. Inhibition indices were obtained using pronephric cells treated with the supernatant obtained from 2-day cultures of Con A with normal leucocytes, followed by removal of the Con A by Sephadex G-200 gel filtration*

Source of leucocytes used in cultures	Amount of Con A added to 2.5ml cultures:	
	10μg	20μg
Blood	*0.56 ± 0.23	1.16 ± 0.17
Pronephros	1.03 ± 0.21	*0.80 ± 0.08
None	—	0.99 ± 0.02

*Significantly different from control at the 1% probability level.
Note: The most consistent results were obtained using supernatants from cultures incubated for 2 days. For shorter incubation periods the results were more variable, while for 3-day cultures no evidence for soluble inhibitory factors was obtained and some supernatants were even slightly stimulatory. See Secombes (1981). Values are means ± standard error.

Non-Specific Defence Mechanisms

Non-specific immunity involving both cells and soluble factors plays an important role in the defence mechanisms of fish both in the adult and during earlier stages of development (see Fletcher, 1981). Indeed the fish are probably almost entirely dependent on non-specific immunity during the period of free-living existence before their immune system has matured. Passive immunity, transferred from the mother to the fry, has not been demonstrated in fish, through C-reactive protein-like precipitins have been detected in the lumpsucker ova (Fletcher and Baldo, 1976) and lectin-like agglutinins are also present in fish eggs (Anstee *et al.*, 1973). Recently, van Loon *et al.* (1981) demonstrated maternal immunoglobulin in the ova of carp, though it is not known whether this is specific antibody and none has been detected in salmon (Ellis, 1977).

Phagocytosis has been studied by injecting colloidal carbon from as early an age as this procedure is possible in fish, namely in rainbow trout at 4 days post-hatching (Grace, 1981) and in carp at 2 weeks old (Grace *et al.*, 1981). In the trout at day 4, the kidney has not yet acquired a lymphoid population and the spleen anlage has only just appeared. Carbon particles were phagocytosed mostly by free macrophages. These accumulated in the connective tissue, under the skin, in the gut and in the gills and some were also found in the kidney, although not to any great extent at this age. By day 18, the kidney had become efficient in trapping carbon, while in 8-month-old trout, the main sites of localization of phagocytosed material were the spleen, kidney, heart and the macrophages of the blood. The largest amounts were in the kidney, which in trout has a better developed system of melano-macrophage centres than does the spleen (Agius, 1980; Grace, 1981). In young carp of 2 weeks old, the adult pattern of phagocytosis had already been attained, the kidney and spleen rapidly localizing the largest amounts of carbon as in older animals. After 20 days, the phagocytosed material was concentrated in areas where melano-macrophage centres occur in older fish, although little melanin was seen in these young fry.

Role of the Thymus in the
Ontogenetic Development of the Immune System

The fish thymus, particularly that of teleosts, differs from the mammalian thymus in several respects, not only in the surface immunoglobulin of its thymocytes, the poor cortex/medullary distinction, the paucity of Hassall's corpuscles and other epithelial derivatives, and the presence of plasma cells and plaque-forming cells, but also in its anatomical relationships. The teleost thymus starts its development as a thickening of the epithelium in the dorso-anterior part of the pharynx without the distinct separation of any thymic epithelial buds as such. Moreover, instead of losing contact with the pharyngeal epithelium early in ontogeny, the teleost thymus retains this contact and is separated from the pharyngeal lumen by only a single layer of cells (Grace, 1981; Manning, 1981). It is therefore of interest to see whether removal of the thymus has the same effect in fish as in other vertebrates.

Thymectomy operations have been performed on young fish in the tilapia by Sailendri (1973) and in the rainbow trout by Grace (1981) and by Secombes (1981). Thymectomy in trout fry aged 4 to 24 days had no noticeable effect on the lymphocytic population of the kidney, but greatly decreased the numbers of lymphoid cells in the spleen. In trout thymectomized at day 14 post-hatching, the lymphoid cells of both spleen and kidney demonstrated a pyroninophilic and proliferative response to antigenic stimulation when the fish were immunized 1 month after thymectomy and killed 4 to 6 weeks later. This response was, however, less intense than in sham-thymectomized fish. Similarly, a lymphocytic response to allografts occurs in young thymectomized fish but is less intense than in controls.

In adult fish, short-term thymectomy in the tilapia reduced the response to sheep erythrocytes whilst leaving unaltered the response to PVP (poly-

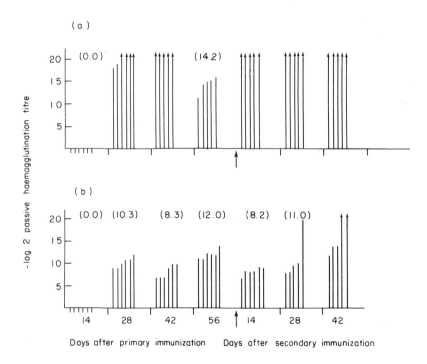

Fig. 3. Antibody production against HGG (human gamma globulin) in trout following adult thymectomy (a) or sham-operation (b). Each column represents one individual with mean values given in parentheses, arrows at the top of these columns indicate that the titre exceeded well 20. Bold arrow denotes the time of the booster immunization.

M. J. MANNING *ET AL.*

vinylpyrrolidone) (Jayaraman *et al.*, 1979). In mammals, these are thymus-dependent and thymus-independent antigens respectively. Adult thymectomy had no effect on either first-set or second-set rejection of skin allografts in rainbow trout (Grace, 1981). It did, however, affect antibody production in carp and trout (Secombes, 1981) in a way which provides tentative evidence for a suppressive role of the thymus in antibody formation in fish. Thus in carp immunized 4 weeks after adult thymectomy, serum antibody levels against *Aeromonas salmonicida* were elevated above those of sham-operated fish at day 7 of the response, returning to normal values at subsequent stages. Similarly, in rainbow trout short-term adult thymectomy resulted in elevated titres in the response to HGG both in the primary and in the secondary response (Fig. 3), although unlike the results for carp, antibody production against *Aeromonas salmonicida* remained unaffected by thymectomy (Fig. 4).

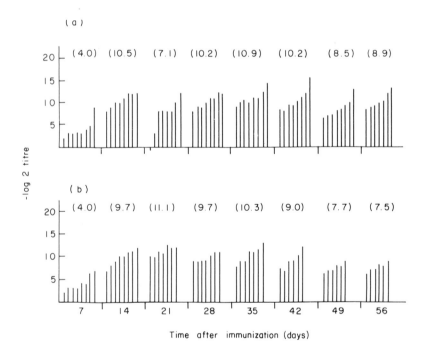

Fig. 4. Antibody production against *Aeromonas salmonicida* in trout following adult thymectomy (a) or sham-operation (b). Each column represents one individual with mean values given in parentheses.

Discussion

One aim in immunizing fish against disease is to produce a good response on secondary exposure. Strong and long-lasting immunological memory is of greater importance than a good primary response, and it has already been demonstrated in carp that high antibody titres following the first injection do not necessarily ensure the best results on subsequent exposure (Rijkers *et al.*, 1980). Also, all three aspects of immunity (non-specific, cell-mediated and humoral) must be considered in order to enhance those components which are likely to be of greatest benefit to the fish. Furthermore, there may be strong incentives for commencing immunization early in development, both to afford protection as soon as possible and for motives of economy and convenience. The criteria for good long-term protection in these circumstances must include a consideration of any possible tolerogenic factors. This involves examination of the type of antigen chosen and of the way in which it is presented, as well as recognition of any potentially adverse environmental conditions (Avtalion, 1981). Furthermore, the schedule for immunization should be related to the state of immunocompetence of the young fish so that the antigen can be used to prime the immune system at an age when it can act effectively to induce a good secondary response.

From the evidence presented here, albeit somewhat tentatively, it seems that in carp and rainbow trout non-specific immunity is soon supplemented by the rapidly developing cell-mediated component of the immune system, although the relative importance of these two forms of defence, and how they interact, remains to be determined. In these cell-mediated reactions, memory can be induced as early as the second week of life and is effective in 1-month-old fish. The humoral antibody component of immunity takes longer to mature, however, and states of non-responsiveness can be induced to certain antigens. In our experiments, young fish responded better to formalin-killed *Aeromonas salmonicida* organisms (which were not tolerogenic) than to foreign proteins, but whether this is a comparison between particulate and soluble antigens or between those that are thymus-independent and those that are thymus-dependent respectively (see Secombes, 1981) is not clear. That the latter may be the case is suggested by the finding that early immunization with the thymus-dependent antigen SRBC can also lead to a state of non-responsiveness in carp; also by the results of Etlinger *et al.* (1979) who obtained good responses using thymus-independent antigens in young trout. Evidence that suppressor cells occur in fish (Lopez *et al.*, 1974; Avtalion *et al.*, 1980), together with our present preliminary work on enhanced antibody production in thymectomized adults suggests that some of the mechanisms which regulate immunological reactivity and tolerance in mammals may also be present in fish.

Acknowledgments

The work from our laboratory was supported by a research grant (GR3/3297) from the Natural Environment Research Council and by a Science Research Council CASE award (to C.J.S.).

References

Anstee, D. J., Holt, P. H. and Pardoe, G. I. (1973). Agglutinins from fish ova defining blood groups B and P. *Vox Sang, Basel* **25**, 347–360.

Agius, C. (1980). Phylogenetic development of melano-macrophage centres in fish. *Journal of Zoology, London* **191**, 11–31.

Avtalion, R. R. (1981). Induction of immunological tolerance in carp and its possible implication in seasonal diseases of fish. *In* "Immunology and Immunization of Fish" (Ed. W. B. van Muiswinkel). *Developmental and Comparative Immunology* suppl. 2 (in press).

Avtalion, R. R., Wishkovsky, A. and Katz, D. (1980). Regulatory effect of temperature on specific suppression and enhancement of the humoral response in fish. *In* "Phylogeny of Immunological Memory" (Ed. M. J. Manning), pp.113–121. Elsevier/North Holland Biomedical Press, Amsterdam.

Botham, J. W. and Manning, M. J. (1981). Histogenesis of the lymphoid organs in the carp *Cyprinus carpio* L. and the ontogenetic development of allograft reactivity. *Journal of Fish Biology* **19**, 403–414.

Botham, J. W., Grace, M. F. and Manning, M. J. (1980). Ontogeny of first set and second set alloimmune reactivity in fishes. *In* "Phylogeny of Immunological Memory" (Ed. M. J. Manning), pp.83–92. Elsevier/North Holland Biomedical Press, Amsterdam.

Dorson, M. (1974). Production d'anticorps précipitants anti-dinitrophénol chez les alevins de truite Arc-en-ciel (*Salmo gairdneri*) immunisés à l'âge d'une mois. *C.r.Acadamie Science, Paris* **278**, 3151–3152.

Ellis, A. E. (1977). Ontogeny of the immune response in *Salmo salar*. Histogenesis of the lymphoid organs and appearance of membrane immunoglobulin and mixed leucocyte reactivity. *In* "Developmental Immunobiology" (Eds. J. B. Solomon and J. D. Horton), pp.225–231. Elsevier/North Holland Biomedical Press, Amsterdam.

Etlinger, H. M., Chiller, J. M. and Hodgins, H. O. (1979). Evolution of the lymphoid system IV. Murine T-independent but not T-dependent antigens are very immunogenic in rainbow trout *Salmo gairdneri*. *Cellular Immunology* **47**, 400–406.

Fletcher, T. C. (1981). Non-specific defence mechanisms of fish. *In* "Immunology and Immunization of Fish" (Ed. W. B. van Muiswinkel). *Developmental and Comparative Immunology* suppl. 2 (in press).

Fletcher, T. C. and Baldo, B. A. (1976). C-reactive protein like precipitins in lumpsucker (*Cyclopterus lumpus* L.) gametes. *Experientia* **32**, 1192-1201.

Grace, M. F. (1981). The Functional Histogenesis of the Immune System in Rainbow Trout, *Salmo gairdneri* Richardson 1836. Ph.D. Thesis, University of Hull.

Grace, M. F. and Manning, M. J. (1980). Histogenesis of the lymphoid organs in rainbow trout, *Salmo gairdneri* Rich. 1836. *Developmental and Comparative Immunology* **4**, 255-264.

Grace, M. F., Botham, J. W. and Manning, M. J. (1981). Ontogeny of lymphoid organ function in fish. *In* "Aspects of Comparative and Developmental Immunology 1" (Ed. J. B. Solomon), pp.467-468. Pergamon Press, New York and Oxford.

Jayaraman, S., Mohan, R. and Muthukkaruppan, Vr. (1979). Relationship between migration inhibition and plaque-forming cell responses to sheep erythrocytes in the teleost, *Tilapia mossambica*. *Developmental and Comparative Immunology* **3**, 67-75.

Kallman, K. D. and Gordon, M. (1957). Transplantation of fins in Xiphophorin fishes. *Annals of the New York Academy of Science* **71**, 307-318.

Khalifa, K. A. and Post, G. (1976). Immune response of advanced rainbow trout fry to *Aeromonas liquefaciens*. *Progressive Fish Culturist* **38**, 66-68.

Lopez, D. M., Sigel, M. M. and Lee, J. C. (1974). Phylogenetic studies on T cells. Lymphocytes of the shark with differential response to phytohaemagglutinin and concanavalin A. *Cellular Immunology* **10**, 287-293.

Manning, M. J. (1981). A comparative view of the thymus in vertebrates. *In* "The Thymus Gland" (Ed. M. D. Kendall), pp.7-20. Symposium No. 1 of the Anatomical Society, Academic Press, London.

Manning, M. J., Grace, M. F. and Secombes, C. J. (1981). Ontogenetic aspects of tolerance and immunity in carp and rainbow trout: Studies on the role of the thymus. *In* "Immunology and Immunization of Fish" (Ed. W. B. van Muiswinkel (in press). *Developmental and Comparative Immunology* suppl. 2.

McKinney, E. C., Ortiz, G., Lee, J. C., Sigel, M. M., Lopez, D. M., Epstein, R. S. and McLeod, T. F. (1976). Lymphocytes of fish: multipotential or specialized? *In* "Phylogeny of Thymus and Bone Marrow — Bursa Cells" (Eds. R. K. Wright and E. L. Cooper), pp.73-82. Elsevier/North Holland Biomedical Press, Amsterdam.

Morrow, W. J. W. (1978). The Immune Response of the Dogfish *Scyliorhinus canicula* L. Ph.D. Thesis, Plymouth Polytechnic (CNAA).

O'Neill, J. G. (1978). The Immune Response in Teleosts: The Effects of Temperature and Heavy Metals. Ph.D. Thesis, Trent Polytechnic, Nottingham (CNAA).

Paterson, W. D. and Fryer, J. L. (1974). Immune response of juvenile coho salmon (*Oncorhynchus kisutch*) to *Aeromonas salmonicida* cells administered intraperitoneally in Freund's Complete Adjuvant. *Journal of the Fisheries Research Board, Canada* **31**, 1751-1755.

Rijkers, G. T. and van Muiswinkel, W. B. (1977). The immune system of cyprinid fish. The development of cellular and humoral responsiveness in the rosy barb (*Barbus conchonius*). *In* "Developmental Immunobiology" (Eds. J. B. Solomon and J. D. Horton), pp.233-240. Elsevier/North Holland Biomedical Press, Amsterdam.

Rijkers, G. T., Frederix-Wolters, L. M. H. and van Muiswinkel, W. B. (1980). The immune system of cyprinid fish: The effect of antigen dose and route of administration on the development of immunological memory in carp (*Cyprinus carpio*). *In* "Phylogeny of Immunological Memory" (Ed. M. J. Manning), pp.93–102. Elsevier/North Holland Biomedical Press, Amsterdam.

Sailendri, K. (1973). Studies on the Development of Lymphoid Organs and Immune Responses in the Teleost, *Tilapia mossambica* (Peters). Ph.D. Thesis, Madurai University, India.

Secombes, C. J. (1981). Comparative Studies on the Structure and Function of Teleost Lymphoid Organs. Ph.D. Thesis, University of Hull.

Secombes, C. J. and Manning, M. J. (1980). Comparative studies on the immune system of fishes and amphibians: antigen localization in the carp *Cyprinus carpio* L. *Journal of Fish Diseases* **3**, 399–412.

Secombes, C. J. and Manning, M. J. (1981). Histological changes in lymphoid organis of carp following injection of soluble or particulate antigens. *In* "Immunology and Immunization of Fish" (Ed. W. B. van Muiswinkel). *Developmental and Comparative Immunology* suppl. 2 (in press).

Serero, M. and Avtalion, R. R. (1978). Regulatory effect of temperature and antigen upon immunity in ectothermic vertebrates III. Establishment of immunological suppression in fish. *Developmental and Comparative Immunology* **2**, 87–94.

Triplett, E. L. and Barrymore, S. (1960). Tissue specificity in embryonic and adult *Cymatogaster aggregata* studied by scale transplantation. *Biological Bulletin* **118**, 463–471.

van Loon, J. J. A., van Oosterom, R. and van Muiswinkel, W. B. (1981). Development of the immune system in carp (*Cyprinus carpio*). *In* "Aspects of Comparative and Developmental Immunology 1" (Ed. J. B. Solomon), pp.469–470. Pergamon Press, New York and Oxford.

3

The Development of Bacterial Vaccines
for Fish

P. D. WARD

Wellcome Research Laboratories
Langley Court, Beckenham, Kent, England

Introduction

Although severe epizootics are known in wild fish populations, for example a disease in white perch (*Roccus americanus*) in the Chesapeake Bay area of U.S.A. caused by a *Pasteurella*-like organism (Sniesko *et al.*, 1964) and a disease caused by a similar *Pasteurella*-like organism in menhaden and mullet in Galveston Bay (Lewis *et al.*, 1970) it is fair to say that the major problems caused by bacterial diseases in fish are seen in farmed fish. As happened with other intensively farmed species, the high stocking density necessary for financial success on a fish farm provides an ideal environment for the transmission of diseases. Losses due to seasonal outbreaks of disease can be enormous, necessitating the institution of control measures immediately an outbreak is confirmed.

Until recently, the only methods available for treating fish have been therapeutic based on the use of chemicals and antibiotics. Chemicals suffer from the limitation that they rely on a differential toxicity and the therapeutic index, the differences between the therapeutic and toxic doses, is very low. Antibiotics, in general, are not toxic to the host but prolonged or repeated applications may cause resistance to develop in the target organism making further treatment much more difficult. Where treatment is effective, it is not usually started until an outbreak of disease has been confirmed by which time a significant proportion of the fish might be infected. The cost of treatment then includes not only the cost of the antibiotic but also the cost to the farmer of the dead fish since a proportion of the infected fish will not be cured. This happens because infected fish are often anorexic and they do not eat enough of the medicated food provided. In light of this, alternative strategies of disease control have been sought.

Vaccination against bacterial diseases is a well established practice in

47

most systems of animal husbandry. It has the advantage over therapeutic antibiotic treatment of being applied prophylactically. Protection provoked by vaccination is usually long lasting; animals require only one or two doses to protect them over a full season of exposure and it suffers none of the problems of resistance or residue accumulation which may arise with anti-biotics. In the long term, therefore, if vaccines are available they are likely to be the method of choice for protecting fish against bacterial diseases.

The Concept of Immunizing Fish

Vaccination will be an effective way of protecting fish from disease only if it is possible to provoke a protective immune response in the host against the pathogen involved.

The Immune Response in Fish

The phylogeny of the immune response throughout the animal kingdom has been the subject of intense study for several years and the work prior to 1976 is comprehensively reviewed by Marchalonis (1977).

For details of the immune response of fish, the reader is referred to the chapters by Manning and Ellis in this volume. Suffice it to say here that fish, over a certain size/age threshold, are capable of mounting both antibody mediated and cellular immune responses. The role of these responses in the protection of fish against pathogenic micro-organisms is in most cases not yet clear. For example, there appears to be no direct relationship between the antibody response of rainbow trout (*Salmo gairdneri*) to antigens derived from the bacterium *Vibrio anguillarum*, as measured by bacterial agglutination, passive haemagglutination or complement fixation, and the capacity of the fish to resist challenge (Horne, M. T., unpublished results). Likewise, the role of cellular immunity is not understood since the necessary investigations have not been performed.

In spite of the lack of information on the precise mechanisms of protective immunity in fish, it has been shown on numerous occasions that fish can be protected against bacterial diseases by immunization. Commercial vaccines to combat infections by *Yersinia ruckeri* (Wildlife Vaccines, Colorado 80033, U.S.A.) and *Vibrio anguillarum* (Wildlife Vaccines and Biomed Laboratories, Washington 98122, U.S.A.) are available and experimental vaccines against *Aeromonas salmonicida* (Duff, 1942; Krantz *et al.*, 1964), *Pseudomonas anguilliseptica* (Nakai and Muroga, 1979) and *Renibacterium salmoninarum* (Paterson *et al.*, 1981) have all been claimed to be effective against laboratory challenge.

Vaccine Delivery Systems

Vaccines are usually delivered by injection but alternatives have been developed. For example, some *Escherichia coli* vaccines are administered orally after adsorption on to feedstuff and live *Bordetella* vaccines are administered by inhalation. In the aquatic environment other options are open and the four major delivery systems available will now be discussed.

Intraperitoneal injection. Intraperitoneal injection of antigens is an effective way of provoking an antibody response in fish (Clem and Sigel, 1963). It suffers, however, from numerous drawbacks which limit its potential use in the field. It is time consuming, labour intensive and consequently expensive to administer to the large numbers of fish held on farms. Fish must be anaesthetized before they can be injected; this stresses them, producing effects that could significantly affect their ability to mount optimal immune responses. For safe handling and injection, fish would have to be of reasonable size; it would not be possible to contemplate vaccination of small fry by injection. Because of these limitations it is likely that injection of vaccine will be used only in fish of sufficiently high unit value to absorb the cost of the procedure. For example, salmon smolts were injected with a *Vibrio anguillarum* vaccine and a high level of protection was obtained (Sawyer and Strout, 1977).

Direct immersion. Immersion of fish in antigen solutions emerged as a potential commercial process following the work of Amend (1976) and Antipa and Amend (1977). These workers developed a hyperosmotic immersion technique where prior to immersion in antigen solution fish were dipped for a short time in a hyperosmotic salt solution. This step, it was suggested, enhanced the uptake of antigen. Subsequently, it was found that immersing the fish in the vaccine was sufficient exposure to immunize (Gould *et al.*, 1979). Although this method is not free of stressing manipulations, it has the advantage that it can easily be adapted to vaccinate large numbers of fish and it can be used to vaccinate fry of any size above the critical size for immune responsiveness.

Spray vaccination. This can be seen as a variant of direct immersion where antigen is sprayed under pressure on to the fish as they are propelled along a shallow channel (U.S. Patent 4223014).

Oral vaccination. Presentation to fish of antigen absorbed on to food is potentially the most useful method of vaccination available. It is non-stressing, it can be used to vaccinate fish of any size and requires no extra labour or time than normal farm husbandry. It does, however, suffer from a few limitations. To obtain effective immunity it is necessary to give a large number of doses of antigen (Fryer *et al.*, 1976), the total amount of antigen needed is very much greater than that needed in the methods already described and the immunity which oral vaccination provokes is not as long lasting as that provoked by injection. If, however, it can be shown to cover the period of risk then it would still be useful.

As will be apparent, the route of administration chosen will depend on a balance of factors, including assessment of each method in relation to the pathology of the disease in question.

Identification of Disease Problems and Potential Vaccines

The starting point for developing any vaccine is the recognition by the farming and veterinary services that a disease problem exists. In the case of a bacterial disease a putative causative agent will be isolated. Definitive proof of the causative role of such an isolate must rest on proving Koch's postulates in the target species. If it is possible to provoke a disease similar in all respects to the natural disease and to re-isolate the organism from the infected animal then it can be assumed that the organism isolated is the causative agent.

At this stage scientific developments can proceed along a number of lines and it becomes necessary to obtain a commercial appraisal of the potential of a vaccine against the disease in question.

Scientific Investigation

This can be conveniently divided into the areas listed below.

Disease pathology. This must be investigated in order to establish the site and mechanism of infection. Such investigations may well indicate the point in the infectious process at which acquired immunity could be effective and thus suggest possible approaches to a vaccine. This approach is typified by the development of vaccines against colibacillosis in piglets. Histological and genetic studies showed that infecting *E. coli* adhere to the mucosal surface of the anterior small intestine and that this adhesion was mediated by a surface antigen, K88 (Jones and Rutter, 1972). A vaccine which stimulated antibodies against the K88 antigen inhibited the adhesion of *E. coli* to the mucosa, thus stopping colonization and disease (Jones and Rutter, 1974).

The organism. In vitro studies contribute towards an understanding of the role of the causative organism in the disease process. The production of toxins, if any, should be investigated, the antigenic composition of the cell wall or capsule if present should be analysed and the number of antigenic types which exist in the field should be determined. This latter information will provide an estimate of the likely number of components which any future vaccine will need to give adequate cover in the field.

With a view ultimately to production of a vaccine, the cultural requirements of the organism should be established. The influence on growth of conditions including temperature, medium, dissolved gases and incubation time should be investigated to ensure that all are optimized.

Laboratory challenge system. To enable experimental vaccine formulations to be tested a good challenge system is necessary. Ideally this should be in the target animal. This is not a problem with farmed fish species. The system developed should approximate as closely as possible to the mode of infection in the field and above all it must be reproducible.

The challenge should aim to produce >80% morbidity or mortality in challenged fish on a time scale similar to the natural disease. For fish the most appropriate route of infection is via the water but some workers use intraperitoneal injection since in this way it is easier to quantitate the challenge.

Choice of antigens and vaccine formulation. With the establishment of an effective, reproducible laboratory challenge and information from the other fields mentioned, testing of potential vaccines can begin.

For some organisms there will be a number of approaches to protection and the likely candidates will have been defined by investigations of the disease pathology. It may be possible to provoke a protective antibacterial immunity or alternatively, as with *E. coli* in piglets, an anti-adhesin may be the preferred course. Thirdly, if toxin-mediated damage appears to be the major problem then a vaccine which produces effective antitoxic antibodies may be effective. In this case, vaccinated fish may be asymptomatic but carrying a high bacterial load and the effect of this on future performance should be considered.

As well as the choice of antigens the need for adjuvants must also be considered. Incorporation of adjuvants into vaccines can produce reactogenic products. In most cases a balance must be struck between providing effective levels of immunity and minimal reactivity. In fish, the response to intraperitoneal vaccination would seem the only one likely to be modified by an adjuvant, so care should be taken to ensure that lesions in this cavity are minimal. The possible use of adjuvants in dip or spray vaccines does not seem to have been investigated.

As the formulation of the vaccine becomes clearer the dose of antigen and the timing and frequency of administration will be investigated in relation to the duration of protection, the aim being to produce immunity over the complete season of risk with the minimum number of administrations of antigen.

Commercial Considerations

Concurrent with the laboratory investigations of the disease, the commercial prospects of vaccines must be considered. The potential of new vaccines must be clearly defined very early in any development since production requires the allocation of research and development facilities and production plant ranging from fermenters to packaging equipment. This requires a minimum level of profitability.

It is the role of the marketing capability within an organization to produce data on potential markets for new products, on the cost of the disease to the industry and from this the likely selling price of a vaccine, and finally, to estimate the available market share and overall profitability. Such data are collected from as wide a base as possible, specially commissioned surveys are able to give state of the art information and indicate future trends, local information is obtained from veterinary services and also by contact with individual farmers.

Throughout this commercial appraisal, constant communications between the scientific and commercial functions is vital, for if commercial considerations indicate that it is unwise to continue development work there must be an agreed termination. If, however, the future for a product appears good, then the level of scientific manning must be considered to optimize the rate of progress.

Production and Testing

Once an effective vaccine has been developed on a laboratory scale, it must be scaled up for production. This primarily involves changing from fermenters of up to 10 litre capacity to fermenters of up to 1500 litre capacity. Not only does the size change but often the construction material is different. These differences, plus those that develop from differences in tank geometry and aeration method, make the adaptation of technique an individual process for each fermenter.

The success of transfer can finally be judged by showing that in the experimental challenge system used to test laboratory formulations the production material performs at least as well.

Testing

Regulations set up by the licensing authorities ensure that only vaccines which are safe and effective are launched on to the market.

Initial field-testing. In the U.K. the first phase of testing a new vaccine requires the issue of an Animal Test Certificate. This enables the holder to field-test a vaccine preparation which has been shown to be safe and efficacious in the target species under laboratory conditions.

These trials should be performed in populations of fish where there is a reasonable expectation of a natural challenge. Control and experimental fish should be identically treated ensuring that the contents of each holding unit be it tank, pond or floating net cage contains a number from each group. Only in this way can indeterminate non-specific environmental effects be excluded. To ensure that the vaccine is performing in the field as well as it did in the laboratory, arrangements should be made to monitor the immune response by an appropriate method and to challenge a number of vaccinated fish in the laboratory setting. In this way, it may prove possible to establish a set of non-destructive criteria which will indicate whether fish have been effectively immunized.

This field-trial stage is an appropriate time to assess the effect of vaccination on the performance of the treated population. It should prove possible to assess food conversion rates, growth rates and need for antibiotic–chemical treatment in vaccinated and control groups to ensure that treated fish perform better than controls. An effective vaccine which concurrently reduces growth rate or food conversion is not likely to be a successful product.

Product Licence

Trials performed under the aegis of an Animal Test Certificate should provide sufficient data on efficacy to proceed to a submission for a Product Licence. There is at present no mention of fish vaccines in the British Veterinary Codex 1965 (B.Vet.C) or the Supplement (B.Vet.C. Suppl.) published in 1970. However, the majority of the requirements described for other vaccines appear directly applicable to fish. In the list below deviations from the Codex will be indicated.

Sterility. Vaccines submitted for sale should be sterile. The standard test detailed in the B.Vet.C. Suppl. pp.269–271 would appear to be directly applicable to fish vaccines.

These tests require media which will support aerobic and/or anaerobic growth to be inoculated with samples taken from production batches of vaccines. No growth should occur under any conditions. In the event of growth occurring, there is the possibility of re-testing the vaccine twice. If after three tests there is still a question over the sterility the batch must not be passed. The test also specifies the number of samples which must be tested from production runs of various sizes; this is to ensure that a statistically significant sample is taken.

Safety. The B.Vet.C. Suppl. prescribes that 'A minimum of two healthy susceptible animals of at least one of the species in which the vaccine is intended to be used are each injected by the route recommended by the manufacturer for field use with twice the appropriate vaccinating dose and observed for an appropriate period of not less than 7 days. No abnormal reactions should develop.'.

This test would appear directly applicable to fish only when vaccines intended for intraperitoneal injection are tested and even then it is important that the size of fish to be used is specified. Our experience indicates that different sizes of fish respond to the same vaccine in different ways. Regulations should ensure that the smallest fish likely to be vaccinated is safe.

With vaccines intended for use as a direct immersion bath the requirement of 'twice the recommended dose' could best be complied with by making up the immersion suspension at twice the recommended concentration and immersing the fish for the stated time. Again the size should be the minimum size recommended for vaccination and the use of compressed oxygen to maintain the dissolved oxygen levels should be considered.

Freedom from abnormal toxicity. The B.Vet.C. Suppl. lays out the following test for vaccines:

(i) Two healthy mice, each weighing 18–22g are each injected sub-cutaneously with 0.5ml of the vaccine and observed for 5 days; no abnormal reaction develops.
(ii) Two healthy guinea pigs, each weighing 250–400g are each injected intraperitoneally with at least 2ml of the vaccine and observed for 10 days; no abnormal reaction develops.

As stated, these tests exclude 'abnormal toxicity' from the vaccine; they are, however, drawn up to ensure that vaccines are safe for use in homoeothermic animals. One of their aims is to exclude the toxicity derived from excessive endotoxin contamination of vaccines. Fish being poikilothermic do not respond to endotoxins in the same way as do homoeotherms. Investigations have shown that fish are refractory to the toxic effects of endotoxins derived from Gram-negative bacteria. Preparations with a mouse LD50 of 21.6mg kg^{-1} were tolerated to a level of >714mg kg^{-1} by fish. Thus these tests would seem inapplicable to fish vaccines. Our suggestion is that fish vaccines be subjected to one test to ensure safety and freedom from abnormal toxicity and it should be drawn up along the lines suggested for the safety test. This suggestion has been accepted by the U.K. Licensing Authority for at least one vaccine.

Potency. The B.Vet.C. and Supplement do not specify any tests for fish vaccines. The following suggested tests are drawn up on the basis of treating the fish to be vaccinated as a population and not as individuals. Herd immunity will, therefore, be the aim of vaccination and the requirements for protection in potency tests will reflect this.

For vaccines to be administered by intraperitoneal injection groups of 50 fish of the recommended size of a susceptible species should be acclimatized to water temperatures in the range where an effective immune response can be expected, 10–15°C for salmonids. They should be anaesthetized, injected with the recommended vaccine dose and 28 days later challenged with a single LD90 dose of a virulent strain of the causative organism. Saline-injected controls should also be challenged. All fish should be kept for 10 days. Vaccinated fish should show a relative per cent survival (RPS) of >70%. RPS is defined as:

$$1 - \frac{\% \text{ Mortality of Vaccinated Fish}}{\% \text{ Mortality of Controls}} \times 100$$

For vaccines to be administered by direct immersion, groups of 50 fish of the recommended size of a susceptible species should be acclimatized to a water temperature in the range where an effective immune response can be expected, 10–15°C for salmonids. They should be immersed in the recommended concentration of vaccine for the appropriate time; control fish should be manipulated in the same way. Twenty eight days later all groups should be challenged by dipping in a culture of virulent organisms adjusted to produce a control mortality of 80–100% in 8–10 days. Vaccinated fish should show an RPS of >70%.

It will be clear from reading these tests that they will not cover all the situations which arise. However, they do suggest lower limits to the acceptable levels of immunity.

At the outset of manufacture, a vaccine should be set aside for use as a standard for future comparison. As experience in testing widens it will become possible to establish National and Working Standards whereby further production batches can be judged.

Stability. Although no test is laid down in the regulations, it is necessary to provide data which show that the vaccine retains its potency for the maximum recommended storage period.

Presentation. The presentation of the vaccine must be specified. Consideration should be given to the composition of containers (glass or plastic), the size of the pack (for fish this is almost certain to be multidose packs) and the documentation to be included with the product.

If a product complies with all these requirements then it is granted a product licence and it can be marketed.

After-Sales Service

The responsibility of vaccine manufacturers does not end with the sale of the approved vaccine. In spite of all the precautions taken during manufacture and testing, there will inevitably be cases of adverse reactions to the vaccines or apparent breakdown of the protection conferred. All these instances must be investigated to try to ensure that the underlying cause is identified to preclude a recurrence in the case of reactions or to check that the condition giving rise to the apparent breakdown is indeed caused by the organism against which the vaccine should confer protection. Investigation of these instances can give rise to the identification of new serotypes not covered by those blended into the vaccine; in which case it may be necessary to modify the vaccine by including the new serotype. It may, however, identify an organism giving rise to a new epizootic with the potential for a new vaccine.

The ultimate acceptability of any vaccine depends on the users assessment of the financial gain accuring from vaccination. Factors contributing to this include a better conversion rate, a higher growth rate, a larger number of fish raised to market size and lower therapy costs. All these must be monitored to ensure that the vaccine is fulfilling its potential.

Conclusions

As fish farming spreads to encompass new species and new environments, so the range of bacterial diseases encountered will grow. Vaccination has been shown to be an effective way of protecting fish against bacterial diseases and consequently the number of vaccines will increase. Ultimately combination vaccines will be developed to immunize against a range of conditions; these will include not only bacterial diseases but viral diseases and possibly parasite infections as well.

References

Amend, D. F. (1976). Prevention and control of viral diseases of salmonids. *Journal of the Fisheries Research Board of Canada* 33, 1059–1066.

Antipa, R. and Amend, D. F. (1977). Immunization of Pacific salmon: Comparison of intraperitoneal injection and hyperosmotic infiltration of *Vibrio anguillarum* and *Aeromonas salmonicida* bacterins. *Journal of the Fisheries Research Board of Canada* 34, 203–208.

Clem, L. W. and Sigel, M. M. (1963). Comparative immunochemical and immunological reactions in marine fishes with soluble viral and bacterial antigens. *Federation Proceedings* 22, 1138–1144.

Duff, D. C. B. (1942). The oral immunization of trout against *Bacterium salmonicida*. *Journal of Immunology* 44, 87–94.

Fryer, J. L., Rohovec, J. S., Tebbit, G. L., McMichael, J. S. and Pilcher, K. S. (1976). Vaccination for control of infectious diseases in Pacific salmon. *Fish Pathology* 10, 155–164.

Gould, R . W., Antipa, R. and Amend, D. F. (1979). Immersion vaccination of sockeye salmon (*Onchorhynchus nerka*) with two pathogenic strains of *Vibrio anguillarum*. *Journal of the Fisheries Research Board of Canada* 36, 222–225.

Jones, G. W. and Rutter, J. M. (1972). Role of the K88 antigen in the pathogenesis of neonatal diarrhoea caused by *Escherichia coli* in piglets. *Infection and Immunity* 6, 918–927.

Jones, G. W. and Rutter, J. M. (1974). Contribution of the K88 antigen of *Escherichia coli* to enteropathogenicity: Protection against disease by neutralizing the adhesive activity of K88 antigen. *American Journal of Clinical Nutrition* 27, 1414–1449.

Krantz, G. E., Reddecliff, J. M. and Heist, C. E. (1964). Immune response of trout to *Aeromonas salmonicida*. Part I. Development of agglutinating antibodies and protective immunity. *Progressive Fish Culturist* 26, 3–10.

Lewis, D. H., Grumbles, L. C., McConnell, S. and Flowers, A. I. (1970). *Pasteurella*-like bacteria from an epizootic in menhaden and mullet in Galveston Bay. *Journal of Wildlife Disease* 6, 160–163.

Marchalonis, J. J. (1977). "Immunity in Evolution". Edward Arnold Ltd. ISBN 0 7131 2657 4, London.

Nakai, T. and Muroga, K. (1979). Studies on Red Spot Disease of pond-cultured eels. V. Immune response of the Japanese eel to the causative bacterium *Pseudomonas anguilliseptica*. *Bulletin of the Japanese Society of Scientific Fisheries* 45, 817–821.

Paterson, W. D., Desoutels, D. and Weber, J. M. (1981). The immune response of

Atlantic salmon, *Salmo salar* to the causative agent of bacterial kidney disease *Renibacterium salmoninarum*. *Journal of Fish Diseases* **4/2**, 99–11.

Sawyer, E. S. and Strout, R. G. (1977). Survival and growth of vaccinated, medicated and untreated Coho salmon (*Onchorhynchus kisutch*) exposed to *Vibrio anguillarum*. *Aquaculture* **10**, 311–315.

Sneisko, S., Bullock, G., Hollis, E. and Boone, J. G. (1964). *Pasteurella sp.* from an epizootic of white perch (*Roccus americanus*) in Chesapeake Bay tidewater areas. *Journal of Bacteriology* **88**, 1814–1815.

4

Newly Discovered Viruses and Viral Diseases of Fishes, 1977–1981

KEN WOLF

Fish and Wildlife Service,
National Fish Health Research Laboratory,
Kearneysville, West Virginia 25430 U.S.A.

Introduction

The first fish virus was isolated in 1957 and reported 3 years later; however, the history of fish virology can be traced back much farther. In the first text on fish diseases (Hofer, 1904), Konrad Gesner was credited with describing fish pox in the year 1563. Hofer attributed fish pox to a primary internal myxosporidan infection, but his student Plehn (1924) prophetically attributed fish pox and lymphocystis to "ultramicroscopic" organisms. In the interim, Weissenberg (1914) had reported the first of his studies of lymphocystis disease and correctly interpreted the cells' distinctive inclusions as being of viral origin; however, proof of the viral aetiology of lymphocystis disease waited for nearly 50 years.

Since the first isolation of a fish virus was reported, knowledge of the subject has accumulated rapidly and is expected to continue in that mode for at least the next decade or two. There exists a sizeable sequence of reviews of fish virology. Accordingly, the present work encompasses the more recently discovered agents and their diseases or neoplasms—more specifically, it is restricted to selection of literature appearing during 1977–1981.

Nigrelli (1952), who compiled the first review of fish viral diseases, suggested a viral aetiology for fish pox, lymphocystis, and certain lympho-sarcomas and papillomas. Although his review predated isolation of virus, he also mentioned several other conditions that later were found to involve virus. Watson (1954) was next to review the subject and seven of the eight diseases he discussed were later found to have an associated if not causal virus.

Ten years elapsed before the next review but by that time two agents had been isolated—the viruses of infectious pancreatic necrosis and viral haemorrhagic septicemia (Wolf, 1964). Two years later, the grunt fin agent and lymphocystis virus had been isolated; electron microscopy showed evidence of several other agents, and still other candidate conditions were postulated as having a viral aetiology (Wolf, 1966).

The renowned fish pathologist Schäperclaus (1969), who published a comprehensive review of fish viral diseases—established and putative—included nearly 20 such conditions. The next review, which was only partial and covered the period of 1966 to 1971, included seven specific viral infections confirmed during that period and offered electron micrographs, as well as data, or speculations, for nine other viral conditions (Wolf, 1972).

Liversidge and Munro (1978) discussed the fish viral diseases in *Fish Pathology*, the most recent and comprehensive English language text on fish diseases. In Europe, Schäperclaus (1979) similarly covered the subject in his German language two-volume fourth edition of *Fischkrankheiten*. Another of the recent reviews concerned the biochemical, biophysical and biological properties of the fish viruses and provided an overview of the diseases (McAllister, 1979). More recently, Pilcher and Fryer (1980) reviewed the viral diseases of fish through 1978, and the same year Ahne and Wolf (1980) published their illustrated German language review. Wolf and Mann (1980), who published a tabular survey with key references, showed that at least 17 viruses had been isolated and that at least 15 others were recognized by electron microscopy.

The fish viruses can best be characterized as representative vertebrate viruses. Although many are as yet ungrouped, others clearly possess the attributes of major viral groups. In fish there are now seven known rhabdoviruses, seven herpesviruses, and several iridoviruses. Several reviews of herpesviruses have included the agents from fish; the most recent and comprehensive is that of Wolf (1981).

General comments on the newly recognized viruses from fishes are in order. Since the last listing (Wolf and Mann, 1980) aquarium species have been found with two new agents—a rhabdovirus isolated from a cichlid and an icosahedral agent, thus far only visualized, but also from a cichlid. Both caused significant mortality among the victims.

Herpesvirus salmonis and *Oncorhynchus masou* virus (OMV) are clearly virulent for young salmonids of susceptible species, but OMV is especially noteworthy for it has all indications of being oncogenic—the first virus of fish origin to be so designated. At the other extreme, the reovirus of the chum salmon (*Oncorhynchus keta*) and the calicivirus of the opaleye (*Girella nigricans*) are thus far completely without evidence of virulence for the fish species of origin; they are probably not fish viruses in the usual sense. The calicivirus is a significant pathogen among homoeotherms, but the role of the reovirus is unknown.

The herpesviruses of fishes are growing in number, and the agent from walleyes (*Stizostedion vitreum vitreum*) is a likely candidate for tumour induction, albeit a benign condition. New herpesviruses have been found in salmonids, and seen in cod (*Gadus macrocephalus*) and turbot (*Scophthalmus maximus*). Four of the seven fish herpesviruses now known have been isolated.

Although it remains to be isolated, and thus correctly identified, the adenovirus-like agent seen in cod cell nuclei is the first evidence of a representative of this group in fish. While their role as fish pathogens is dubious, the calicivirus of the opaleye and the reovirus of the chum salmon are also "firsts".

It will be interesting in the years ahead to see how many of the agents thus far only visualized—or completely unknown—are eventually isolated. Word of mouth has already brought new agents to the horizon—first reports have yet to appear.

Viruses Isolated from Fish Hosts

Carp Gill Necrosis Virus

Definition. Carp gill necrosis virus is a large cytoplasmic iridovirus-like agent reported isolated in Russia from carp (presumably *Cyprinus carpio*) having gill necrosis (Popkova and Shchelkunov, 1978).

Viral properties. The agent was isolated from gills and kidneys of 1- to 3-year-old carp. When materials were inoculated onto FHM cells and incubated at 28°C, almost all showed cytopathic effects (CPE) on original inoculation. Thereafter, passage of most materials was accompanied by a decrease in and eventually a loss of, ability to induce cytopathic effects. One isolant, however, showed increased cytopathic effects with transfer and was passaged 10 times.

Fish were sampled from four carp farms, and virus was isolated from two populations of fish with gill necrosis. Negatively stained culture medium clearly showed icosahedra with a diameter of 200–210nm. Experimental infections with the agent isolated were not reported.

Chum Salmon Virus

Definition. The chum salmon virus (CSV) is a new member of the family Reoviridae, encountered but once during a 1978 virological examination of 60 kidney and spleen samples from sexually mature chum salmon (*Oncorhynchus keta*) returning to a hatchery in Hokkaido, Japan. The agent is hepatotropic and replicates in, but causes no mortality among, several salmonids tested (Winton *et al.*, 1981).

Viral properties. Chum salmon virus is a 75nm doubly encapsidated icosahedral particle that is acid- and chloroform-stable. Particles have 20 peripheral capsomeres and no envelope. The genome is double-stranded RNA consisting of 10 segments, and has a buoyant density of 1.33–1.36 g ml^{-1}. As in certain of the reoviruses, alpha-chymotrypsin treatment of CSV removes the outer capsid. That action results in a particle size of 50–55nm with an overall enhanced infectivity; unheated control virus having a titre of 5×10^7 TCID$_{50}$ ml^{-1} and the chymotrypsin-treated portion having a titre of 6.3×10^8 TCID$_{50}$ ml^{-1}. Infectivity is not neutralized by antiserum against IPNV (infectious pancreatic necrosis virus). Serological comparisons with reovirus antisera have not been reported. Chum salmon virus is labile at 56°C for 1 hour, and it does not agglutinate human Type 0 erythrocytes; in all other attributes it shares the characteristics of the reovirus group.

Chum salmon virus is replicated by all of the widely used fish cell lines, but the CHH-1 (chum salmon) and CHSE-214 lines yield the highest titres —about 10^6 TCID$_{50}$ ml^{-1}. The STE-137, KO-6, LBF-2, BF-2, WC-1 and EPC lines give titres of at least 10^4 TCID$_{50}$, whereas FHM, RTG-2 and BB yield only 10^2 TCID$_{50}$ ml^{-1}.

The temperature range for replication is 10–20°C, the optimum being 15°C.

The effect of CSV in susceptible cells such as CHSE-214 consists of focal fusion of cells that eventually envelops the entire cell sheet. Stained with acridine orange, the cytoplasm of syncytial masses shows green inclusion bodies.

Signs and pathological changes. The virus was isolated from a spawning run of adults that were presumably normal in behaviour and appearance. Infectivity trials were later carried out with culture-grown virus and fry of the source species, chum salmon, as well as fry of chinook salmon (*O. tschawytscha*) and kokanee (*O. nerka*). Fry were injected intra-peritoneally with 10^4 TCID$_{50}$ virus then held at 12°C for 42 days. Other fry of the same species were similarly injected and samples were titrated for viral infectivity during the 42-day period. Still other fry were sampled and fixed for histological examination.

Neither gross signs of disease nor significant mortality occurred after injection of virus. However, virus was replicated by the fry of all three species—slowly in chinook salmon and more actively in kokanee and chum salmon. The titre in chum salmon reached a peak 21 days post-injection and was about 100 times greater than input. Lesser amounts were produced by kokanee and chinook salmon fry, but at the end of 42 days the titres were all about the same, 10 times greater than input.

Histopathological changes were found in the livers of the chum and chinook salmon fry. Focal necrosis was found in chum salmon, beginning about day 8 and increased in extent and severity by day 14. By day 21, however, there was evidence of healing. Chinook fry showed a similar but less severe involvement; no changes were found in the kokanee.

Virus could not be demonstrated in electron micrographs of liver lesions.

Cod (Atlantic) Ulcus Syndrome Viruses

Definition. The cod ulcus syndrome is a viral associated subacute to chronic progressive ulcerating condition in the skin of Atlantic cod (*Gadus morhua*) taken from certain of Denmark's coastal waters. Indications are that the condition leads to significant mortality.

Viral properties. Two different viruses have been found in and isolated from affected cod — a rhabdovirus having a mean diameter of 55nm and a length of 175nm, and a cytoplasmic icosahedral agent having a mean diameter of 145–150nm and a nucleoid measuring about 100nm (Jensen *et al.*, 1979). Although Rivers' postulates have not been fulfilled, the evidence tends to indicate that the icosahedral agent, presumably an iridovirus, is causal (N. J. Jensen and J. L. Larsen, personal communication).

Neither virus produced a cytopathic effect in original inoculated cultures; instead, several passages had to be made and differences in cell response became evident. The BF-2, FHM, and RTG-2 cell lines showed no viral effects during four passages. The rhabdovirus did best in the pike sarcoma (PS) line of Ljungberg in which it gave a titre of about 1×10^5 $TCID_{50}$ ml^{-1}. The PS cells enlarged and sloughed after 3 to 4 days incubation at 15°C. The EPC line showed a weak response to the rhabdovirus and very low titre after a week of incubation. However, this line was preferred for the iridovirus, for it showed viral effects as early as 20 hours post infection and yielded a maximal titre of about 1×10^5 $TCID_{50}$ ml^{-1}. Infected cells rounded and produced a cytoplasmic inclusion that stained green with acridine orange thereby giving presumptive evidence of double stranded nucleic acid — possibly DNA.

Signs and pathological changes. Larsen and Jensen (1979) and Jensen and Larsen (1979) described and illustrated five stages in the course of the disease: (1) papulo-vesicular, (2) erosive, (3) early ulcerative, (4) late ulcerative and (5) healing. The determinations were made from lesions on wild fish that were captured, rather than from lesions that were experimentally induced.

The external signs of stage one consist of multiple dermal papules 2 to 8mm in diameter and 1 to 3mm thick. Some are slightly haemorrhagic, and the usual progression is to hemispherical vesicles containing serous fluid.

Stage two is erosive and exhibits crater-like perforations of the skin and raised edges. Central epithelium and connective tissue are lost and the lesions are grey to yellow with a pink cast.

Stage three early ulcerations are concave with a red margin of hyperplastic tissue, and the centres may be grey and necrotic.

Stage four, late ulceration, consists of one or more ulcers 2 to 8cm in diameter, the most severe of which penetrate the abdominal wall. Large ulcers are believed to develop from individual earlier lesions or from fusion of lesions.

Stage five, observed in late autumn, is considered a recovery or healing stage. However, the authors considered healing to be most common after stages one and two. Newly healed lesions are whitish scars without pigment cells or scales.

The appearance of internal organs of fish with the ulcus syndrome has not been described.

Jensen and Larsen (1979) also described and illustrated the histopathological findings of the ulcus syndrome.

Stage one lesions are confined to the stratum compactum and the tissues above it. The epithelium is rough but intact and the stratum spongiosum is oedematous. Scale pockets contain accumulated fluid and show granulocytic infiltration. Hyperaemia and haemorrhages may also be present.

In stage two, the oedema and infiltration involve the underlying musculature. Epidermis has been lost from the centres of the lesions and margins are thickened. The loose connective tissue is strongly infiltrated.

Oedema is conspicuous in the stratum compactum of stage three lesions but the tissue is usually not perforate. The loose connective tissue above the stratum compactum shows distended capillaries and well vascularized and infiltrated granulation tissue. In some cases the stratum compactum is breached and the underlying musculature exposed.

In stage four the stratum compactum is typically breached and the granulation tissue thicker than in stage three. Exposed musculature is oedematous, necrotic and infiltrated.

In the healing stage, the lesion is covered with epithelium and fibroblasts have replaced infiltrating cells.

Aetiology. Larsen and Jensen (1979), who investigated the bacteriological aspects of the ulcus syndrome, examined 350 cod with skin lesions and found 178 that had bacterial infections of the lesions themselves; the rest were described as "sterile skin alterations". Evidence against a systemic bacteraemia was found in that bacteria could be cultured from only 9% of the cod kidneys. *Vibrio anguillarum* was the predominant organism cultured, but attempts to reproduce the syndrome by applying *V. anguillarum* to scarified skin or injecting it intraperitoneally were unsuccessful (N. J. Jensen and J. L. Larsen, personal communication) justifies rejection of a bacterial etiology for the ulcus syndrome.

The possibility of a viral aetiology arose when filtrates of homogenized papules from a pool of seven cod yielded an icosahedral cytoplasmic virus and a rhabdovirus (Jensen *et al.*, 1979). However, subsequent virological examination of 33 individuals yielded only one with virus, again an icosahedral agent.

Rivers' postulated have not been fulfilled for the ulcus syndrome; however, some experimental results suggest that the condition is infectious and, moreover, that virus is involved (N. J. Jensen and J. L. Larsen, personal communication). Cohabitation of six healthy cod with four that bore stage one lesions resulted in 100% induction within 11 days. Also, some evidence of transmission was found when papule homogenates were applied to scarified skin or were decontaminated by filtration and injected intraperitoneally.

The most suggestive evidence was obtained with the icosahedron — presumably an iridovirus — following intracardial inoculation of the virus, eight of 36 cods so inoculated developed early stage ulcus syndrome. However, one of the controls also did. Inasmuch as the test fish were taken from the wild, their health history was completely unknown. Similar transmission work with specific pathogen-free or immunosuppressed fish could be highly informative.

Golden Shiner Virus

Definition. The golden shiner virus (GSV) is a double-stranded RNA agent isolated from and mildly pathogenic for the bait minnow, *Notemigonus crysoleucas* (Plumb *et al.*, 1979). It has been isolated in America's midsouth region.

Viral properties. The GSV is a 70nm icosahedron that is ether-, acid- (pH 3.0) and alkaline-stable (pH 10.0) and whose infectivity persists after it is heated at 50°C for 30 minutes. Replication occurs in the cytoplasm and is not inhibited by iododeoxyuridine and neither DNAase nor RNAase significantly reduces its infectivity. Infected FHM cells stained with acridine orange show apple green fluorescence in the cytoplasm. Accordingly, the genome is presumed to be double-stranded RNA.

In vitro replication occurs in the range of 20–30°C, the optimum being about 25°C. At 30°C, a one-step growth curve shows a lag phase of 2–4 hours; thereafter, exponential replication occurs for 13–16 hours. Peak titres of about $10^{6.5}$ $TCID_{50}$ are reached at about 24 hours; beyond that time the infectivity of cell-associated virus persists, whereas that of released virus begins to decrease.

Thus far, only the FHM cell line will support growth of GSV; BB, CCO and RTG-2 lines have been found to be refractory. Infection of FHM cells results in focal vacuolation and development of syncytia. Cytopathic effects begin as early as 16–18 hours post-inoculation and by 24 hours cell sheets begin to contract and debris is released. Cell sheet regeneration and overgrowth often occur, and unless cultures are examined regularly the cytopathic effect may be overlooked.

Electron microscopy of infected FHM cells shows cytoplasmic virions predominantly in paracrystalline array and only infrequently occurring individually. Clusters of virus are surrounded by distinct areas of hyalinization.

Isolations of virus are made from filter-decontaminated homogenates of visceral organs, and the agent is serologically identified with specific rabbit antiserum in neutralization test (Schwedler and Plumb, 1980). Though GSV shares many of the characteristics of IPNV, cross-neutralization tests show that the two are wholly unrelated. While GSV is similar to reoviruses, no serological comparisons have been made.

Signs and pathological changes. Available information on the effects of GSV is rather sparse, for outbreaks have been infrequent, and only a limited amount of experimental infection work has been carried out. The initial isolation was made in 1977 from one of three groups of golden shiners submitted for virological examination because of undue mortality. A second isolation was made the following year.

Summer temperatures and crowding in ponds seem to favour the appearance of GSV, and result in a low chronic mortality. Plumb *et al.* (1979) mentioned one case in which a virus resembling GSV was isolated from a tank population of 12,000 minnows that sustained 75% mortality.

Affected golden shiners were listless and swam near the surface; they dived when disturbed but soon returned to the top. As a result of haemorrhages in the dorsal musculature, the back became reddish. Petechia also occurred in the cornea, in ventral body surfaces and internally in visceral fat and intestinal mucosa.

Histopathological studies have yet to be reported.

Intraperitoneal injection of young golden shiners (6–8cm long) with about $10^{4.5}$ TCID$_{50}$ third passage virus resulted in one successful attempt in which three of five fish died during a matter of 7–13 days. Virus was reisolated from the viscera. In a second trial with 20 fish injected with sixth passage virus, no signs of clinical disease developed and there was no mortality during the ensuing 3 weeks. Periodic virological assay showed that virus was recoverable from the viscera of sample fish but that the amount decreased with time.

Herpesvirus Salmonis

Definition. Herpesvirus salmonis is a salmonid pathogen isolated from ovarian fluids of post-spawning rainbow trout (*Salmo gairdneri*) at a single location in America's Pacific Northwest (Wolf *et al.*, 1978). In an experimental situation, culture-grown *H. salmonis* produces subacute to acute systemic disease and mortality in young rainbow trout. A similar virus, termed NeVTA, has been isolated in Japan (Sano, 1976).

Viral properties. Herpesvirus salmonis has the size, shape, capsomere number, nuclear origin and cytoplasmic envelopment and maturation typical of members of the herpesvirus group (Wolf *et al.*, 1978). Viral DNA has a buoyant density of 1.709 and a guanosine-cytosine value of 50%. *Herpesvirus salmonis* does not haemagglutinate. It is consistently replicated by susceptible cells at 5 and 10°C, but only inconsistently at 15°C, and not at all at higher temperatures.

The virus is replicated with cytopathic effects consisting of cell fusion followed by lysis, but only by salmonid cell lines such as RTG-2 and CHSE-214. Non-salmonid fish cells are refractory. It is suggested that cell culture infections are best initiated and that titres attained are highest if the virus is adsorbed for 2 hours at 10°C.

Near-optimal replication occurs at 10°C and at that temperature a one-step growth curve requires more than 4 days. New virus first appears at about 24 hours; at that time syncytia also become evident. Exponential growth follows until about 60 hours and peak titres are reached at 4 to 5 days. Released virus then attains a level of about 5×10^4 p.f.u. (plaque-forming units) ml^{-1} and cell-associated virus is about 10-fold greater at 3×10^5 p.f.u. ml^{-1}.

Cytopathic effects in cell cultures begin with rounding and increased refractility. The dominant change is syncytium formation, followed by syncytial contraction and limited lysis. Stained cells show basophilia, margination of chromatin, and Cowdry Type A intranuclear inclusions.

Infectivity of *H. salmonis* is not degraded by three cycles of freezing and thawing, but the agent is somewhat labile if frozen at pH 7.6 or greater. At 4°C, virus in culture medium without serum loses more than 99% of its infectivity within 3 weeks. Suggested storage is at $-80°C$, best preservation being in infective cell culture medium containing 10% serum. The response to lyophilization is unknown.

Injected intraperitoneally into rainbow trout, the virus produces 50–100% mortality in fry and in fingerlings less than 6 months old, kept at 6–9°C. T. Kimura (personal communication) found that fry of chum salmon (*O. keta*) injected with *H. salmonis* began to die after about 2 weeks at 10°C, and that virus could be recovered from them. Yearling rainbow trout are refractory as are young Atlantic salmon (*Salmo salar*), brown trout (*S. trutta*), brook trout (*Salvelinus fontinalis*) and yearling kokanee (*Oncorhynchus nerka*). It is worth noting that NeVTA, a herpesvirus from salmonids, was isolated from a landlocked Japanese population of *O. nerka*; however, *H. salmonis* could not even be reisolated from a land-locked North American form of *O. nerka* at the completion of the infectivity trials.

Virological assays of rainbow trout fry that were moribund or dead after experimental infection showed that kidneys were the prime target organs and that they harboured about 10^6 $TCID_{50}$ per gram of tissue; stomach and liver contained more than 10^4 $TCID_{50}$ g^{-1} and the intestines more than 10^3 $TCID_{50}$ g^{-1} (Wolf and Smith, 1981). Because of the small size of the fry it was impractical to assay other tissues.

Although the infection can be experimentally induced by intraperitoneal or intramuscular injection, attempts to achieve transmission by holding young susceptible rainbow trout fry with dead or moribund fingerlings have failed.

Signs and pathological changes. Behaviour changes, the first signs to appear in young trout experimentally inoculated with *H. salmonis*, are noted at about 3 weeks post-injection. Victims are anorexic and lethargic, and though some lose motor stability they remain capable of brief erratic swimming if alarmed.

Thick white mucoid casts trail from the vent of some fry. Many victims darken appreciably and develop a distended abdomen. Exophthalmia, at times extreme, is common and the eyes may show haemorrhages. Fin bases may also be slightly haemorrhagic and gills are typically pale.

Internally, the general picture is one of visceral pallor with slight to relatively copious amounts of ascitic fluid that can be fibrinous or gelatinous. The stomach is devoid of food and appears whitish. If food is present in the digestive tract, it is in the posterior intestine or rectal area. The liver is pale-to-mottled or haemorrhagic and its texture is friable.

Kidneys are usually pale but not noticeably enlarged. Limited haematological examination shows that peripheral blood from moribund specimens contains abnormal numbers of immature erythrocytes and blast cells of indeterminate nature.

Marked histopathological changes are to be found in the kidneys, respiratory tissues, heart, digestive tract and liver (Wolf and Smith, 1981). Syncytia have been found in pancreatic acinar tissue and are considered to be pathognomonic.

Renal haematopoietic tissue shows some hyperplasia and general oedema. Glomeruli are slightly oedematous but not otherwise affected, but posterior haematopoietic tissue and renal tubules show light-to-moderate necrosis and the lumens of some tubules may contain serous material. The kidneys of fish are prime targets for a number of bacterial and viral pathogens — *H. salmonis* among them.

The liver is also a significant target tissue and shows oedema, necrosis and haemorrhage or congestion. Hepatocytes surrounding central veins remain normal, but focal vacuolation, at times heavy, occurred elsewhere with accompanying diffuse necrosis. Liver margins show haemorrhage and moderate-to-extreme sinusoidal dilation.

Despite the amount of virus often present in the stomach, that organ is not consistently altered. Oedema around the cardiac glands and tunica propria and focal necrosis of the muscularis occurs in about half the specimens; the rest show essentially normal tissues. The intestines also harboured significant amounts of virus and that fact could be related to marked necrosis, mucosal sloughing and focal leucocytic infiltration of the submucosa of the posterior intestine. Sloughed mucosal tissue is believed to constitute much of the cast material that trails from the vent of some victims.

The heart of most specimens is grossly necrotic and oedematous. Leucocytic infiltration is pronounced and exterior portions show localized haemorrhages. Muscle fibres show loss of striation and, on occasion, hyaline necrosis. Respiratory tissues are also affected. Gill epithelium is oedematous and hypertrophied. Separation of lamellar epithelium is found, as is haemorrhage, in some specimens. Pseudobranchs are consistently altered with oedema that ranges from slight to extreme. Some nuclei are hypertrophied and margination of chromatin is present in some. Slight-to-moderate necrosis is present in local areas. Spleens are moderately oedematous and extensively congested.

Slight changes occur in the eyes, brain and skeletal muscle. Testes are invariably normal but some ovaries show oedema, some inflammation, necrosis of interstitial tissue and atresia of ova.

Host and geographical range. Herpesvirus salmonis was isolated from captive rainbow trout brood stock in a single facility and presumptive isolations were made during several preceding years. The brood fish were disposed of, but for a period of 2 years stations that had received their eggs were carefully examined for presence of the virus. *Herpesvirus salmonis* has not been found again in America. If the virus had been in or on eggs from the source brood stock, disinfection procedures may have inactivated it. Alternatively, water temperatures at recipient facilities that were favourable for salmonids may have been inimical to infection by the cold-requiring virus.

It is uncertain whether *H. salmonis* is the same agent as the one that Sano (1976) designated as NeVTA. Certainly, NeVTA is a herpesvirus and its maximal titre in RTG-2 cells is similar to that of *H. salmonis*. The Japanese agent also induces syncytium formation *in vitro* but neither margination of chromatin nor intranuclear inclusions are mentioned; instead, infected cells show eosinophilic cytoplasmic inclusions. Histopathological changes in rainbow trout experimentally infected with *H. salmonis* and in Japanese *O. nerka* naturally infected with NeVTA are similar in a few aspects but notably different in others. The Japanese *O. nerka* had granular degeneration of skeletal muscle, leakage of proteinaceous material into Bowman's capsule and vacuolation of pancreatic acinar cells. Both species showed swelling and loss of gill epithelium, but the Japanese agent was notable in that syncytia were found in renal interstitial cells.

Critical serological comparisons of the two viruses need to be made. Perhaps NeVTA is identical with the Japanese *Oncorhynchus masou* virus. Where did *H. salmonis* come from and why was it not found elsewhere?

Menhaden (Atlantic) Spinning Disease Virus

Definition. The virus of Atlantic menhaden (*Brevoortia tyrannus*) "spinning disease" is an agent resembling infectious pancreatic necrosis virus (IPNV); it is isolated, rather unusually, from specimens afflicted with the disease in Chesapeake Bay on the eastern coast of the United States. Spinning disease has been known for at least 25 years and, in the absence of evidence for a parasitic or microbial cause, viral isolations and limited experimental transmission work implicate the menhaden agent as causal (Stevens *et al.*, 1980).

Viral properties. Limited characterization has shown that the menhaden agent has the major biological, physical and chemical properties of IPNV, and that it is completely neutralized by polyvalent anti-IPNV serum. However, reciprocal neutralization of IPNV with spinning disease virus antiserum has not been reported, nor has serum from victim menhaden been tested for virus neutralizing activity.

The described effects of the menhaden virus in cell cultures deviate in a significant way from those usually encountered with IPNV. The menhaden virus was isolated on the MK cell line, which is of menhaden kidney origin. The cytopathic effect was described and illustrated as consisting of cellular vacuolation and the presence of "numerous cytoplasmic inclusions". A lytic phase did not occur on primary inoculation. When original cultures were sonicated and used to inoculate fresh cultures, a general lysis resulted.

Apparently, and in contrast to IPNV of salmonid origin, the menhaden virus cannot be isolated using common fish cell lines such as BF-2, CHSE-214 and RTG-2, but once grown in the MK cells it can be replicated in other fish cell lines, and with cytopathic effects.

At the time of this writing, the MK cell line has apparently lost its susceptibility to the menhaden agent.

Signs and pathological changes. The terminal behaviour of naturally affected fish is described as "loss of coordinated movement and erratic swimming behaviour". Experimentally infected menhaden of two different sized groups developed signs of spinning disease and showed haemorrhages in fin bases and eyes, and along the body. Darkened pigmentation followed, and was followed in turn by circular swimming and death. Virus was reisolated from the fish that had been injected but not from the single control fish that also died.

Histopathological studies have not been reported.

Oncorhynchus Masou Virus

Definition. Oncorhynchus masou virus (OMV) is a herpesvirus occurring in populations of masu salmon on Hokkaido, Japan. It is pathogenic for the young of *O. masou* and several other salmonid species; among survivors a sequela is the development of squamous cell epidermal papillomas (Kimura *et al.*, 1981a, b).

Viral properties. That OMV is a herpesvirus is clearly shown by its size, shape, capsomere number, mode of replication from nucleus to cytoplasm and inhibition by iododeoxyuridine, phosphonacetate and acycloguanosine at 50 μg ml^{-1}. The virus is ether- and acid-labile, it does not haem-agglutinate, and its infectivity passes membranes of 450nm but not 100 or

220nm, mean pore diameter. As could be expected for a salmonid herpesvirus, OMV is replicated by RTG-2, CHSE-214, KO-6 and other salmonid
cell lines, but not by FHM, SBK, EPC, BB, and other lines from non-
salmonid species. Replication occurs at temperatures of 5 to 18°C but not at
25°C. Optimal growth is considered to occur at 15°C, and the maximal titre
—about $10^6\,TCID_{50}\,ml^{-1}$—is attained at 9 days.

The *in vitro* cytopathic effects begin with rounding followed by
syncytium formation and terminal lysis. The changes occur within 5–7 days.
Stained cell sheets show small eosinophilic cytoplasmic inclusions.

The OMV tends to be labile in storage at temperatures of $-20°C$, 99.9%
of its infectivity being lost at 17 days. When held at 15°C, all infectivity is
lost within 17 days. At $-80°C$, however, infectivity is preserved for at least
6 months.

Kimura *et al.* (1981b) found that OMV is serologically distinct from
Herpesvirus salmonis.

The OMV is infectious to susceptible salmonids that are simply immersed
in a virus suspension of $100\ TCID_{50}\ ml^{-1}$ for 1 hour at 10°C. Young chum
salmon (*O. keta*), kokanee (*O. nerka*), coho salmon (*O. kisutch*) and
rainbow trout (*Salmo gairdneri*) are all susceptible. Experimental work with
O. masou, the species of origin, has not been reported—possibly because
available specimens have been exposed by vertical transmission.

Work with young chum salmon shows that susceptibility differs with age;
older fish are the more resistant, and 3-month-old fry the most susceptible.
Among 80 day fry, mortality begins at 11–12 days and reaches 60% by 65
days. Fry that are 150 days old show first mortality at 20 days and only 35%
die in the following 4 months. Fingerlings of 240 days are resistant to
disease by comparable immersion plus intraperitoneal injection of 200
$TCID_{50}$. Virus is readily recoverable from fish that die, and the mean titre is
about $10^6\,TCID_{50}$ per gram of body weight.

One of the most significant findings is that a 60% incidence of epidermal
tumours occurs among the fish that survive infection with OMV.

Signs and pathological changes. Kimura *et al.* (1981b) described affected
fish as anorexic but showing no agonal or abnormal swimming. Some show
exophthalmia or petechia, especially under the jaw.

Internally, livers are mottled with white, and in advanced cases the liver is
pearly white. The spleen of some is swollen, but kidneys appear normal.
The digestive tract is empty.

As could be expected from its gross appearance, the liver shows marked
pathological changes. Multiple foci of severe necrosis are found and
syncytia are present. Partial necrosis occurs in some spleens and cardiac
muscle is oedematous. In contrast to infection of young rainbow trout

with *H. salmonis*, pancreatic and kidney tissues of fish with OMV are normal.

Electron microscopy of infected liver sections shows large numbers of hepatocytes with intranuclear capsids and nucleocapsids. However, there is no evidence of the fibrillar strands found in cells infected with *H. salmonis* or channel catfish virus.

Kimura *et al.* (1981a), who reported on their investigation of the oncogenic nature of OMV, first noticed tumours among chum salmon, survivors of OMV, on the 130th day after infection; by the 250th day the incidence had reached 60%. The most frequent site of tumour formation was about the mouth; in decreasing frequency, the caudal fin, gill cover, and eyes were involved and one of 52 fish was found with a renal tumour 10.5 months after infection.

Histologically, the tumours were composed of abnormally proliferating squamous epithelial cells in papillomatous array and supported by fine connective tissue stroma. Mitoses were abundant. Regardless of their location, the features of the tumours were similar; any differences could probably be attributed to age of development. The renal tumour, however, though also consisting of epithelial cells, showed internal necrosis and displacement of normal kidney tissue. Accordingly, the authors suggested that the tumours are malignant.

Electron microscopy showed variability in the size of tumour nuclei and loose intercellular connections, but no virus. On the other hand, viral recovery attempted on organs and tumours of 11 specimens was successful in two. Virus was recovered from a necrotic tumour tissue sample in one case and from a degenerating primary culture of tumour cells in the other.

Survivors of experimental infection were bled and their sera tested for neutralizing activity against 100 $TCID_{50}$ of OMV. The titre of uninfected control fish was less than 1:20. In contrast, the titre of fish with tumours was 1:160 and of non-tumourous survivors, 1:320.

Observations on tumour induction were repeated the year after the initial findings. Again, the incidence was 50–60% and the time of first appearance 110–130 days. The work also showed that tumours were inducible in coho salmon that survived infection.

The work with OMV is the most convincing case to date of tumour induction by a fish virus.

Opaleye Calicivirus (San Miguel Sea Lion Virus)

Definition. The opaleye calicivirus is a *bona fide* mammalian pathogen better known as San Miguel sea lion virus (SMSV). It occurs in, and is replicated by, the opaleye (*Girella nigricans*), a small marine perch-like fish

from California's coastal waters. The opaleye has been implicated in a
nematode–fish–marine mammal cycle for the SMSV calicivirus (Smith *et al.*, 1980a, b).

Viral properties. Caliciviruses are small icosahedral RNA members of
Picornaviridae. Several serotypes have been isolated from the opaleye,
SMSV 5-7. Calicivirus was isolated from two of 30 visceral homogenates
from individual fish, from a single spleen homogenate and from one of 15
fish whose internal tissues were virologically assayed individually.
Isolations were made on the Vero cell line of African green monkey kidney
origin, incubated at 37°C. Initial titres were not given, presumably because
cytopathic effects were not seen during the first three passages.

Experimentally, calicivirus has been shown to replicate in opaleye spleen
to the extent of $10^{7.5}$ TCID$_{50}$ g^{-1} (Smith *et al.*, 1980b).

Signs and pathological changes. Although replicated by the opaleye,
histopathological examination of fish tissues has not been carried out. The
greater significance of the virus lies in its effects on mammals.

Smith *et al.* (1980b) reported that the fish isolant SMSV type 7 has
"produced a disease condition identical to vesicular exanthema in
experimentally infected swine". More recently, fur seal pups were
experimentally infected with SMSV-5 and became diseased in one of nine
cases with a vesicular lesion (Smith *et al.*, 1980a).

During the period 1932–1959, outbreaks of calicivirus-caused vesicular
exanthema of swine occurred first in California and then spread throughout
the U.S.A. The virus was believed to have been transported in contaminated
garbage. In 1972, the virus was found in the California sea lion (*Zalophus
californianus*) and later in other marine pinnipeds.

Most serotypes of calicivirus have been isolated in southern California,
thus leading to the suggestion that the state is a "possible focus of
calicivirus activity". Inasmuch as the opaleye is an intermediate host to a
nematode lung worm that parasitizes the California sea lion, there exists a
biological connection for transmission of the virus from the fish to marine
mammals. Smith *et al.* (1980a, b) postulated that the opaleye may be a
reservoir for the virus of vesicular exanthema of swine and that opaleye
calicivirus is the first viral pathogen of a terrestrial mammal that has a
marine fish as a natural reservoir.

Rio Grande Perch (Cichlid) Rhabdovirus

Definition. The Rio Grande perch rhabdovirus is a newly discovered
agent isolated from a shipment of specimens of the North American

(Mexican) cichlid *Cichlasoma cyanoguttatum* that died following an acute but otherwise undefined disease course (Malsberger and Lautenslager, 1980).

Viral properties. The virus is ether-sensitive and its replication is not inhibited by either actinomycin D or bromodeoxyuridine. Replication with cytopathic effect occurs at 23 and 33°C, but other temperatures have not been reported. The FHM cell line yields 3×10^6 p.f.u. ml^{-1} at 23°C and 1×10^7 p.f.u. ml^{-1} at 33°C. The RTG-2 cell line yields 1×10^6 p.f.u. ml^{-1} and the BB line less than 1×10^2 p.f.u. ml^{-1}. Cytopathic effects of the more susceptible lines, BF-2 and FHM, appeared within 2 days after the original inoculation. The agent has typical rhabdovirus morphology but free virions show a rounded rather than the more usual flat base. By virtue of its origin and ability to replicate at 33°C, the virus seems not to be one of the previously recognized fish rhabdoviruses. However, serological tests will surely be made.

Signs and pathological changes. The isolation was made from specimens of a shipment of 50 fish, all of which quickly developed acute disease signs and died within a week of receipt. Tests for pathogenicity were made in convict cichlids (*C. nigrofasciatum*), a species native to Central America. Of 10 specimens, each inoculated with 0.1ml of virus containing 4×10^7 p.f.u. ml^{-1}, eight died during days 3 to 5 but two survived for 14 days. Signs and features of the disease have not been reported.

Host and geographical range. The demonstrated lethality of the Rio Grande perch virus for a second species of the genus *Cichlasoma* supports speculation made for the pathological potential of this agent. It seems reasonable to expect that other cichlids might be similarly susceptible to this rhabdovirus—an agent from a group not particularly noted for high host specificity.

Walleye Herpesvirus

Definition. The walleye herpesvirus is a new agent with characteristics of the nominal virus group, isolated in Canada from a single adult walleye (*Stizostedion vitreum vitreum*) afflicted with epidermal hyperplasia.

Viral properties. Original isolation was on the WO line of walleye ovarian origin, but subsequently other walleye cell lines — WC-1 and We-2 — also proved to be susceptible (Kelly *et al.*, 1980a). As could be expected, the percid herpesvirus was not replicated in non-percid cell lines: CHSE-214, BB, FHM and RTG-2.

The agent is ether-labile and its replication is inhibited by iododeoxy-uridine, bromodeoxyuridine and phosphonacetate. Thymidine reverses the inhibition of the pyrmidine analogues. In susceptible cells replication occurs at 4–15°C but not at 20°C. Cytopathic effect is evident as syncytium formation followed by lysis. At 15°C, 10 to 13 days are required for plaque formation and maximal titre is 10^5 p.f.u. ml^{-1}.

Micrographs have not been published, but Kelly *et al.* (1980b) reported that numerous incomplete intranuclear virions were found in hyperplastic epidermis from an affected walleye and that morphologically identical particles were later found in infected WO cell cultures. Although size of the agent was not given, infectivity passed membranes with mean pore diameters of 200nm, but was retained on 100nm membranes.

The walleye herpesvirus is distinctly different from previously reported walleye viruses: lymphocystis and the C-type particles associated with dermal sarcoma and epidermal hyperplasia occurring in other geographic areas.

Signs and pathological changes. The subject specimen was merely described as having epidermal hyperplasia. No claim was made that the virus causes hyperplasia. The authors noted, however, that the prevalence of hyperplasia was greatest in Spring and declined thereafter. They noted further that tagging studies indicated that the condition is unlikely to contribute to post-spawning mortality (Kelly *et al.*, 1980b).

Visualized Viruses and Virus-like Forms

Bullhead (Brown) Papilloma Virus-Like Agent

Definition. The brown bullhead papilloma virus-like agent is a small spherical form occurring abundantly in the nuclei and cytoplasm of papillomatous epidermal cells examined from a single frozen specimen of brown bullhead (*Ictalurus nebulosus*) taken from a lake in New York (Edwards *et al.*, 1977).

Viral properties. The particles have a mean diameter of 50nm, a dense core, and an enclosing double membrane interpreted by the authors as the capsid. Particles were abundant in dilated cisternae of the nuclear membrane and in vesicles of the endoplasmic reticulum. No particles were found budding from the plasma membrane, and the agent has not been isolated.

Signs and pathological changes. The subject fish was one of four with skin papillomas among seven specimens taken. The component cells were predominantly fusiform epidermal cells with pleomorphic nuclei and vesiculated cytoplasm attributed to proliferating endoplasmic reticulum membranes.

Cichlid (Ramirez' Dwarf) Virus

Definition. Ramirez' dwarf cichlid virus is an agent that has yet to be isolated, but that has been unequivocally visualized in, and is putatively the cause of, an acute disease with 100% morbidity and high mortality among the South American tropical fish *Apistogramma ramirezi* (Leibovitz and Riis, 1980a, b).

Viral properties. Icosahedral virus occurs in arrays in a reticulated cytoplasmic matrix in spleen cells. Virion size ranges from 100 to 130nm. Other details have yet to be determined.

Signs and pathological changes. Newly imported affected cichlids were submitted for examination within 3 days after arrival in the United States. Victims were inappetent, pale and showed respiratory distress and signs of weakness. Haemorrhages were present in the skin and iris; as the disease progressed, degenerative changes of the eye increased and the iris developed an irregular outline. Transient scoliosis that occurred was attributed to muscle spasms. Respiration became slow and shallow before death. The disease ran its course in 3 to 4 weeks and mortality ranged from 40 to 80%.

Internally, the visceral mass was contracted. The digestive tract lacked food but contained a clear mucoid fluid. Spleen size was three to 10 times normal and the organ was pale, as were the liver and kidneys. Bacteriological cultures of kidneys, liver and spleen were negative.

Histopathological examination revealed degenerative changes in spleen, intestines, liver, kidneys, pancreas and eyes. Extensive areas of focal necrosis and occasional petechial haemorrhages were found in the affected organs. Early in the course of the disease, spleen cells showed abundant cytoplasmic inclusions, but inclusions were less frequent later. At early stages, affected spleen cells were swollen and basophilic and had ill-defined cell membranes. Late-stage cells had remnant cell and nuclear membranes, a small eosinophilic cytoplasmic inclusion, and generally few other cellular components. Ocular changes consisted of mononuclear infiltration of the retrobulbar sinus; there were focal haemorrhages displaying fibrin networks. Viral inclusions, however, were not found.

Host and geographical range. Thus far, the only host known is *A. ramirezi* and, because the affected fish were diseased on receipt, it seems logical to conclude that the virus originates in South America. Leibovitz and Riis (1980a, b), authors of the sole reports on the virus, correctly pointed out that other cichlid fishes — aquarium species and food fishes — may also be susceptible to the virus. They further advised dealers in fishes to employ quarantine and other hygienic procedures in their operations.

Cod (Atlantic) Adenovirus-like Agent

Definition. The cod adenovirus-like agent is an icosahedral intranuclear virus visualized in cells of epidermal plaques of *Gadus morhua* taken in the Baltic Sea (Jensen and Bloch, 1980).

Viral properties. Icosahedral virions measuring 77nm from apex to apex were found in the nucleus of a few scattered cells in the outermost layers of abnormally proliferated epithelium. Fine fibres, 20–25nm long, projected from, or connected corners of, many virions with the stained nucleoplasm. Virions displayed a lightly stained 10nm capsid-like structure surrounding a more intensely stained inner component or nucleoid.

Signs and pathological changes. Subject Atlantic cod were taken from Danish waters and showed flat transparent circular lesions or plaques at various places on the body, but particularly in caudal regions. The plaques were slightly raised and were 3–20nm in diameter. On death of the fish, the lesions became opaque and white.

Histologically, the lesions were epidermal and had a thickness about four times that of the normal skin, but mucous cells were smaller and fewer. Cells of the germinal layer were somewhat shorter than normal and, beneath the basement layer, the vascularity was greater than normal.

Electron microscopy showed that the epithelial cells were generally normal in appearance.

Cod (Pacific) Herpesvirus-like Agent

Definition. The cod herpesvirus-like agent is an entity described, but not yet illustrated, within nuclei and cytoplasm of abnormal giant cells of Pacific cod (*Gadus macrocephalus*) taken in the Bering Sea (McArn *et al.*, 1978; McCain *et al.*, 1979).

Viral properties. Virus-like particles measuring 80–110nm in diameter and in apparent various stages of development were present in the nuclei of the giant or hypertrophied cells. In herpesvirus-like fashion, larger particles measuring 120 × 170nm were present in the cytoplasm (McArn *et al.*, 1978).

Signs and pathological changes. The cod had two kinds of pathological skin conditions, prominent ulcers and pale, raised circular spots 1–15mm in diameter. The raised lesions contained hypertrophied cells that resembled lymphocystis and epitheliocystis cells, but the giant cells were of epithelial origin, did not contain Bedsonia, and had an outer coat of PAS-positive material. McCain *et al.* (1979) termed the raised spots "ring-like lesions" and noted that they measured as much as 50mm in diameter. In lieu of the term "giant hypertrophied cells" used by McArn *et al.* (1978), McCain *et al.* (1979) described the distinctive feature of the histopathology as "cyst-like bodies". The cysts had vacuolated basophilic centres surrounded by an eosinophilic margin. The margin contained eosinophilic bodies, which were also diffusely scattered throughout the basophilic centres. Inflammatory cells in the stratum spongiosum near some cysts were considered suggestive of the presence of an infectious agent. McCain *et al.* (1979) referred to the preliminary electron microscopic examination of McArn *et al.* (1978) that revealed a "herpes-like virus" in the cysts.

Superficially, the ring-like lesions resemble those described by N. J. Jensen and B. Bloch (personal communication) in Atlantic cod (*Gadus morhua*). However, histological features of the lesions of the two cods differ as does the size of virus particles in the nucleus.

Platyfish Virus-like Particles

Definition. The platyfish virus-like particles are intranuclear and intra-cytoplasmic forms induced in melanoma and neuroblastoma cells following intramuscular injection of xiphophorine hybrid poeciliid fish with 200µg bromodeoxyuridine (Kollinger *et al.*, 1979).

Viral properties. In all, four kinds of virus-like particles were described and illustrated by Kollinger *et al.* (1979). Two kinds of particles were induced in melanoma tissue—40–50nm particles in the cytoplasm and intercellular spaces and 25–30nm particles in cell nuclei. Some intranuclear particles were arranged in paracrystalline array. The authors noted that, by their size, shape and arrangement, the particles resembled papovaviruses of the polyoma type. The third and fourth kinds of particles were cytoplasmic in occurrence in neuroblastoma cells and both measured 100nm. One form was ring-shaped with an outer membranous envelope and a core of little contrast. The other had an eccentric electron-dense core and occurred mostly in intracellular vacuoles. In contrast to those in melanoma cells, the forms seen in neuroblastoma cells were solitary and scarce. The authors noted the similarity of neuroblastoma forms to B and C-type virus particles.

No virus-like particles were found in control melanoma or neuroblastoma cells, i.e. in neoplasms of fish not injected with bromodeoxyuridine.

Induction of endogenous mammalian virus with halogenated pyrimidines or inhibitors of protein synthesis is well documented (Aaronson and Dunn, 1974).

Rainbow Trout Intraerythrocytic Virus-like Form

Definition. The intraerythrocytic entity of rainbow trout is a virus-like particle found in cytoplasmic vesicles in erythrocytes of Donaldson strain *Salmo gairdneri* suffering from a haemorrhagic disorder (Landolt *et al.*, 1977).

Viral properties. The agent is spherical and uniformly about 80–90nm in diameter. The outer margin is relatively more electron-dense than interior portions. Attempts at isolation in FHM and RTG-2 cells have not been successful.

Signs and pathological changes. Typically, adult females are affected and they show exsanguinating haemorrhage and hypoxia prior to sudden death. Internally there are massive subcapsular haematomas or blood in the body cavity. Histologically, there is diffuse necrotic hepatitis, eosinophilic cytoplasmic inclusions in hepatocytes and renal tubular epithelium, and disseminated intravascular coagulation and dystrophy of skeletal muscle.

Haematological findings show unusually abundant circulating immature erythrocytes and frequent basophilic cytoplasmic inclusions in erythrocytes.

Electron micrographs show membrane-bound inclusions of about 1000nm, containing amorphous material but no viral particles, in the cytoplasm. Viral particles are to be found in 900nm cytoplasmic vesicles.

Salmon (Atlantic) Papillomatosis Virus-like Agent

Definition. Atlantic salmon papillomatosis is a fairly common benign plaque-like proliferation of epidermis that occurs transiently in 2-year-old parr and occasionally in young adult *Salmo salar*. Some evidence suggests the presence of an associated virus.

Viral properties. Evidence for an infectious nature and more specifically for viral involvement is less than conclusive. Wiren (1971) noted that attempts to transmit the condition were not successful, and Chronwall (1976) was unable to find evidence of virus in the electron microscopy phase of his study. On the other hand, Carlisle (1977) described and illustrated virus-like particles that were 125–150nm in diameter and had an internal electron dense "nucleoid" 70–95nm in diameter. The particles were found in degenerating epidermal cells or near the plasma membrane of intact cells. Carlisle prepared homogenates of papillomata, kidneys and spleens and inoculated cultures of the fibroblastic AS cell line of Atlantic salmon origin. Four passages were carried out but no evidence of virus isolation was obtained. Primary cultures were made of papilloma cells but they could not be continued as a cell line.

Signs and pathological changes. Carlisle and Roberts (1977) described the lesions as smooth white plaques, 2–5mm thick and up to 4cm in diameter, and occurring in multiples on the fins or on the body posterior to the head. Lesions first appear late in summer but seldom persist through winter. Although the prevalence may reach 50%, the papillomatosis apparently is usually without serious impact on the fish.

Histologically the lesions consist of stratified squamous epithelium 5–15 times thicker than normal epidermis. Mucous cells are less frequent than in normal skin and mitoses are moderately more frequent. Thick lesions usually show a central stalk of fibrovascular dermis. Some lesions show eosinophilic cytoplasmic inclusions especially in degenerating cells. Host response to the lesions varied from hyperaemia and a few migrating leucocytes to massive lymphocytic infiltration. Termination of the condition is attributed to a cell-mediated response that results in sloughing and, with few exceptions, uncomplicated epithelialization.

According to Carlisle (1977), the nuclei of tumour cells showed conspicuous clumping and margination of chromatin—features not noted by Chronwall (1976).

The condition merits additional study to resolve the question of viral involvement.

Salmon (Atlantic) Swim Bladder Fibrosarcoma Virus

Definition. Atlantic salmon swim bladder fibrosarcoma virus is unequivocally a viral agent, abundantly present in the subject neoplastic tissue in *Salmo salar.*

Viral properties. Virions do not occur in the cytoplasm but rather at the cell surface where they bud into extracellular space as mature particles with a diameter of about 120nm (Duncan, 1978). The agent has not been isolated and its role in tumour induction remains to be demonstrated.

Signs and pathological changes. The condition occurred at an incidence of nearly 5% among a population of 500 salmon in cage culture in Scotland. Although external lesions were absent, affected specimens could often be recognized by their sluggishness and poor condition. Internally, obvious hard nodular neoplasms involved the swim bladder—sometimes throughout its length—and protruded into the body cavity. The largest masses were anteriorly, but there were no invasions, metastases or adhesions (McKnight, 1978).

Histologically the tumours arose at the junction of the inner smooth muscle layer and the areolar tissue zone. The tumours consisted of well-differentiated bundles of elongate spindle cells. Mitoses were common and, though tumour growth was mainly outward with the vascularized areas, ischaemic necrosis occurred internally. Definitively, the tumour was identified as a leiomyosarcoma.

Sea Bream Papilloma Virus-like Agent

Definition. The sea bream papilloma agent is a virus-like form visualized in cells of a benign maxillary neoplasm occurring in the gilthead sea bream (*Sparus auratus*) taken from Spanish waters (Gutierrez *et al.*, 1977).

Viral properties. Particles measure 35–65nm and occur singly or in small groups in the cytoplasm. Some forms appear to bud from a membrane and, internally, an occasional form has electron-dense material resembling a nucleoid. Many of the particles show an array of regular knob-like projections from their surfaces. Attempts at isolation were not reported.

Signs and pathological changes. Tumours were found on seven of 39 fish, they were papillomatous in appearance and interfered with feeding. Histologically, the growths were said to be fibroepithelial and their basement membranes were intact. Other features of the histology were not reported except that there was no evidence of invasion or metastasis.

Sucker (White) Papilloma Virus

Definition. The white sucker papilloma virus is a C-type particle abundantly present in papillomatous epidermal growths from the body of *Catostomus commersoni* taken from North America's Great Lakes (Sonstegard, 1977a, b).

Viral properties. The viral particles have a mean diameter of about 100nm, bud from cytoplasmic membranes, and occur as aggregates in inter-cellular spaces. The presence of reverse transcriptase suggests that the virus has a causal role in the occurrence of the tumour, but attempts at experimental induction have thus far been unproductive. *In vitro* transformation of RTG-2, FHM, BB and BF-2 cell lines by tumour preparations have similarly failed to occur.

Signs and pathological changes. The tumours seem not to affect the behaviour of the fish. Tumour texture is firm and the colour is white to pinkish-white. There is no evidence of invasiveness or metastasis; the condition is considered benign. In the upper Great Lakes the overall frequency of tumours has been less than 1%, but in heavily polluted areas of Lake Ontario the incidences have been as high as 30 and 50%.

Tumours are first seen when fish reach sexual maturity at about 4 years; thereafter, they increase in size and frequency and probably persist for life.

Turbot Herpesvirus Infection

Definition. Herpesvirus infection of turbot (*Scophthalmus maximus*) is an enzootic and superficial condition characterized by the presence of specific giant cells in skin and gill epithelium of young fish in the wild and apparently in intense husbandry. In husbandry, there is evidence that the condition can result in mortality.

Viral properties. The pathognomonic giant cells contain neither parasite nor microorganism; instead, they contain an agent with the size, shape and apparent mode of replication of herpesvirus. Although the agent has yet to be isolated, it has been given the provisional name of *Herpesvirus scophthalmi* (Buchanan *et al.*, 1978).

Viral capsids, some naked and some with a nucleoid, are found at times in paracrystalline aggregates in giant cell nuclei. Particle size is about 100nm and cores or nucleoids are about 25–30nm. As in typical herpesvirus replication, enveloped particles (200–220nm in diameter) are found only in the cytoplasm and extracellularly. Envelopes are trilaminar and in some cases show an outer fringe of 18nm petal-like spikes reminiscent of those of coronavirus (Buchanan and Madeley, 1978).

Signs and pathological changes. Richards and Buchanan (1978) described affected fish as anorexic and lethargic and as offering little resistance when netted. When an affected fish lay on the bottom, its head and tail were raised—an abnormal posture for a flatfish. Other external features were lacking, as were internal signs of the condition.

Histopathological examination reveals pathognomonic giant cells in the epithelium of skin and gills (Richards and Buchanan, 1978). The giant cells range in size from 9 × 15μm to 70 × 130μm and occur individually in light infections or to a depth of several layers in heavy infections. Giant cells are more numerous in the skin of the upper than of the lower side of the fish. Most giant cells have a single nucleus that can occupy most of the cell but, in some cases, the cells are multinucleated and their fusion is postulated to result in giant nuclei. Giant nuclei measure up to 75μm and are typically densely basophilic, Feulgen-positive and PAS—negative. Some nuclei have a Feulgen-negative inclusion or a dense eosinophilic area surrounding a less eosinophilic central area. Moribund specimens have crypt-like depressions in the skin where giant cells were postulated to have been lost or sloughed.

As in the skin, the frequency of giant cells in the gills can range from light to heavy. In light infections the giant cells occur between lamellae, and the tips of the lamellae may fuse in response. However, the host response to heavy occurrence results in several lamellae being fused and in the surrounding malpighian cells being hyperplastic. Vascular stasis and fibrinous thrombosis can occur and, overall, functional respiratory surface is reduced.

Mortality has typically followed handling, transport, temperature fluctuations, or high chlorine levels in the nuclear generating plant effluent used to rear the fish. Perhaps virus is causal, but stress may also be involved.

Host and geographical range. Thus far, only young-of-the-year turbot in waters off Scotland and Wales are known to be infected.

An Ulcerative Dermal Necrosis (UDN)-like Disease and Virus-like Particles

Lounatmaa and Janatuinen (1978) investigated a UDN-like disease of landlocked Atlantic salmon (*Salmo salar*) and brown trout (*S. trutta*) at a facility in Finland. They found virus-like particles in lesion cells from the landlocked salmon. The particles were described and illustrated as compact and electron-dense. They occurred singly, in free groups, and membrane-enclosed groups in the cytoplasm. Particles were circular to hexagonal in outline and measured a uniform 30–33nm in diameter.

The role of the particles in the disease process was not determined and although the authors favour a viral nature for the particles, they offer an alternative identification of glycogen granules.

Proposed Withdrawals from Listings of Fish Viruses

Kidney Tumour Agent

More than 20 years ago, multiple tumour-like lesions were found in the aquarium fish *Pristella riddlei*. The tumours were transmitted to other aquarium species, notably the guppy, *Lebistes reticulatus*, by feeding and by injection of what was claimed to be cell-free filtrates. Kidneys were the primary target organs for the agent, but heart, intestine, testes and musculature were secondarily affected, presumably by spread through the circulatory system. The agent—postulated to be a virus—was lost in a laboratory accident and has not been reported since (Wessing and von Bargen, 1959).

Beckwith and Malsberger (1980) recently reopened the case of the kidney tumour agent and attempted to isolate the causal agent. In answer to an advertisement for tumourous tropical fish they received a specimen of *Brachydanio rerio* with an abdominal mass that proved, on sectioning, to be compatible with the description of Wessing and von Bargen (1959). Cell-free tumour extract proved to be infectious for another aquarium species *B. albolineatus*, and in a chronic course produced new tumours. However, neither cell-culture assay of tumour extract nor electron microscopy of tumours and inoculated cell cultures showed evidence of virus.

Histologically, both the original and the experimental tumours proved to be granulomas, in some cases with necrotic centres. Accordingly, when acid-fast staining was applied it revealed the presence of acid-fast bacilli that were later cultured and identified as *Mycobacterium fortuitum*. It has been well documented in homoeotherms that cell-free fractions of tubercle bacilli can induce granulomas in animals with mycobacterial infections. Accordingly, the contention of Beckwith and Malsberger (1980) that the kidney tumour agent reported by Wessing and von Bargen (1959) is in reality a mycobacterial component seems well justified.

Grunt Fin Agent

About 20 years ago cell cultures were initiated from fin tissue of the blue-striped grunt (*Haemulon sciurus*), a North American marine fish. Two years later a single culture in 65th passage showed focal necrosis that ultimately destroyed the entire cell sheet and proved to be an infectious agent. The agent has since been referred to as the grunt fin agent or GFA (Clem *et al.*, 1964). It is not pathogenic for newborn mice, chick embryos or adults of *H. sciurus* or *H. album*. There are no reports of a second encounter with GFA or agents that in any way resemble it. In addition, although GFA has been deposited with the American Type Culture Collection and designated VR683, there have been few requests for the agent and no new reports have been published since that of Beasley and Sigel (1968).

The GFA has some characteristics of virus, but the possibility of it being a mycoplasma cannot be excluded. At best, electron microscopy of thin sections of infected cell and pelleted material is only superficially suggestive of virus.

The agent is ether-sensitive and completely inactivated by heating at 45°C for 15 minutes. The halogenated uridine derivatives do not inhibit its growth, and it has not agglutinated erythrocytes from guinea pigs, man or fishes. It cannot be grown on bacteriological media, KB, HeLa, RTG-2 or goldfish fin cells, but it is replicated by the GF line in which it was first recognized and by primary grunt fin, liver and ovary cultures. Beasley *et al.* (1966), Beasley and Sigel (1968), and Sigel *et al.* (1968) reported the ability of GFA to cause chronic infection and the carrier state in GF cells. They noted that superinfection with IPNV was possible but that the yield was far less than normal, due to the presence of an interferon-like product induced by GFA.

Too few characteristics of GFA have been determined to establish that it is or is not a virus. Compared with bona fide fish viruses, a notable hiatus has occurred in the history of literature on the agent. The viral nature can be considered as suspect and it is hoped that the present discussion will stimulate definitive investigations.

Acknowledgments

I thank P. E. McAllister for review of this manuscript. P. H. Eschmeyer provided skilled editorial review and advice. R. K. Kelly gave a valued reading that revealed several important reports not in my compilation of references.

References

Aaronson, S. A. and Dunn, C. Y. (1974). High frequency C-type virus induction by inhibitors of protein synthesis. *Science* **183**, 422–424.

Ahne, W. and Wolf, K. (1980). Viruserkrankungen der Fische. *In* "Krankheiten und Schädigungen der Fische" 2nd edition (Ed. H. H. Reichenbach-Klinke), pp.56–105. Gustav Fisher Verlag, Stuttgart and New York.

Beasley, A. R. and Sigel, M. M. (1968). Interferon production in cold-blooded vertebrates. *In Vitro* **3**, 154–165.

Beasley, A. R., Sigel, M. M. and Clem, L. W. (1966). Latent infection in marine fish tissue cultures. *Proceedings of the Society for Experimental Biology and Medicine* **121**, 1169–1174.

Beckwith, D. G. and Malsberger, R. G. (1980). Kidney tumor virus—tumor or mycobacterial tubercle? *Journal of Fish Diseases* **3**, 339–348.

Buchanan, J. S. and Madeley, C. R. (1978). Studies on *Herpesvirus scophthalmi* infection of turbot *Scophthalmus maximus* (L.) ultrastructural observations. *Journal of Fish Diseases* **1**, 283–295.

Buchanan, J. S., Richards, R. H. and Sommerville, C. (1978). A herpes-type virus from turbot (*Scophthalmus maximus* L.). *The Veterinary Record* **102**, 527–528.

Carlisle, J. C. (1977). An epidermal papilloma of the Atlantic salmon II: ultrastructure and etiology. *Journal of Wildlife Diseases* **13**, 235–239.

Carlisle, J. C. and Roberts, R. J. (1977). An epidermal papilloma of the Atlantic salmon I: epizootiology, pathology and immunology. *Journal of Wildlife Diseases* **13**, 230–234.

Chronwall, B. (1976). Epidermal papillomas in *Salmo salar* L.: a histological description. *Zoon* **4**, 109–114.

Clem, L. W., Sigel, M. M. and Friis, R. R. (1964). An orphan virus isolated in marine fish cell tissue culture. *Annals of the New York Academy of Sciences* **126**, 343–361.

Duncan, I. B. (1978). Evidence for an oncovirus in swimbladder fibrosarcoma of Atlantic salmon *Salmo salar* L. *Journal of Fish Diseases* **1**, 127–131.

Edwards, M. R., Samsonoff, W. A. and Kuzia, E. J. (1977). Papilloma-like viruses from catfish. *Fish Health News* **6**, 94–95.

Gutierrez, M., Crespo, J. P. and Arias, A. (1977). Particulas virus-like en un tumor en boca de dorada, *Sparus aurata* L. *Investigaciones Pesqueras* **41**, 331–336.

Hofer, B. (1904). "Handbuch der Fischkrankheiten." Verlag der Allgemein Fischerei-Zeitung, B. Heller, Munchen.

Jensen, N. J. and Bloch, B. (1980). Adenovirus-like particles associated with epidermal hyperplasia in cod (*Gadus morhua*). *Nordisk Veterinaermedicin* **32**, 173–175.

Jensen, N. J. and Larsen, J. L. (1979). The ulcus syndrome in cod (*Gadus morhua*) I. A pathological and histopathological study. *Nordisk Veterinaermedicin* **31**, 221–228.

Jensen, N. J., Bloch, B. and Larsen, J. L. (1979). The ulcus-syndrome in cod (*Gadus morhua*) III. A preliminary virological report. *Nordisk Veterinaermedicin* **31**, 436–442.

Kelly, R. K., Nielson, O. and Yamamoto, T. (1980a). A new herpes-like virus (HLV) of fish (*Stizostedion vitreum vitreum*). *In Vitro* **16**, 255.

Kelly, R. K., Nielsen, O., Campbell, J. S. and Yamamoto, T. (1980b). Current status of lymphocystis, dermal sarcoma/fibroma and related diseases in walleye, *Stizostedion vitreum vitreum*, in western Canada. In *Proceedings of the 4th Biennial Fish Health Section and Fish Disease Workshops*, mimeographed. (Available from: F. Meyer, National Fishery Research Laboratory, La Crosse, Wisconsin 54601 U.S.A.).

Kimura, T., Yoshimizu, M. and Tanaka, M. (1981a). Studies on a new virus (OMV) from *Oncorhynchus masou* II. Oncogenic nature. *Fish Pathology* **15**, 149–153.

Kimura, T., Yoshimizu, M., Tanaka, M. and Sannohe, H. (1981b). Studies on a new virus (OMV) from *Oncorhynchus masou* I. Characteristics and pathogenicity. *Fish Pathology* **15**, 143–147.

Kollinger, G., Schwab, M. and Anders, F. (1979). Virus-like particles induced by bromodeoxyuridine in melanoma and neuroblastoma in Xiphophorus. *Journal of Cancer Research and Clinical Oncology* **95**, 239–246.

Landolt, M. L., MacMillan, J. R. and Patterson, M. (1977). Detection of an intraerythrocytic virus in rainbow trout. *Fish Health News* **6**, 4–6.

Larsen, J. L. and Jensen, N. J. (1979). The ulcus syndrome in cod (*Gadus morhua*) II. A bacteriological investigation. *Nordisk Veterinaermedicin* **31**, 289–296.

Leibovitz, L. and Riis, R. C. (1980a). A viral disease of aquarium fish. *Journal of the American Veterinary Medical Association* **177**, 414–416.

Leibovitz, L. and Riis, R. C. (1980b). A new viral disease of aquarium fish. *Fish Health News* **9**(1), iv–vi.

Liversidge, J. and Munro, A. L. S. (1978). The virology of teleosts. *In* "Fish Pathology" (Ed. R. J. Roberts), pp.114–143. Bailliere Tindall, London.

Lounatmaa, K. and Janatuinen, J. (1978). Electron microscopy of an ulcerative dermal necrosis (UDN)-like salmon disease in Finland. *Journal of Fish Diseases* **1**, 369–375.

Malsberger, R. G. and Lautenslager, G. (1980). Fish viruses: rhabdovirus isolated from a species of the family Cichlidae. *Fish Health News* **9**(2), i–ii.

McAllister, P. E. (1979). Fish viruses and viral infections. *In* "Comprehensive Virology" (Eds. H. Fraenkel-Conrat and R. R. Wagner), Vol. 14, pp.401–470. Plenum Publishing Corp., New York.

McArn, G. E., McCain, B. and Wellings, S. R. (1978). Skin lesions and associated virus in Pacific cod (*Gadus macrocephalus*) in the Bering Sea. *Federation Proceedings* **37**, 937.

McCain, B. B., Gronlund, W. D., Myers, M. S. and Wellings, S. R. (1979). Tumors and microbial diseases of marine fishes in Alaskan waters. *Journal of Fish Diseases* **2**, 111–130.

McKnight, I. J. (1978). Sarcoma of the swimbladder of Atlantic salmon (*Salmo salar* L.). *Aquaculture* **13**, 55–60.

Nigrelli, R. F. (1952). Virus and tumors in fishes. *Annals of the New York Academy of Sciences* **54**, 1076–1092.

Pilcher, K. S. and Fryer, J. L. (1980). The viral diseases of fish: a review through 1978. *In* "CRC Critical Reviews in Microbiology" (Ed. H. D. Isenberg), Vol. 7, pp.287–364, Vol. 8, pp.1–25, CRC Press, Inc., Boca Raton, Florida.

Plehn, M. (1924). "Praktikum der Fischkrankheiten." E. Schweizerbart'sche Verlasbuchhandlung, Stuttgart.

Plumb, J. A., Bowser, P. R., Grizzle, J. M. and Mitchell, A. J. (1979). Fish viruses: a double-stranded RNA icosahedral virus from a North American cyprinid. *Journal of the Fisheries Research Board of Canada* **36**, 1390–1394.

Popkova, T. I. and Schelkunov, I. S. (1978). Isolation of virus from carp afflicted with gill necrosis. (Vedelenie virusa ot karpov, bol'nykh zhabernym nekrozom.) *VNIIPRKH, Rybnoe Khozyaistvo* **4**, 34–38. In Russian. (Translation by M. E. Markiw.)

Richards, R. H. and Buchanan, J. S. (1978). Studies on *Herpesvirus scophthalmi* infection of turbot *Scophthalmus maximus* (L.): histopathological observations. *Journal of Fish Diseases* **1**, 251–258.

Sano, T. (1976). Viral diseases of cultured fishes in Japan. *Fish Pathology* **10**, 221–226.

Schäperclaus, W. (1969). Virusinfektionen bei Fischen. *In* "Handbuch der Virus-infektionen bei Tieren" (Ed. H. Röhrer), pp.1067–1141. Gustav Fischer Verlag, Jena.

Schäperclaus, W., Editor. (1979). "Fischkrankheiten", 4th Edition. 2 Vols. Akademie-Verlag, Berlin, DDR.

Schwedler, T. E. and Plumb, J. A. (1980). Fish viruses: serologic comparison of the golden shiner and infectious pancreatic necrosis viruses. *Journal of Wildlife Diseases* 16, 597–599.

Sigel, M. M., Russel, W. J., Jensen, J. A. and Beasley, A. R. (1968). Natural immunity in marine fishes. *Bulletin de l'Office International des Epizooties* 69, 1349–1351.

Smith, A. W., Skilling, D. E. and Brown, R. J. (1980a). Preliminary investigation of a possible lungworm (*Parafilaroides decorus*), fish (*Girella nigricans*), and marine mammal (*Callorhinus ursinus*) cycle for San Miguel sea lion virus Type 5. *American Journal of Veterinary Research* 41, 1846–1850.

Smith, A. W., Skilling, D. E., Dardiri, A. H. and Latham, A. B. (1980b). Calicivirus pathogenic for swine: a new serotype isolated from opaleye *Girella nigricans*, an ocean fish. *Science* 209(4459), 940–941.

Sonstegard, R. A. (1977a). Environmental carcinogenesis studies in fishes of the Great Lakes of North America. *Annals of the New York Academy of Sciences* 298, 261–269.

Sonstegard, R. A. (1977b). The potential utility of fishes as indicator organisms for environmental carcinogens. *In* "Wastewater Renovation and Reuse" (Ed. F. M. D'Itri), pp.561–577. Marcel Dekker, New York.

Stevens, E. B., Newman, M. W., Zachary, A. L. and Hetrick, F. M. (1980). A viral etiology for the annual spring epizootics of Atlantic menhaden *Brevoortia tyrannus* (Latrobe) in Chesapeake Bay. *Journal of Fish Diseases* 3, 387–398.

Watson, S. W. (1954). Virus diseases of fish. *Transactions of the American Fisheries Society* 83, 331–341.

Weissenberg, R. (1914). Über infektiöse Zellhypertrophie bei Fischen (Lymphocystiserkrankung). *Sitzungsberichte der königlich preussischen Akademie der Wissenschaften., Phys-Math K1.23*, 792–804.

Wessing, A. and von Bargen, G. (1959). Untersuchungen über einen virusbedingten Tumor bei Fischen. *Archiv für die gesamte Virusforschung* 9, 521–536.

Winton, J. R., Lannan, C. N., Fryer, J. L. and Kimura, T. (1981). Isolation of a new reovirus from chum salmon in Japan. *Fish Pathology* 15, 155–162.

Wiren, B. (1971). Vartsjuka hos lax (*Salmo salar* L.) Histologiska studier over epidermala papillom hos odlad lax. *Laxforsknings Institutet Meddelande* 7, 9 pages.

Wolf, K. (1964). Characteristics of viruses found in fishes. *Developments in Industrial Microbiology* 5, 139–148.

Wolf, K. (1966). The fish viruses. *In* "Advances in Virus Research" (Eds. K. M. Smith and M. A. Lauffer), Vol. 12, pp.35–101. Academic Press, New York and London.

Wolf, K. (1972). Advances in fish virology: a review 1966–1971. *In* "Symposia of the Zoological Society of London" (Ed. L. E. Mawdesley-Thomas), No. 30, pp.305–331. Academic Press, London.

Wolf, K. (1981). Biology and properties of fish and reptilian herpesviruses. *In* "Comprehensive Virology Series II" (Ed. B. Roizman), Vol. 3, In press. Plenum Press, New York.

Wolf, K. and Mann, J. A. (1980). Poikilotherm vertebrate cell lines and viruses: a current listing for fishes. *In Vitro* 16, 168–179.

Wolf, K. and Smith, C. E. (1981). *Herpesvirus salmonis*: pathological changes in experimentally infected rainbow trout fry. *Journal of Fish Diseases* **4**, 445–457.

Wolf, K., Darlington, R. W., Taylor, W. G., Quimby, M. C. and Nagabayashi, T. (1978). *Herpesvirus salmonis*: characterization of a new pathogen of rainbow trout. *Journal of Virology* **27**, 659–666.

5

Infectious Pancreatic Necrosis Virus
and Its Virulence

B. J. HILL

*Ministry of Agriculture, Fisheries and Food, Directorate of Fisheries Research,
Fish Diseases Laboratory, The Nothe, Weymouth, Dorset, U.K.*

Introduction

Infectious pancreatic necrosis (IPN) is an acute, highly contagious viral disease, primarily of young salmonid fish held under intensive rearing conditions. The first recorded cases of the disease were almost certainly those reported from Canada in 1940 by M'Gonigle (1941), who described the condition in brook trout (*Salvelinus fontinalis*) fry as an "acute catarrhal enteritis". Outbreaks of a clinically identical disease in brook trout hatcheries in the eastern U.S.A. in 1954 were investigated by Wood *et al.* (1955) whose transmission experiments and histopathological examination of the condition led them to classify it as an "infectious pancreatic necrosis" and to suggest a viral aetiology. Snieszko *et al.* (1957, 1959) confirmed the infectious nature of the disease and reported possible outbreaks in fingerlings of rainbow trout (*Salmo gairdneri*), Atlantic salmon (*Salmo salar*) and brown trout (*Salmo trutta*). The viral nature of IPN was confirmed soon after by Wolf *et al.* (1960), who isolated the virus in fish tissue cultures and reproduced the disease in experimentally infected brook trout fry.

Subsequent virological investigations into mortalities in fish hatcheries revealed that IPN was also present in the western areas of the U.S.A., where several salmonid species were affected (Parisot *et al.*, 1963). A few years later, a survey by MacKelvie and Artsob (1969) demonstrated the widespread presence of IPN in fish culture stations in the Canadian Maritime Provinces. Elsewhere, the first report of IPN in Europe came in 1965 with an outbreak of the disease in rainbow trout in France (Besse and de Kinkelin, 1965), since when its presence has been demonstrated in at least

10 European countries, including Scandinavia and the British Isles (for example, see Jorgensen and Bregnballe, 1969; Ball *et al.*, 1971; Ljungberg and Jorgensen, 1972; Schlotfeldt *et al.*, 1975; Hastein and Krogsrud, 1976). In Japan, the "unknown disease" of rainbow trout fry, which had been the cause of major epizootics in the 1960s, was demonstrated to be IPN by Sano (1971a, b). Further investigations (Sano, 1972a) revealed that a large proportion of rainbow trout hatcheries in Japan were affected by the disease.

With its presence in most, if not all, the major trout-farming countries of Europe, North America and Japan, IPN has a greater geographical distribution than any of the other known serious virus diseases of fish.

Host Range

Salmonid Species

Although originally observed in brook trout, outbreaks of IPN are now most commonly reported in rainbow trout, probably a reflection more of the wider cultivation of the latter species rather than of a higher susceptibility to infection. The disease has also been observed in hatchery-reared cutthroat trout (*Salmo clarki*) (Parisot *et al.*, 1963) and "Amago" (*Oncorhynchus rhodurus macrostomus*) (Sano and Yamazaki, 1973) and the susceptibility of "Himemasu" (landlocked form of *Oncorhynchus nerka*) to IPN has been demonstrated by experimental infection (Sano, 1973).

Natural infections with IPN virus have been observed in several other salmonid species, namely, Atlantic salmon (*Salmo salar*) and brown trout (*Salmo trutta*) (MacKelvie and Artsob, 1969), Coho salmon (*Oncorhynchus kisutch*) (Wolf and Pettijohn, 1970), Arctic char (*Salvelinus alpinus*) (Ljungberg and Jorgensen, 1972), Japanese char (*Salvelinus pluvius*) (T. Kimura, personal communication) and Danube salmon (*Hucho hucho*) (Ahne, 1980). However, with the exception of Atlantic salmon and brown trout, there has been no report of clinical IPN disease in these species.

Non-salmonid Species

Although IPN is generally regarded as a disease of salmonid fish, there has been mounting evidence during the past decade that IPN virus is also able to infect a wide variety of non-salmonid fish, including some marine species. In most cases, classification of these viruses as strains of IPN virus has been on the basis of neutralization with antisera against reference serotypes of

IPN virus. For some isolates, additional evidence has come from biophysical/biochemical characterization studies.

The first indication of a non-salmonid host came with the isolation of the virus from a natural population of apparently healthy white suckers (*Catastomus commersoni*) in the outlet channel of an IPN-affected hatchery in Canada (Sonstegard *et al.*, 1972). Later, during routine diagnostic investigations into mortalities in natural populations of fish in a lake in England in 1973/74, IPN virus was isolated on several occasions from carp (*Cyprinus carpio*), roach (*Rutilus rutilus*), bream (*Abramis brama*), crucian carp (*Carassius carassius*) and perch (*Perca fluviatilis*) (B. J. Hill and K. Way, unpublished observations). However, there was no evidence to indicate that infection with these viruses was the cause of disease in the host species. In experimental infections, all isolates, except that from perch, proved pathogenic to some degree for rainbow trout fry, producing characteristic clinical signs of IPN.

Munro *et al.* (1976) reported detection of IPN virus in minnows (*Phoxinus phoxinus*), perch (*Perca fluviatilis*) and lamprey (*Lampetra fluviatilis*) resident in a fresh-water loch in Scotland which received the effluent from a trout farm with a history of IPN disease. In this case also, the infected fish showed no signs of clinical disease.

In Germany, Ahne (1978, 1980) has reported the frequent isolation of IPN virus from moribund pike (*Esox lucius*) fry with a haemorrhagic disease, but the extent to which the virus contributed to the clinical disease was not determined. Experimental infections of pike fry failed to reproduce the disease, nor did the virus produce IPN in experimentally infected rainbow trout fry. Ahne (1980) also reported non-clinical infections of IPN virus in natural populations of grayling (*Thymallus thymallus*), barbel (*Barbus barbus*) and carp (*Cyprinus carpio*), and has since obtained further isolates of IPN virus from nase (*Chondrostoma nasus*), silver bream (*Blicca bjoernka*), gudgeon (*Gobio gobio*) and rudd (*Scardinius erythrophthalmus*) (personal communication). More recently, similar infections have been described in goldfish (*Carassius auratus*), bream (*Abramis brama*) and discuss fish (*Symphysodon discus*) in Northern Ireland (Adair and Ferguson, 1981). In addition, experimental infection of the zebra fish (*Brachydano rerio*) with IPN virus and vertical transfer via the egg has been demonstrated by Seeley *et al.* (1977).

Further to these examples of non-clinical infections, there have been recent reports of specific diseases in non-salmonid fish caused by IPN or "IPN-like" viruses. In Japan, Sano (1976) and Sano *et al.* (1981) have reported the isolation of a virus associated with major annual epizootics in farmed populations of European eels (*Anguilla anguilla*) and Japanese eels (*Anguilla japonica*). The virus, first isolated from European eels and designated EVE (eel virus European), was found to be morphologically indistinguishable from IPN virus and related serologically to a French strain of IPN virus. Infectivity trials confirmed that the virus was pathogenic for young Japanese eels, but it appeared to be avirulent for rainbow trout fry. Subsequently, an IPN virus of the Sp serotype was isolated from apparently healthy European elvers in France (Castric and Chastel, 1980). However, in contrast with the results for Japanese eels, experimental infections failed to produce significant mortalities or any clinical signs of disease in young European eels, but did produce typical IPN disease in young rainbow trout fry. More recently, a strain of the second European serotype (Ab) of IPN virus has been isolated from farmed European eels in England (Hudson *et al.*, 1981), but this isolate has also proved non-pathogenic for European elvers under experimental conditions (B. J. Hill and R. F. Williams, unpublished observations).

A virus has been isolated recently in England from diseased cyprinids (carp) which has the typical *in vitro* properties of IPN virus but which shows no antigenic relationship in neutralization tests (B. J. Hill and K. Way, unpublished observations). The virus is , however, neutralized by antiserum against Tellina virus (TV-1), the reference strain of serogroup II of the "IPN-like" viruses which have been isolated from marine shellfish (see below). It is not known yet whether the carp isolate is pathogenic for carp or whether it produces IPN in rainbow trout fry.

Diseases in marine fish are now being associated with viruses which are indistinguishable from IPN virus in their *in vitro* properties. Stephens *et al.* (1980) investigating the cause of large-scale annual epizootics of "spinning disease" in natural populations of the Atlantic menhaden (*Brevoortia tyrannus*) in Chesapeake Bay on the East Coast of the U.S.A., isolated from the brains of diseased fish a virus with typical biological, biophysical and biochemical properties of IPN virus. In addition, the isolate was completely neutralized by a polyvalent antiserum against IPN virus. The authors ·claimed success in reproducing the "spinning disease" in experimentally inoculated menhaden, but further tests with cloned or purified virus are required to confirm that the isolate is the true aetiological agent of the disease. In France, a virus identified in neutralization tests as belonging to the Sp serotype of IPN virus has been isolated from moribund 4–6-week-old hatchery reared sea bass (*Dicentrarchus labrax*) larvae in outbreaks of a severe disease on the Mediterranean coast in which cumulative mortalities may reach 90–100% (J-R. Bonami and B. J. Hill, unpublished observations). Preliminary experimental infectivity tests have indicated that both the sea bass and menhaden isolates are infectious but non-pathogenic for rainbow trout fry (B. J. Hill and K. Way, unpublished observations). A similar virus has been isolated from diseased hatchery-reared sea bass larvae on the Atlantic coast of France (J. Castric, personal communication), where other isolates have also been isolated from abnormal eggs of turbot (*Scophthalmus maximus*) and Dover sole (*Solea solea*).

Marine Shellfish

Viruses which are biochemically, biophysically and serologically indistinguishable from IPN virus have been isolated from a variety of marine shellfish from around the coast of Britain and the east coast of Canada (Hill, 1976a, b; Underwood *et al.*, 1977; Dobos *et al.*, 1979). The list of isolates and host species is gradually extending and currently comprises: tellina (*Tellina tenuis*), flat oyster (*Ostrea edulis*), Pacific oyster (*Crassostrea gigas*), American oyster (*Crassostrea virginica*), hard clam (*Mercenaria mercenaria*), mussel (*Mytilus edulis*), limpet (*Patella vulgata*), common periwinkle (*Littorina littoria*) and the shore crab (*Carcinus maenas*). Three isolates (two from tellina and one from flat oyster) show no antigenic relationship to IPN virus, but cross-react with each other in neutralization tests and appear to represent a distinct serogroup. As mentioned above, an isolate from carp also falls into this serogroup. Results of infectivity tests have been variable, but at least eight of the shellfish isolates appear pathogenic to rainbow trout fry in which they produce typical signs of IPN disease. In infectivity experiments with flat oysters and Pacific oysters some of the isolates have caused mild-to-moderate pathological lesions (Hill and Alderman, 1979), but the results have been inconsistent and a firm conclusion on the significance of these viruses for their shellfish hosts cannot yet be drawn. Furthermore, it remains unresolved whether these viruses are truly infecting their hosts or are merely contaminating the host tissues as a result of ingestion of infected or contaminated material.

The reports outlined above clearly demonstrate that IPN virus (or, perhaps more strictly speaking, the group of viruses to which IPN virus belongs) has an extremely wide host range involving fresh-water and marine fish and quite possibly marine shellfish also.

Characteristics of IPN Virus

Of all the fish viruses, IPN virus has been by far the most thoroughly characterized. Detailed studies on the biochemical and biophysical properties of the virion and its genome have been published in several reports (Cohen *et al.*, 1973; Dobos, 1976; Underwood *et al.*, 1977;

Dobos *et al.*, 1977, 1979; Macdonald and Yamamoto, 1977; Macdonald *et al.*, 1977; Chang *et al.*, 1978; Dobos *et al.*, 1979).

In negatively-stained preparations, purified IPN virus has icosahedral symmetry and a diameter of 59nm (Fig. 1). A single capsid of IPN virus is composed of 180 structural sub-units shared by 92 pentagonal and

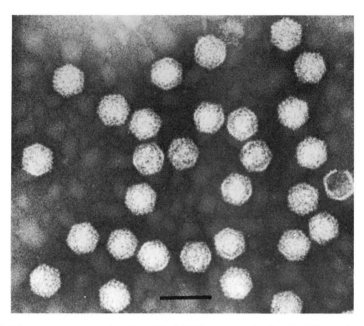

Fig. 1. Electron micrograph of purified IPN virus stained with 2% methylamine tungstate. Bar = 100nm.

hexagonal capsomers. The virion has a sedimentation coefficient of 430–440S, a molecular weight of about 55×10^6 and a buoyant density of 1.32–1.33 g ml^{-1} in CsCl. By polyacrylamide-gel electrophoresis analysis, IPN virus contains four polypeptides of approximate molecular weight 90,000, 60,000, 29,000 and 27,000 in the proportion 3:24:17:15. The genome, which represents 8.7% of the total virion mass, comprises two segments of double-stranded RNA of approximate molecular weight 2.2×10^6 and 2.4×10^6, each with a GC content of 54%.

The serology of IPN virus is complex. Cross-neutralization tests reveal that there are several serotypes of IPN virus, although they all cross-react and there is quite a wide antigenic diversity amongst strains within each serotype (Wolf and Quimby, 1971; Jorgensen and Kehlet, 1971; Lientz and Springer, 1973). Comprehensive cross-neutralization studies currently being carried out indicate that there are four serotypes in Europe which can be readily differentiated from the three (or four) serotypes present in North America (B. J. Hill and K. Way, unpublished observations).

Although for many years the IPN virus group has been referred to as "reo-like viruses", the biophysical and biochemical properties of the viruses, as determined above, do not allow them to be included within the Reoviridae with its current definition. It has therefore been suggested that they should be regarded as representing a new family and a suggested name has been "Birnaviridae" (Dobos *et al.*, 1979). However, official acceptance of this suggestion will have to await the deliberations of the ICTV. It is interesting to note that two non-aquatic viruses with bi-segmented double-stranded RNA genomes (infectious bursal disease virus of chickens and virus X of *Drosophila melanogaster*), although showing no antigenic relationship, have all the general physico-chemical features of the IPN group of viruses (Nick *et al.*, 1976; Todd and McNulty, 1979; Teninges, 1979; Dobos *et al.*, 1979).

Characteristics of IPN Disease

Although, as described above, infections with viruses indistinguishable from IPN virus have been reported for many species of fish (and possibly shellfish), infectious pancreatic necrosis disease *per se* appears to be a condition specific to a few salmonid species. The clinical disease has been observed only under circumstances of hatchery cultivation of fish. To date, there have been no reports of epizootics of IPN disease in wild juvenile salmonids, although this could merely be a reflection of the difficulty in monitoring the health of such populations.

In hatchery populations, a sudden and usually progressive increase in the daily mortalities, particularly in the faster growing individuals, is often the first sign of an outbreak. The cumulative mortalities due to IPN disease vary considerably between different outbreaks. In the worst situation an epizootic may persist for many weeks and the cumulative mortality reach 90% or more. However, losses are usually much lower than this in commercial hatcheries and may even be hardly significant (Jorgensen and Bregnballe, 1969; Jorgensen and Kehlet, 1971; Munro and Duncan, 1977). Virus levels in the visceral organs reach a peak of 10^7–10^9 infectious particles g^{-1} and large quantities of virus are excreted by moribund fry via intestinal discharges. The concentration of infectious virus in the water during an IPN epizootic in a commercial hatchery has been recorded as high as 10^5 $TCID_{50}$ ml^{-1} (Desautels and MacKelvie, 1975). Horizontal transmission readily takes place via the contaminated water or by cannibalism.

An important feature of IPN is the marked increase in resistance of the host with age, the most susceptible fish being early feeding fry, and high resistance being reached by the age of 5–6 months. Rare cases of the disease have, however, been recorded in yearling fish (Elazhary *et al.*, 1976). An IPN syndrome in 6–11-month-old fingerling rainbow trout was reported by Roberts and McKnight (1976), who concluded it to be a stress-induced recrudescence of acute IPN in fish which had survived an outbreak of the disease as fry.

It has been generally observed that fish surviving an acute IPN infection at the fry stage may have significantly reduced growth rates (McKnight and Roberts, 1976; Munro and Duncan, 1977).

Clinical Signs

The clinical signs of IPN disease include darkened pigmentation, a pronounced distended abdomen and, most typically, a cork-screwing and spiralling swimming motion in severely moribund fish. Exophthalmia may be present. Internally, there is frequently a large amount of whitish mucus and sloughed epithelial cells within the lumen of the stomach and intestine. There may also be signs of petechial haemorrhages over the anterior visceral mass and the liver and spleen are often enlarged and pale.

Histopathology

As the name of the disease suggests, the pancreas is the major target organ in IPN. Severe necrosis of the pancreatic acinar cells occurs, together with nuclear piknosis, karyorrhexis and occasional intracytoplasmic inclusions. Islet tissue may or may not be affected. The mucosa of the pylorus, pyloric caecea and anterior intestine show an acute enteritis in the form of necrosis and sloughing of the epithelium. A comprehensive report of the sequential histopathology of naturally-occurring IPN has been given by McKnight and Roberts (1976).

Electron microscopy of infected tissues has revealed large crystalline arrays of virus within the cytoplasm of pancreatic cells showing advanced pathological changes approaching necrosis (Lightner and Post, 1969; Ball *et al.*, 1971).

Carrier State and Vertical Transmission

Most, if not all, survivors of an IPN outbreak become non-clinical carriers, probably for life, and excrete various quantities of virus in their faeces and in their seminal or ovarian fluids when spawning (Wolf *et al.*, 1968; Billi and Wolf, 1969; Frantsi and Savan, 1971a). The virus is also detectable in the visceral organs of carriers, particularly the kidney. The incidence and persistence of the carrier state has been found to be higher in brook trout than in rainbow trout (Wolf *et al.*, 1968; Yamamoto, 1974, 1975a, b; Yamamoto and Kilistoff, 1979). It has been claimed that decreases in the amount of virus in the tissues of carriers appears to correlate with an increase in circulating antibody and that the antibody response in brook trout is much less than that in rainbow trout and consequently the carrier state persists longer (Yamamoto, 1975a, b). However, evidence has been presented that shows no correlation between the neutralizing titre of the serum of carrier brook trout and rainbow trout and the virus titres in the organs (Reno, 1976; Reno *et al.*, 1978).

More recently, it has been speculated that defective interfering particles may play a major role in determining the persistence of the carrier state for IPN. It has been demonstrated that IPN virus can produce defective interfering particles in cells *in vitro* which interfere with the production of homologous standard infectious virus (Nicholson and Dunn, 1974; Macdonald, 1978) and lead to persistent infection in tissue cultures (Macdonald and Kennedy, 1979; Hedrick *et al.*, 1978). Furthermore, Nicholson and Dexter (1975) described the possible interference in the isolation of IPN virus from carrier fish due to the presence of defective interfering particles in the host tissues. Hedrick *et al.* (1978) suggested that the ability of IPN virus to persist in carrier trout may be the result of the balance between defective interfering particles and complete infectious virion production in the host and that the variation in infectious virus released from carrier trout may be due to variations in defective interfering particle concentrations.

During the earliest investigations into IPN it was suggested that there was evidence for vertical transmission of the disease (Snieszko *et al.*, 1957). Further work has shown that eggs from female carriers are infected or intimately contaminated with the virus which cannot be removed by surface disinfection techniques effective for other fish viruses and that vertical transmission to the offspring readily takes place (Wolf *et al.*, 1963; Bullock *et al.*, 1976; Fijan and Giorgetti, 1978). Not only does this result in "recycling" of IPN disease on those affected farms which maintain their own brood stocks but, through the practice of trading in fish eggs, it is also a major cause of the spread of disease to new sites.

Other Diseases Involving IPN or "IPN-like" Viruses

IPN, as described above, appears to be a disease restricted to a few salmonid species and has not been recorded in any of the large number of non-salmonid fish species found infected with an IPN virus or an "IPN-like" virus. In the few cases where a disease has been associated with such virus infections in a non-salmonid fish, the pathology has differed from that of IPN. However, reports of such diseases are only just emerging and, with one exception, pathological details are very scanty.

The disease of Japanese eels which has been described as branchionephritis has occurred annually in eel farms in Japan during the winter months since 1969 and has become one of the most serious in Japanese fish culture (Sano, 1976; Sano *et al.*, 1981). Clinically, moribund fish exhibit spasms or rigidity, a retracted abdomen with occasional diffuse congestion and, in many cases, congestion of the gill and anal fin. Internally there is slight hypertrophy of the kidney and, occasionally, ascitic fluid is found in the abdominal cavity. Histological examination reveals glomerulonephritis, hyaline degeneration of renal tubular epithelial cells, focal necrosis in the renal interstitium and focal necrosis of the spleen and liver. The pancreas, however, appears mainly unaffected. Almost all of these signs have been reproduced in experimental infection of Japanese elvers with the virus, which can be re-isolated from gills, spleens, guts, livers and kidneys of moribund fish. Under experimental conditions, cumulative mortalities in excess of 50% are reached in less than 20 days.

The "spinning disease" of Atlantic menhaden occurs as annual epizootics during the spring months causing massive fish kills, and takes its name from the erratic swimming behaviour of dying fish. In menhaden experimentally infected with the isolated virus, moribund fish show signs of haemorrhages at the base of the fins, in the eyes and along the body, followed by darkened pigmentation, erratic swimming in circles and finally death within 3–5 days (Stephens *et al.*, 1980). Virus can be re-isolated from the brain, pancreas and several other internal organs and also from the blood of experimentally infected fish. No details have yet been published of the histopathology of the disease.

There are insufficient details available at this stage for these non-salmonid diseases to allow comparisons to be made with IPN disease in salmonids. However, in the case of the eel disease, it is clear that there are major differences from IPN of trout, in particular the absence of pancreatic necrosis. Also of interest, is the clinical feature of the menhaden spinning disease which is characteristic of IPN disease in trout, namely the loss of co-ordinated movements and development of erratic swimming behaviour such as spiralling or corkscrewing. This, together with the observed "spasms" in the diseased eels, suggests the possibility that in diseases caused by IPN viruses neurotropism is a common feature, although other aspects of the pathology may differ in different fish species.

Information on the virulence for their hosts of IPN virus or "IPN-like" viruses isolated from shellfish is very limited at the present time. Preliminary studies on the virulence of two viruses from serogroup II (one from *Ostrea edulis* and one from *Tellina tenuis*) for *Ostrea edulis* have indicated that the two virus strains produce a pathological effect on the digestive gland which is more pronounced at 8–10°C than at 16–18°C (Hill and Alderman, 1979). Histopathologically there was a general development of tissue oedema with the maximum effect being observed in the digestive gland where haemocyte infiltration and necrosis of connective tissue occurred. At 8–10°C the maximum effect appeared to be reached between day 20 and day 30 post-inoculation and coincided with the maximum titres of infectious virus extracted from the tissues. It must be emphasized, however, that these results are of a preliminary nature and that further experiments are needed to confirm the observations.

Studies are currently in hand to determine whether the IPN virus isolate from the shore crab is virulent for marine crustacean species. Early results have shown that the virus infects (or persists in) the tissues of the hepato-pancreas for periods of several weeks in experimentally challenged lobster (*Homarus vulgaris*), brown crab (*Cancer pagurus*), spider crab (*Maia squinado*), fiddler crab (*Macropipus puber*) and the shore crab (*Carcinus maenas*), but that it does not appear to cause mortality. The tissues of these animals are presently being studied by histology and electron microscopy to determine whether a true infection is taking place and to what extent, if any, there is an overt lesion.

Factors Affecting the Virulence of IPN Virus

Perhaps not surprisingly in view of its long history, it is to IPN disease in salmonids that most of the information on factors affecting the virulence of IPN virus relates. It is a general observation that the severity and cumulative mortalities of IPN infections in trout hatcheries can vary considerably from as high as 90% or more to insignificance. Infections of IPN are frequently noted in trout fry populations without any clinical evidence of the disease or mortalities. It is generally accepted that the virulence of IPN virus infections in salmonids depends on a combination of a number of factors relating to the host, the virus and the environment.

Host Factors

Species. The virulence of IPN virus depends to a great extent on the particular host species it infects. Within the salmonids, there are marked differences between species in the degree of susceptibility to IPN disease.

From general observations alone it is clear that brook trout, rainbow trout and (in Japan) amago trout are the species which are most severely affected by IPN. Although there have also been some references to natural occurrences of IPN in Atlantic salmon and brown trout and the virus has been isolated from these species by several workers, the rarity of field cases points to a much lower susceptibility to the disease than that of brook trout and rainbow trout. There have been no case reports of natural clinical IPN in other salmonids (apart from cutthroat trout) despite the detection of a natural virus infection.

Laboratory studies involving experimental challenge with IPN virus could provide useful information on its relative virulence for different species, but few such studies have been carried out. Parisot *et al.* (1963) reported that chinook salmon (*Oncorhynchus tshawytscha*), kokanee salmon (*O. nerka*) and coho salmon (*O. kisutch*) were resistant to the disease when inoculated with an isolate of the virus virulent for brook trout, but no details were given of the age or size of the fish tested. However, Sano (1973) has reported that IPN virus from rainbow trout was almost as equally virulent for two *Oncorhynchus* species, amago (*O. rhodurus*) and himemasu (landlocked form of *O. nerka*) as it was for rainbow trout fry at a mean water temperature of 9°C. In studies on the pathogenesis of IPN in Atlantic salmon, Swanson and Gillespie (1979) have reported that clinical IPN failed to develop in young salmon fry experimentally infected by contaminated water with a rainbow trout isolate despite evidence of virus replication. In contrast, intraperitoneal inoculation of virus into yearling salmon caused pancreatic necrosis without clinical disease.

Studies on the relative susceptibilities of rainbow trout, Atlantic salmon, brown trout and brook trout to IPN viruses isolated from these hosts are being carried out under standardized conditions at the author's laboratory. To date it has been found that both Atlantic salmon and brown trout can develop IPN disease, but that its severity depends upon the virus strain used. With the virus strains from brook trout, rainbow trout and salmon, brook trout were more susceptible than salmon, which were more susceptible than brown trout. However, the virus strain from brown trout was most virulent for salmon, less virulent for brown trout and least virulent for brook trout. There was some evidence of different degrees of host specificity for the viruses isolated from different hosts.

From general observations in the field it has been speculated that even for a particular fish species such as rainbow trout, there may be differing degrees of susceptibility between different strains. Published evidence, however, is very scanty and limited to that of Elazhary *et al.* (1976).

Apart from the cases of diseases in menhaden, Japanese eels and sea bass larvae, very little is known about the virulence of IPN virus for non-salmonid fish species. Simple laboratory challenge experiments in the fry of non-salmonid species from which the virus has been isolated could provide much useful information on this little-understood aspect of IPN virus.

Age. For IPN of trout, the important influence of the age of the host on the virulence of the virus infection has been recognized since the first field observations of M'Gonigle (1941). With the exception of the rare cases reported in older fish, susceptibility to IPN disease decreases steadily with age and it is generally accepted that resistance to the disease is reached by the age of 5–6 months for the susceptible salmonid species. Fish older than this can be infected by the virus, but show no clinical signs of disease even following intraperitoneal injection. Such fish develop a transient non-clinical infection which results in high levels of neutralizing antibody and, ultimately, loss of virus from the fish tissues (Wolf and Quimby, 1969). This is consistent with the field observations that, in older fish exposed naturally to IPN virus, the infection is transient and the carrier state not established. Consequently, when the original source of contamination is removed there is a decline in the prevalence of infection in the fish population.

Laboratory studies on the effect of age on susceptibility to IPN disease in salmonids have been few but do confirm the field observations. Frantsi and Savan (1971b) in experimental infections of brook trout obtained cumulative mortalities of 85% in 1-month-old fish, 73% in 2-month-old fish, 45% in 4-month-old fish and negligible mortalities in 6-month-old fish within a 60-day observation period. More recently, Dorson and Torchy (1981) made a similar study on the effect of age on the increase in resistance of rainbow trout to IPN. Cumulative mortalities within 2 months of infection decreased steadily from 70% in fish infected when 1 or 2 weeks old to a negligible percentage in fish infected when 20 weeks old. A graph of cumulative mortality against age at the time of infection shows an almost linear relationship. The authors concluded that using mortality as a criterion, rainbow trout ceased to be susceptible to IPN when 15–20 weeks old even though they may be actively infected by the virus following exposure. (It was also of interest to note that fry which had not yet started feeding could develop the disease, and that the survivors could not be considered immunologically tolerant as previously suggested (Wolf and Quimby, 1969).

The reason for the virtual linear decrease in susceptibility (as measured by mortalities) to IPN disease with increasing age remains unclear. A reflection of the developing immune system is a possibility that has been considered, but Munro and Duncan (1977) have pointed out that the susceptibility of young fish to IPN disease is unlikely to be simply due to a poor immune responsiveness because large numbers of lymphocytes coated with immunoglobulin have been found to appear 1–2 weeks after first feeding.

Environmental Factors

It is generally recognized that IPN virus infections in hatchery populations of susceptible brook trout and rainbow trout fry frequently occur without producing mortalities or clinical disease (for example, see Jorgensen and Bregnballe, 1969; Munro and Duncan, 1977). In one such case in brook trout fry it was shown (Sonstegard and McDermott, 1971) that the virus involved was not avirulent as might be thought, but was capable of inducing heavy mortalities in other populations of brook trout fry following experimental challenge. Similarly, the author has isolated a strain of IPN virus from apparently healthy rainbow trout fry in a commercial hatchery in England which had experienced no unusual mortalities. The virus not only proved virulent to other rainbow trout fry, but also induced IPN disease and heavy mortalities in the fry from which it originated, after experimental challenge. This demonstrates that an inherently virulent strain of IPN virus may infect susceptible fry without necessarily causing IPN disease. A possible explanation for this is that the hatchery fish had been initially exposed to only a low level of infectious virus and had been able to contain it by their defence mechanisms which had been overwhelmed when subsequently challenged experimentally with a higher infectious dose (10^4 p.f.u. ml^{-1} in the water).

Adverse conditions. The observation of such asymptomatic infections in populations of hatchery-reared fry has led to the general view that the development of clinical IPN in infected fry occurs mainly when fish are under "stress" due to adverse environmental conditions such as poor water quality, overcrowding and handling, all of which are thought to depress the immune responsiveness. Certainly, marked physiological changes in salmonids occur when they are handled or when they are held in high population densities (Wedemeyer, 1976). The depression of the immune response to IPN virus in at least one fish species when held in overcrowded conditions has been demonstrated by Perlmutter *et al.* (1973), who also provided some evidence to link this to release by the fish of immunosuppressive factors into the water. In the field, it has been observed that reduction of the population density of hatchery-reared rainbow trout can lower the mortality in an IPN outbreak (Jorgensen and Bregnballe, 1969) and that "stress" induced by adverse water quality (such as low oxygen content) and transportation causes a marked enhancement of the replication of IPN virus in carrier fish (Frantsi and Savan, 1971a; Roberts and McKnight, 1976).

Such observations have led to the view that employment of good husbandry techniques may significantly reduce the virulence of IPN infections in hatchery reared trout. Laboratory studies on the effect of fish population density per unit change of water could provide useful information for practical application in the field.

Water temperature. Water temperature is an important factor in the development of most fish diseases. Fish are poikilothermic and have a body temperature which is always close to that of their aquatic environment. Farmed trout may experience water temperatures ranging from 4°C or less in winter to 20°C or more in summer. The physiological responses of fish, including the defence mechanisms, are dependent to a great extent on the body temperature. Naturally, fish pathogens, including viruses such as IPN, have optimal temperature ranges for replication. Thus, the outcome of an infection with a pathogen in fish is affected significantly by the water temperature.

In most trout fry hatcheries the water is usually taken from springs or bore-hole supply and the temperature is normally within the range 8–12°C. The majority of natural cases of IPN have therefore been observed within this temperature range. Limited studies have been made to determine the effect of water temperature on the virulence of IPN virus infections as measured by the cumulative mortality. Following experimental infection of brook trout fry with IPN virus, Frantsi and Savan (1971b) obtained cumulative mortalities of 74% at 10°C, 46% at 15.5°C and no mortalities at 4.5°C. They suggested that the low ambient temperatures in some Canadian trout farms during the age period susceptibility of the fry could explain the field observations of few mortalities despite IPN virus infections. Sano (1972b) has, however, reported that in two successive winters, infected rainbow trout fry held at 14°C suffered much higher mortalities than those held at 10.5°C and, in contrast to Frantsi and Savan, observed that mortalities were less at 10.5°C than at the lower temperature of 6°C. More recent work by Dorson and Torchy (1981) with rainbow trout fry has shown that the mortality rate in fry held at 6°C was much less than that at 10°C and was almost totally suppressed at 16°C. The relative degree of susceptibility appeared to be directly related to the number of degree days that had elapsed since hatching. Plotting mortality percentages against degree days gave a straight line. When fry were moved from 10°C to 16°C only 3 days before infection the mortalities ceased early and the cumulative loss was much reduced, but when fish were similarly transferred from 16°C to 10°C the mortalities remained high.

The mechanism of increased resistance to IPN virus at high temperatures remains unknown, but it has been shown that production of interferon and antibody in rainbow trout is enhanced at these temperatures (Dorson and de Kinkelin, 1974a; Maisse and Dorson, 1976).

Virus Factors

Virus strain. In addition to the host and environmental factors, the outcome of an IPN virus infection in trout fry will always depend to a great extent on the inherent virulence of the particular virus strain involved. In Europe it has been reported that under field conditions strains of the Sp serotype consistently cause higher mortalities in rainbow trout fry than do the strains of the Ab serotype (Jorgensen and Kehlet, 1971). This has subsequently been confirmed by general observation. However, relatively little has been reported on the comparative determination of the degrees of virulence existent amongst different trout IPN virus strains under experimental conditions. Sano (1971b) tested the virulence of four IPN virus isolates from Japan for groups of 10-week-old rainbow trout fry under experimental conditions and found that the cumulative mortalities ranged from 15% to 58%. However, no evidence was presented to show that the challenge dose was the same for all groups of fry. Hill and Dixon (1977) reported the use of a standard procedure for IPN virus virulence tests comprising the introduction of virus to a final concentration of 10^4 p.f.u. ml^{-1} into the water of 35 litre tanks containing 300 rainbow trout fry at a temperature of 10–12°C. The daily mortalities were counted and a percentage mortality after 30 days (D_{30}c.m.) was calculated. Comparative tests were carried out on the virulence of IPN virus strains isolated in the U.K. from diseased fry, non-clinical infections of fry as well as salmonid and non-salmonid carriers. It was found that with less than five passes in tissue culture, most of the IPN virus strains of the Sp serotype isolated from trout in the U.K. had approximately equal virulence for 8–10-week-old trout fry with a range of 43–56% D_{30}c.m. irrespective of whether isolated from diseased fry, non-clinically infected fry or from older carriers. An Ab serotype of the virus isolated from a low mortality epizootic in a commercial hatchery was found to have low virulence (about 15% D_{30}c.m.). Of the three IPN virus isolates tested from non-salmonid carriers, one from roach and another from perch were found to have low virulence (10% and 6% D_{30}c.m. respectively), but the third virus (from carp) appeared to be highly virulent (about 60% D_{30}c.m.).

As has been mentioned above, other tests have been carried out to determine the virulence of IPN virus isolates from different salmonid species for the fry of those species. These studies are still in progress, but to date results indicate that, in addition to the overriding differences in degrees of susceptibility of the host species, the degrees of virulence of the virus for the different hosts is dependent upon the original host from which it was isolated.

Challenge dose. Practically nothing is known about the concentration of virus in the water that constitutes an infective dose and the necessary minimum level of challenge to induce overt disease. Limited studies in the author's laboratory have indicated that sub-clinical infections can occur in susceptible trout fry when the concentration of virus in the water at the time of challenge is 10^3 p.f.u. ml^{-1} or lower. However, the results have indicated that the lower limit for inducing clinical disease can differ by a factor of 10-fold or more between different virus strains.

Much more work is necessary in this area before firm conclusions can be drawn.

Effects of growth in tissue culture. Dorson *et al.* (1975, 1978) demonstrated that, after a relatively low number of serial passages through fish tissue cultures, virulent IPN virus develops a sensitivity to neutralization by normal trout serum and at the same time becomes avirulent for trout fry. The neutralization of cell culture adapted (CCA) virus by normal trout serum has been shown to be due to antibody-like non-virus-induced protein which has a sedimentation coefficient of 6S (Jorgensen, 1973; Dorson and de Kinkelin, 1974b). Hill and Dixon (1977) showed that the reduction in virulence from pass level 5 to pass level 11 was slight and independent of the cell line used, but that virus sensitivity to neutralization by normal trout serum (6S sensitivity) developed sooner in some fish cell lines than in others. The phenomenon of development of 6S sensitivity and possible loss of virulence by passage of virus in tissue culture was examined in detail. Three high passage virus strains which were 6S sensitive and avirulent for trout fry, were found to become 6S resistant by serial passage in the presence of increasing strengths of trout serum. The development of 6S resistance coincided with development of virulence for two of the originally avirulent strains, showing that virulence is not necessarily lost permanently by growth in tissue culture and can be regained in tissue culture even after high passage numbers. The third originally avirulent strain did not develop virulence despite becoming 6S resistant, thus showing that 6S resistance does not always indicate virulence. Following plaque cloning of four viruses in the 6S resistant form, serial passage in tissue culture in the absence of trout serum led to the emergence of 6S sensitive virus. This result indicates that 6S sensitive virus does not emerge in tissue culture only by preferential selection on growth rate grounds from an original mixture with 6S resistant virus, but is initially a variant thrown off by clone purified 6S resistant virus. When IPN virus is in its 6S sensitive state after passage in tissue culture it does not induce neutralizing antibody production in trout, either by natural infection or following injection, in contrast to virus in the 6S resistant form which normally does. However, Hill and Dixon (1977) found that infection of rainbow trout with a naturally avirulent strain of IPN virus in its 6S resistant form did not confer immunity as might be expected. The immunocompetence of the fry was demonstrated by injection of formalin-inactivated virulent virus in the 6S resistant form. This result suggests that, in addition to 6S resistance, IPN virus may need to have the virulence factor itself in order to stimulate the defence mechanism in trout fry.

These results demonstrate that in carrying out virulence tests on IPN virus, particularly where relatively small differences in degrees of virulence are being examined, it is absolutely essential that the virus be grown in tissue culture in the presence of normal trout serum to ensure that it is in the 6S resistant form. Most rainbow trout stocks have 6S activity in their serum to some degree and it is advantageous to obtain a serum with high levels of activity so that a dilution of 1:100 can be used routinely in the maintenance medium for tissue culture production of virulent IPN virus.

Chemotherapy. Very few studies have been published on the possible use of chemotherapy to reduce the virulence of IPN virus infections. The work of Economon (1972) suggested that inclusion of polyvinylpyrrolidone-iodine in the diet of brook trout suffering from IPN disease reduced the mortality level by 50%. However, these observations have not been substantiated by other workers. More recently, studies by Migus and Dobos (1980) have shown that virazole (1-D ribofluranosyl-1, 2,4-triazole-3-carboxamide) at concentrations as little as $10\mu g$ ml^{-1} causes a substantial reduction in the yield of IPN virus in infected fish tissue cultures. Subsequent studies by Savan and Dobos (1980) have shown that the mortality rate in 6-week-old rainbow trout infected with IPN virus is reduced only marginally by treatment with a single exposure to virazole, but that doses as high as $400\mu g$ did not result in a marked reduction in the number of deaths. Also, there was no evidence to suggest that higher levels of virazole would necessarily reduce the death rate any further.

Discussion

Although IPN disease appears to be a condition specific to four or possibly five salmonid species, the causative virus is representative of a group of serologically related viruses which, in fact, are found in a wide variety of fish and shellfish species. Indeed, with increasing detection of other host species and in other areas of the world, the virus may become to be regarded as fairly widespread, certainly much more so than at present.

Some of the viruses from non-salmonid fish and even some from shellfish have been found to be pathogenic for rainbow trout fry in which they produce typical IPN, and are therefore justifiably called IPN virus. However, other isolates, which although serologically indistinguishable from IPN virus, have been found to be avirulent for rainbow trout. The question may be asked — is it justified to refer to such isolates as IPN virus? Little yet is known of the virulence of these isolates for their non-salmonid fish hosts or their shellfish hosts, nor indeed whether, conversely, typical trout isolates causing IPN disease have the capacity to be pathogenic for any non-salmonid fish, either freshwater or marine. Further research in this area may eventually reveal that viruses within this group have ranges of different hosts for which they are virulent, perhaps with some strains having different ranges. Equally, it may be found that this group of viruses divides conveniently into separate sub-groups on the basis of the type of host for which their virulence is limited, for example salmonids, eels, marine fish, and possibly molluscs and crustacea. Alternatively, they may form sub-groups on the basis of the specific type of pathology produced irrespective of the host involved. Should the latter be the case, then it would seem correct to restrict the name IPN virus to those strains specifically producing pancreatic necrosis. At the present time, however, there is some confusion in the literature with respect to the use of the term "IPN virus". Some authors use it in a generic sense for any isolate serologically related to reference strains of IPN virus, whereas others use the term "IPN-like" virus for any isolate from a non-salmonid host, even though in all *in vitro* tests it has all the properties characteristic of IPN virus.

Such problems arise when viruses are named after the original specific disease with which they were associated and which is subsequently used as the reference for other related viruses discovered later. Placing the whole of the IPN virus group within a genus with a name based upon the general biochemical and biophysical properties will eventually help to obviate this problem of terminology.

References

Adair, B. M. and Ferguson, H. W. (1981). Isolation of infectious pancreatic necrosis (IPN) virus from non-salmonid fish. *Journal of Fish Diseases* 4, 69–76.
Ahne, W. (1978). Isolation and characterization of infectious pancreatic necrosis virus from pike (*Esox lucius*). *Archives of Virology* 58, 65–69.

Ahne, W. (1980). Vorkommen des Virus der Infektiösen Pankreasnekrose der Forellen (IPN) bei verschiedenen Fischarten. *Berliner und Münchener Tierärztliche Wochenschrift* **93**(1), 14–16.

Ball, H. J., Munro, A. L. S., Ellis, A., Elson, K. G. R., Hodgkiss, W. and McFarlane, I. S. (1971). Infectious pancreatic necrosis in rainbow trout in Scotland. *Nature, London* **234**, 417–418.

Besse, P. and Kinkelin, P. de. (1965). Sur l'existence en France de la nécrose pancréatique de la truite arc-en-ciel (*Salmo gairdneri*). *Bulletin de l'Academie Vétérinaire* **38**, 185–190.

Billi, J. L. and Wolf, K. (1969). Quantitative comparison of peritoneal washes and faeces for detecting infectious pancreatic necrosis (IPN) virus in carrier brook trout. *Journal of the Fisheries Research Board of Canada* **26**, 1459–1465.

Bullock, G. L., Rucker, R. R., Amend, D., Wolf, K. and Stuckey, H. M. (1976). Infectious pancreatic necrosis: transmission with iodine-treated and non-treated eggs of brook trout (*Salvelinus fontinalis*). *Journal of the Fisheries Research Board of Canada* **33**, 1197–1198.

Castric, J. and Chastel, C. (1980). Isolation and characterization attempts of three viruses from European eel, *Anguilla anguilla*: preliminary results. *Annales de Virologie (Institut Pasteur)* **131E**, 435–448.

Chang, N., Macdonald, R. D. and Yamamoto, T. (1978). Purification of infectious pancreatic necrosis virus and comparison of polypeptide composition of different isolates. *Canadian Journal of Microbiology* **24**, 19–27.

Cohen, A., Poinsard, A. and Scherrer, R. (1973). Physico-chemical properties and morphological features of infectious pancreatic necrosis virus. *Journal of General Virology* **21**, 485–498.

Desautels, D. and MacKelvie, R. M. (1975). Practical aspects of survival and destruction of infectious pancreatic necrosis virus. *Journal of the Fisheries Research Board of Canada* **32**, 523–531.

Dobos, P. (1976). Size and structure of the genome of infectious pancreatic necrosis virus. *Nucleic Acids Research* **3**(8), 1903–1924.

Dobos, P., Hallett, R., Kells, D. T. C., Sorensen, O. and Rowe, D. (1977). Biophysical studies of infectious pancreatic necrosis virus. *Journal of Virology* **22**(1), 150–159.

Dobos, P., Hill, B. J., Hallett, R., Kells, D. T. C., Becht, H. and Teninges, D. (1979). Biophysical and biochemical characterization of five animal viruses with bisegmented double-stranded RNA genomes. *Journal of Virology* **32**(2), 593–605.

Dorson, M. and Kinkelin, P. de. (1974a). Mortalité et production d'intérferon circulant chez la truite arc-en-ciel après infection experimentale avec le virus d'Egtved: influence de la témperature. *Annales de Recherches Vététinaires* **5**, 365–372.

Dorson, M. and Kinkelin, P. de. (1974b). Nécrose pancréatique infectieuse des salmonidés: existence dans le sérum de truites indemnes d'une molécule 6S neutralisant spécifiquement le virus. *Comptes rendus de l'Académie des Sciences Série D* **278**, 785–788.

Dorson, M. and Torchy, C. (1981). The influence of fish age and water temperature on mortalities of rainbow trout, *Salmo gairdneri* Richardson, caused by a European strain of infectious pancreatic necrosis virus. *Journal of Fish Diseases* **4**, 213–221.

Dorson, M., Kinkelin, P. de and Torchy, C. (1975). Virus de la nécrose pancréatique infectieuse: acquisition de la sensibilité au facteur neutralisant de sérum de truite après passages successifs en culture cellulaire. *Comptes rendus de l'Académie des Sciences Série D* **281**, 1435–1438.

Dorson, M., Castric, J. and Torchy, C. (1978). Infectious pancreatic necrosis virus of salmonids: biological and antigenic features of a pathogenic strain and of a non-pathogenic variant selected in RTG cells. *Journal of Fish Diseases* **1**, 309–320.

Economon, P. P. (1972). Polyvinylpyrrolidone-iodine as a control for infectious pancreatic necrosis of brook trout. *FAO/EIFAC 72/SC II — Symposium 59*.

Elazhary, M. A. S. Y., Lagace, A., Cousineau, G., Roy, R. S., Berthiaume, L., Paulhus, R. and Frechette, J. L. (1976). Outbreak of infectious pancreatic necrosis in yearling brook trout (*Salvelinus fontinalis*). *Journal of the Fisheries Research Board of Canada* **33**, 2621–2625.

Fijan, N. N. and Giorgetti, G. (1978). Infectious pancreatic necrosis: isolation of virus from eyed eggs of rainbow trout, *Salmo gairdneri* Richardson. *Journal of Fish Diseases* **1**, 269–270.

Frantsi, C. and Savan, M. (1971a). Infectious pancreatic necrosis virus: comparative frequencies of isolation from faeces and organs of brook trout (*Salvelinus fontinalis*). *Journal of the Fisheries Research Board of Canada* **28**, 1064–1065.

Frantsi, C. and Savan, M. (1971b). Infectious pancreatic necrosis virus — temperature and age factors in mortality. *Journal of Wildlife Diseases* **7**, 249–255.

Hastein, T. and Krogsrud, J. (1976). Infectious pancreatic necrosis. First isolation of virus from fish in Norway. *Acta veterinaria scandinavia* **17**, 109–111.

Hedrick, R. P., Leong, J. C. and Fryer, J. L. (1978). Persistent infections in salmonid fish cells with infectious pancreatic necrosis virus (IPNV). *Journal of Fish Diseases* **1**, 297–308.

Hill, B. J. (1976a). Properties of a virus isolated from the bivalve mollusc *Tellina tenuis* (da Costa). *In* "Wildlife Diseases" (Ed. L. A. Page), pp.445–452. Plenum Press, New York and London.

Hill, B. J. (1976b). Molluscan viruses: their occurrence, culture and relationships. *In* "Proceedings of the First International Colloquium on Invertebrate Pathology", pp.25–29. Queens University Press, Kingston, Canada.

Hill, B. J. and Alderman, D. J. (1979). Observations on the experimental infection of *Ostrea edulis* with two molluscan viruses. *Haliotis* **8**, 297–299.

Hill, B. J. and Dixon, P. F. (1977). Studies on IPN virulence and immunization. *Bulletin de l'Office International des Epizooties* **87**, 425–427.

Hudson, E. B., Bucke, D. and Forrest, A. (1981). Isolation of infectious pancreatic necrosis virus from eels, *Anguilla anguilla* L., in the United Kingdom. *Journal of Fish Diseases* **4**, 429–431.

Jorgensen, P. E. V. (1973). The nature and biological activity of IPN virus neutralizing antibodies in normal and immunized rainbow trout (*Salmo gairdneri*). *Archiv für die Gesamte Virusforschung* **42**, 9–20.

Jorgensen, P. E. V. and Bregnballe, F. (1969). Infectious pancreatic necrosis in rainbow trout (*Salmo gairdneri*) in Denmark. *Nordisk veterinaermedicin* **21**, 142–148.

Jorgensen, P. E. V. and Kehlet, N. P. (1971). Infectious pancreatic necrosis (IPN) viruses in Danish rainbow trout: their serological and pathogenic properties. *Nordisk veterinaermedicin* **23**, 568–575.

Lientz, J. C. and Springer, J. E. (1973). Neutralization tests on infectious pancreatic necrosis virus with polyvalent antiserum. *Journal of Wildlife Diseases* **9**, 120–124.

Lightner, D. and Post, G. (1969). Morphological characteristics of infectious pancreatic necrosis virus in trout pancreatic tissue. *Journal of the Fisheries Research Board of Canada* **26**, 2247–2250.

Ljungberg, O. and Jorgensen, P. E. V. (1972). Infectious pancreatic necrosis of salmonids in Swedish fish farms. *EIFAC 72/SC II—Symposium 14.*

Macdonald, R. D. (1978). Ringed plaque formation in infectious pancreatic necrosis virus correlates with defective interfering particle production. *Journal of General Virology* **41**, 623–628.

Macdonald, R. D. and Kennedy, J. C. (1979). Infectious pancreatic necrosis virus persistently infects chinook salmon embryo cells independent of interferon. *Virology* **95**, 260–264.

Macdonald, R. D. and Yamamoto, T. (1977). The structure of infectious pancreatic necrosis virus RNA. *Journal of General Virology* **34**, 235–247.

Macdonald, R. D., Roy, K. L., Yamamoto, T. and Chang, N. (1977). Oligonucleotide fingerprints of the RNAs from infectious pancreatic necrosis virus. *Archives of Virology* **54**, 373–377.

MacKelvie, R. M. and Artsob, H. (1969). Infectious pancreatic necrosis virus in young salmonids of the Canadian Maritime Provinces. *Journal of the Fisheries Research Board of Canada* **26**, 3259–3262.

McKnight, I. M. and Roberts, R. J. (1976). The pathology of infectious pancreatic necrosis. I. The sequential histopathology of the naturally-occurring condition. *British Veterinary Journal* **132**, 76–85.

Maisse, G. and Dorson, M. (1976). Production d'agglutinines anti *Aeromonas salmonicida* par la truite arc-en-ciel. Influence de la température, d'un adjuvant et d'un immunodepresseur. *Annales de Recherches Vétérinaires* **7**, 307–313.

M'Gonigle, R. H. (1941). Acute catarrhal enteritis of salmonid fingerlings. *Transactions of the American Fisheries Society* **70**, 297–303.

Migus, D. O. and Dobos, P. (1980). Effect of ribavirin on the replication of infectious pancreatic necrosis virus in fish cell cultures. *Journal of General Virology* **47**, 47–57.

Munro, A. L. S. and Duncan, I. B. (1977). Current problems in the study of the biology of infectious pancreatic necrosis virus and the management of the disease it causes in cultivated salmonid fish. *In* "Aquatic Microbiology" (Eds. F. A. Skinner and J. M. Shewan), pp.325–337. Academic Press, London.

Munro, A. L. S., Liversidge, J. and Elson, K. G. R. (1976). The distribution and prevalence of infectious pancreatic necrosis virus in wild fish in Loch Awe. *Proceedings of the Royal Society of Edinburgh (B)* **75**, 223–232.

Nicholson, B. L. and Dexter, R. (1975). Possible interference in the isolation of IPN virus from carrier fish. *Journal of the Fisheries Research Board of Canada* **32**, 1437–1439.

Nicholson, B. L. and Dunn, J. (1974). Homologous interference in trout and Atlantic salmon cell cultures infected with infectious pancreatic necrosis virus. *Journal of Virology* **14**, 180–182.

Nick, H., Cursiefen, D. and Becht, H. (1976). Structural and growth characteristics of infectious bursal disease virus. *Journal of Virology* **18**, 227–234.

Parisot, T. J., Yasutake, W. T. and Bressler, V. (1963). A new geographic and host record for infectious pancreatic necrosis. *Transactions of the American Fisheries Society* **91**, 63–66.

Perlmutter, A., Sarot, D. A., Yu, M-L., Filazzola, R. J. and Seeley, R. J. (1973). The effect of crowding on the immune response of the blue gourami, *Trichogaster trichopterus*, to infectious pancreatic necrosis (IPN) virus. *Life Sciences* **13**, 363–375.

Reno, P. W. (1976). Qualitative and quantitative aspects of the infectious pancreatic necrosis virus (IPNV) carrier state in trout. Ph.D. Thesis. University of Guelph, Guelph, Ontario, Canada.

Reno, P. W., Darley, S. and Savan, M. (1978). Infectious pancreatic necrosis: experimental induction of the carrier state in trout. *Journal of the Fisheries Research Board of Canada* **35**, 1451–1456.

Roberts, R. J. and McKnight, I. J. (1976). The pathology of infectious pancreatic necrosis. II. Stress-mediated recurrence. *British Veterinary Journal* **132**, 209–213.

Sano, T. (1971a). Studies on viral diseases of Japanese fishes. I. Infectious pancreatic necrosis of rainbow trout: first isolation from epizootics in Japan. *Bulletin of the Japanese Society of Scientific Fisheries* **37**, 495–498.

Sano, T. (1971b). Studies on viral diseases of Japanese fishes. II. Infectious pancreatic necrosis of rainbow trout: pathogenicity of the isolants. *Bulletin of the Japanese Society of Scientific Fisheries* **37**, 499–503.

Sano, T. (1972a). Studies on viral diseases of Japanese fishes. III. Infectious pancreatic necrosis of rainbow trout: geographical and seasonal distribution in Japan. *Bulletin of the Japanese Society of Scientific Fisheries* **38**, 313–316.

Sano, T. (1972b). Experience paper on current preventative approach to infectious pancreatic necrosis (IPN) in Japan. *FAO/EIFAC 72/SC II — Symposium 17.*

Sano, T. (1973). Studies on viral diseases of Japanese fishes. IV. Infectious pancreatic necrosis of rainbow trout: susceptibility of freshwater salmons of the genus *Oncorhynchus*. *Bulletin of the Japanese Society of Scientific Fisheries* **39**, 117–120.

Sano, T. (1976). Viral diseases of cultured fishes in Japan. *Fish Pathology* **10**, 221–226.

Sano, T. and Yamazaki, T. (1973). Studies on viral diseases of Japanese fishes. V. Infectious pancreatic necrosis of Amago trout. *Bulletin of the Japanese Society of Scientific Fisheries* **39**, 477–480.

Sano, T., Okamoto, N. and Nishimura, T. (1981). A new viral epizootic of *Anguilla japonica* Temmink and Schlegel. *Journal of Fish Diseases* **4**, 127–139.

Savan, M. and Dobos, P. (1980). Effect of virazole on rainbow trout, *Salmo gairdneri* Richardson, fry infected with infectious pancreatic necrosis virus. *Journal of Fish Diseases* **3**, 437–440.

Schlotfeldt, H-J., Liesse, B. and Frost, J. W. (1975). Erstisolierung und Identifizierung des Virus der infektiösen Pankreasnekrose (IPN) der Salmoniden in der Bundesrepublik Deutschland. *Berliner und Münchener Tierärztliche Wochenschrift* **88**, 109–111.

Seeley, R. J., Perlmutter, A. and Seeley, V. A. (1977). Inheritance and longevity of infectious pancreatic necrosis virus in the zebra fish, *Brachydanio rerio* (Hamilton-Buchanan). *Applied and Environmental Microbiology* **34**, 50–55.

Snieszko, S. F., Wood, E. M. and Yasutake, W. T. (1957). Infectious pancreatic necrosis in trout. *American Medical Association Archives of Pathology* **63**, 229–233.

Snieszko, S. F., Wolf, K., Camper, J. E. and Pettijohn, L. L. (1959). Infectious nature of pancreatic necrosis. *Transactions of the American Fisheries Society* **88**, 289–293.

Sonstegard, R. A. and McDermott, L. A. (1971). Infectious pancreatic necrosis of salmonids in Ontario. *Journal of the Fisheries Research Board of Canada* **28**, 1350–1351.

Sonstegard, R. A., McDermott, L. A. and Sonstegard, K. S. (1972). Isolation of infectious pancreatic necrosis virus from white suckers (*Catastomus commersoni*). *Nature, London* **236**, 174–175.

Stephens, E. B., Newman, M. W., Zachary, A. L. and Hetrick, F. M. (1980). A viral etiology for the annual spring epizootics of Atlantic menhaden, *Brevoortia tyrannus* (Latrobe) in Chesapeake Bay. *Journal of Fish Diseases* 3, 387–398.

Swanson, R. N. and Gillespie, J. H. (1979). Pathogenesis of infectious pancreatic necrosis in Atlantic salmon (*Salmo salar*). *Journal of the Fisheries Research Board of Canada* 36, 587–591.

Teninges, D. (1979). Protein and RNA composition of the structural components of *Drosophila* X virus. *Journal of General Virology* 45, 641–649.

Todd, D. and McNulty, M. S. (1979). Biochemical studies with infectious bursal disease virus: comparison of some of its properties with infectious pancreatic necrosis virus. *Archives of Virology* 60, 265–277.

Underwood, B. O., Smale, C. J., Brown, F. and Hill, B. J. (1977). Relationship of a virus from *Tellina tenuis* to infectious pancreatic necrosis virus. *Journal of General Virology* 36, 93–109.

Wedemeyer, G. A. (1976). Physiological response of juvenile coho salmon (*Oncorhynchus kisutch*) and rainbow trout (*Salmo gairdneri*) to handling and crowding stress in intensive fish culture. *Journal of the Fisheries Research Board of Canada* 33, 2699–2702.

Wolf, K. and Pettijohn, L. L. (1970). Infectious pancreatic necrosis virus isolated from coho salmon fingerlings. *Progressive fish culturist* 32, 17–18.

Wolf, K. and Quimby, M. C. (1969). Infectious pancreatic necrosis: clinical and immune response of adult trout to inoculation with live virus. *Journal of the Fisheries Research Board of Canada* 26, 2511–2516.

Wolf, K. and Quimby, M. C. (1971). Salmonid viruses: infectious pancreatic necrosis virus. Morphology, pathology and serology of the first European isolations. *Archives für die gesamte Virusforschung* 34, 144–156.

Wolf, K., Snieszko, S. F., Dunbar, C. E. and Pyle, E. (1960). Virus nature of infectious pancreatic necrosis in trout. *Proceedings of the Society for Experimental Biology* 104, 105–108.

Wolf, K., Quimby, M. C. and Bradford, A. D. (1963). Egg-associated transmission of IPN virus of trouts. *Virology* 21, 317–321.

Wolf, K., Quimby, M. C., Carlson, C. P. and Bullock, G. L. (1968). Infectious pancreatic necrosis: selection of virus-free stock from a population of carrier trout. *Journal of the Fisheries Research Board of Canada* 25, 383–391.

Wood, E. M., Snieszko, S. F. and Yasutake, W. T. (1955). Infectious pancreatic necrosis in brook trout. *American Medical Association Archives of Pathology* 60, 26–28.

Yamamoto, T. (1974). Infectious pancreatic necrosis virus occurrence at a hatchery in Alberta. *Journal of the Fisheries Research Board of Canada* 31, 397–402.

Yamamoto, T. (1975a). Frequency of detection and survival of infectious pancreatic necrosis virus in a carrier population of brook trout (*Salvelinus fontinalis*) in a lake. *Journal of the Fisheries Research Board of Canada* 32, 568–570.

Yamamoto, T. (1975b). Infectious pancreatic necrosis (IPN) virus carriers and antibody production in a population of rainbow trout (*Salmo gairdneri*). *Canadian Journal of Microbiology* 21, 1343–1347.

Yamamoto, T. and Kilistoff, J. (1979). Infectious pancreatic necrosis virus: quantification of carriers in lake populations during a six year period. *Journal of the Fisheries Research Board of Canada* 36, 562–567.

6

Virus Diseases of Warm Water Fish

C. AGIUS

*Institute of Aquaculture, University of Stirling,
Stirling, Scotland, U.K.*

Introduction

The advent of fish cell and tissue culture has brought about rapid developments in fish virology in recent years. Not unexpectedly, research interests have focussed mostly on those fish viruses of economic importance with the result that much more is known about salmonid viruses than all other viruses put together. In particular, knowledge of virus diseases in warm water fish is very meagre. Almost certainly this reflects the fact that most of the fish virus research has been carried out in laboratories in Europe and the United States rather than a shortage of viruses of potential pathogenic significance in the warm water environment. In this review it is attempted to summarize the more important literature on diseases of viral aetiology of warm water fish with special emphasis on those viruses that could potentially cause serious losses in tropical and sub-tropical fish farms as stocking densities are increased.

Commercially, warm water aquaculture offers the added attraction of rapid growth rates and in recent years the commercial culture of warm water fish has witnessed an unprecedented expansion especially in the developing world. In all other animal species, intensification of culture has invariably led to the discovery of serious viral pathogens so it is hardly conceivable that warm water fish would be exceptions. Moreover, from the scanty literature that is available, it appears that some warm water fish may well be susceptible to viral diseases commonly isolated from fish cultured in colder waters. Thus, for instance, Uchida and King (1962) suspected that infectious pancreatic necrosis virus was the cause of heavy mortalities of young *Sarotherodon mossambicus* that were being cultured in tanks in Hawaii. Periodic mass mortalities in warm water fish-culture impoundments have been reported by several workers (see, for example, Bardach

115

et al., 1972) but for various reasons proper investigations of these cases have so far been lacking.

Cell Lines

According to a recent review by Wolf and Mann (1980) there are currently in existence and available to investigators some 61 cell lines representing 17 families and 36 donor species or hybrids of teleost fish. Most of the lines are from freshwater or anadromous species and with few exceptions the apparent condition of starting tissue has been normal. Also, with the exception of the lymphosarcoma cells of the muskellunge (*Esox masquinongy*), all fish cell lines were initiated as cultures that required a surface for attachment although recently Lidgerding and Schulz (1979) reported the adaptation of fat-head minnow (FHM) and rainbow trout gonad (RTG-2) cells to stirred suspension culture. Media used routinely for homoeotherm cell culture are universally used, mostly unmodified, for fish cell and tissue culture; these are Eagle's minimal essential medium, Eagle's basal medium, Medium 199 and Liebovitz medium L-15. Foetal bovine serum is added to a concentration of 10% for growth and 2% for maintenance.

Of the existing 61 cell lines, 28 grow optimally at a temperature of 25°C or higher; these represent 10 families and 22 donor species or hybrids of fish. Four of these cell lines are widely used and have been characterized and designated as Certified Cell Lines (CCL). These are the brown bullhead, BB (CCL 59), bluegill fry, BF-2 (CCL 91), goldfish, CAR (CCL 71) and fathead minnow, FHM (CCL 42); they are in the repository of the American Type Culture Collection (ATCC).

Recently, Nakata *et al.* (1980) described the establishment of primary monolayers from the ovaries of the eel *Anguilla japonica*. The primary cells were mainly epithelial-like but on passaging, fibroblast-like cells became dominant. The cells grew optimally at 34°C. Also, Watanabe *et al.* (1981) have reported the initiation of cell lines from kidney tissues of yellowtail (*Seriola quinqueradiata*) and sea bass (*Lateolabrax japonicus*) and from the fry of red sea bream (*Chrysophrys major*). The yellowtail kidney cell line grows best at 25°C and is now in its 64th passage. The sea bass cell line has been subcultured 31 times while the red sea bream cell line has been subcultured 28 times; both these cell lines seem to grow optimally at temperatures between 20 and 25°C.

No cell lines of *Tilapia* origin have so far been reported and in view of the recent expansion of the culture of these fish in many parts of the world especially in Africa, South-East Asia as well as Central and South America, it has become imperative to increase the efforts in this direction. In our laboratory we have attempted several times to initiate cultures from tissue explants and trypsinized cells from most tissues of *Sarotherodon mossambicus, S. aureus, S. niloticus* and the *S. niloticus/S. aureus* hybrids. On some occasions good primary cultures were obtained, especially from the gonads, but these could only be passaged once satisfactorily.

Viruses

Providing that each is a distinct entity (i.e. that it occurs only in one species), the literature on fish virology presently shows that there are at least 32 viruses; of these 17 have been isolated in cell culture, the rest have been seen by electron microscopy (Wolf and Mann, 1980). The best known of the viruses affecting fish in warm water are the channel catfish virus (CCV), spring viraemia of carp virus (SVCV) and lymphocystis virus (LV). Infectious pancreatic necrosis virus (IPNV) is also included in this review for two reasons; it has recently been isolated from a wide variety of non-salmonid fishes and also a number of publications describing successful experimental infections of warm water fish with this virus have appeared in the last decade or so.

Flatfish and eels are now being commercially reared in warmed sea water from the coolant discharge of nuclear power stations. A number of virus diseases in those fish reared at elevated temperatures have been documented in the literature in recent years and these are briefly reviewed in this paper.

Two viruses, the Golden Shiner Virus (GSV) and the Bluegill Virus have been recently described from the United States and the literature on these is also reviewed.

Channel Catfish Virus Disease

CCVD is a highly contagious herpesvirus infection of cultivated channel catfish (*Ictalurus punctatus*) that occurs during the warm part of the year. The disease is almost exclusively restricted to fish under 4 months old and in severe epizootics losses of up to 100% may occur. Survivors of disease outbreaks should be regarded as carriers of the virus.

The virus has only been reported in the southern U.S.A. and Honduras, Central America (Wolf, 1976) in cultivated channel catfish but the fact that it grows in a continuous cell line of brown bullhead (BB) (Fijan *et al.*, 1970) and in two cell lines from the walking catfish (*Clarias batrachus*) (Noga and Hartmann, 1977) suggests that other *Ictalurus* and *Clarias* species may also be potential carriers. Indeed Galla and Hartmann (1974) reported almost total mortality of *Clarias batrachus* when these were injected intraperitoneally or intramuscularly with CCV produced in BB cell cultures.

Recently, Bowser and Plumb (1980a) observed that a permanent cell line derived from channel catfish ovary (CCO) tissue (Bowser, 1978; Bowser and Plumb, 1980b) produced cytopathic effects (CPE) more rapidly and detected CCV at higher dilutions than did the BB cell line. Production of CCV was more rapid in CCO cells than in BB cells, but the peak titres of the two lines were not significantly different.

Plumb *et al.* (1973) studied the survival of the virus under various conditions. They noted that in dead catfish held at 22°C the virus survived for less than 3 days; in infected catfish held at -20°C and -80°C the virus survived at higher titre for a longer time period.

After experimental infection of channel catfish through injection, Plumb (1971) found that the first organs to show virus were the kidneys followed by the intestine, liver, brain and skeletal muscle in that order. In order of descending quantities of virus, Plumb (1971) ranked the tissues as follows: kidneys, intestine, liver, brain and skeletal muscle.

The main clinical signs of the disease in natural outbreaks are loss of equilibrium, spiral movements and hanging vertically in the water (Liversidge and Munro, 1978). Gross pathology includes haemorrhages of gills, skin and internal organs as well as abdominal distension. Histo-pathologically, lesions appear to begin in the posterior kidney but subsequently focal necrotic lesions develop in the liver, the spleen, the digestive tract and pancreatic acinar tissue. There is also observed submucosal oedema and mucosal necrosis of the digestive tract as well as petechial haemorrhages in muscle and dermis (Wolf *et al.*, 1972; Plumb and Gaines, 1975). Major *et al.* (1975) examined naturally infected as well as experimentally infected catfish and observed that the fish from the natural outbreak had the more severe damage. In addition to the previously reported pathological changes, these workers also found that the virus caused degenerative changes in nervous tissue and erythrocytes. Brain neurons were vacuolated and shrunken and surrounding nerve fibres were oedematous. They inferred that the observed brain pathology and related spinal cord involvement coincided with Plumb's (1971) quantification of CCV in brain tissue.

Both naturally and experimentally infected adult catfish were found to produce neutralizing antibody. Plumb (1973) immunized fish with live virus ($\sim 1.5 \times 10^5$ TCID$_{50}$ each) and found that virus neutralizing activity developed reaching a peak at 60 days post-inoculation and then dropping to a low level at 120 days.

Spring Viraemia of Carp (SVC) and Swim Bladder Inflammation (SBI)

A disease complex of carp known as infectious carp dropsy is widespread in Europe even in the relatively warm northern Mediterranean countries but it appears in the warmer Middle East countries only on a small scale and is unknown in the African countries (Sarig, 1971). In 1971, Fijan *et al.* isolated a virus *Rhabdovirus carpio* from 11 epizootics of the acute form of the disease. The virus was observed to multiply and cause a CPE in carp ovary cells, FHM, BF-2, BB and RTG-2 cell lines. Moreover, in FHM cells it was found to grow up to 31°C. Swim-bladder inflammation of cyprinids is also considered by some workers to be part of the same dropsical syndrome.

SBI is a contagious disease that occurs in most European countries where carp are farmed but there is little information as to the range of species which are susceptible. The disease usually develops in young cyprinids with affected fish starting to lose weight, becoming dark and losing balance. Survivors develop abdominal distension, exophthalmos and reduced reflexes. Internally the most remarkable feature is the degeneration of the walls of the swim bladder (Braun, 1974).

Bachman and Ahne (1973, 1974) have isolated a virus from SBI—infected fish that proved to be morphologically and serologically identical to SVC virus. Hill *et al.* (1975) subsequently confirmed that SVC and SBI are serologically indistinguishable. In the same year, however, Ahne (1975) isolated a rhabdovirus from grass carp that was not neutralized by anti-SBI antiserum indicating a new cyprinid rhabdovirus serotype. Since SVC and SBI have generally been considered to be distinct diseases because of the differences in their pathogenesis, seasonal variation and geographical distribution, further studies are required to clarify the situation.

The main clinical signs of SVC are gathering of fish at water outflows, darkening, petechial haemorrhages, loss of balance, exophthalmos and abdominal dropsy. Internally it is common to find a fibrinous peritonitis, petechial haemorrhages over viscera and catarrhal or necrotic enteritis (Liversidge and Munro, 1978).

Ahne (1978) experimentally infected carp *Cyprinus carpio* with SVC virus by direct immersion at 13°C and observed that after entry through the gills where it starts to multiply, the virus spreads via the blood stream to produce viraemia. Target organs are the kidney, liver, spleen, heart and alimentary tract. Clinical signs of the disease with pathological lesions became evident after an incubation period of 7 days. The first deaths occurred at 20 days post-infection; however, no neutralizing antibodies were observed in any of the fish even 1 month post-infection. The virus was observed to be shed with mucus casts and faeces.

Lymphocystis

Lymphocystis is an infectious viral disease of many wild and cultured marine and freshwater fish species. The virus causes hypertrophy of connective tissue cells resulting in macroscopic nodules which are often located on the fins and skin. The small pearl-like tumefactions can occur either singly or in groups. Internal pathology with lymphocystis virus is not common. Although infected fish appear unsightly, the disease is rarely fatal (Templeman, 1965). The cause of the disease appears to be a large virus or group of morphologically similar viruses of probable icosahedral symmetry and containing deoxyribonucleic acid (Kelly and Robertson, 1973). The virus/viruses replicate in the cytoplasm of infected cells and are tentatively classified in the family Iridoviridae or as members of the "icosahedral cytoplasmic deoxyribovirus group" (Fenner, 1976; Wolf, 1976). The virus can be grown in BF-2 and GF cell lines at 23°C. Walker and Hill (1980) observed that lymphocystis virus from bluegill sunfish (*Lepomis macrochirus*) when grown in a cell line that had been established from the fins and caudal tissue of the same fish species gave maximum yield in 21 days at 25°C. Earlier Wolf and Carlson (1965) had observed that in bluegill the time course of infection was very rapid with the lymphocysts doubling in size every 3 days for 28 days prior to degenerating; virus production was observed to be maximal at 30 days. Vaughan (1979) also managed to initiate clinical lesions after experimentally infecting bluegills with the virus.

Early studies had described LV particles as ranging in size from 200 to 250nm in diameter. Koch *et al.* (1976), however, have published electron micrographs of lymphocystis skin lesions from the walleye pike (*Stizo-stedion vitreum*) showing smaller viral particles (65–100nm) intermingled among the large particles and also contained within the latter. Both forms were observed to be associated with a single inclusion body.

Almost simultaneously, Yamamoto *et al.* (1976) reported that light and electron microscopic examination of tumours on walleye from a spawning run revealed the presence of two distinct tumour types. One was characteristic of lymphocystis, consisting of typical enlarged non-neoplastic cells surrounded by hyaline layers and containing many 260nm diameter LV particles in the cytoplasm. The other tumour, referred to as a dermal sarcoma consisted of a solid mass of normal sized cells and contained in the cytoplasm large numbers of 135nm diameter virus particles referred to as walleye dermal sarcoma virus; the latter was similar in appearance to the leukoviruses. These workers could not verify the presence of the two viruses in the one cell and therefore concluded that it is unlikely that they represent different stages of the same agent.

Apart from the species already mentioned, lymphocystis has been described in several others; examples include the cichlid fish *Cichlasoma synspilum* from Guatemala (Weissenberg, 1965), the striped bass *Roccus saxatilis* from Chesapeake Bay (Krantz, 1970), several *Tilapia* species from East Africa (Paperna, 1973), *Anabas testudineus* from India (Thakur and Nasar, 1977), exotic aquarium fishes such as the black-tailed humbug *Dascyllus melanurus* (Lawler *et al.*, 1977), the black crappie *Pomoxis nigromaculatus* (Amin, 1979) and many other warm water species; it has not yet been reported in salmonids.

Infectious Pancreatic Necrosis

IPNV, an as yet unclassified virus (see for example Wolf, 1976; Underwood *et al.*, 1977; Dobos *et al.*, 1979; Wolf and Mann, 1980) is primarily a salmonid virus causing a very serious disease especially at the fry and fingerling stage (Wolf *et al.*, 1960; Wolf, 1966). However, the isolation of the virus from several non-salmonid species including carp, eels and Atlantic menhaden in recent years (see for example Sano, 1976; Wolf, 1976; Stephens *et al.*, 1980; Hudson *et al.*, 1981) coupled with the ability of the virus to multiply in a large number of cell lines, for example, in a swordtail cell line (Kelly and Loh, 1975), in a fathead minnow cell line (Nicholson *et al.*, 1979), in a Walleye cell line (Kelly *et al.*, 1980) and in eel ovary cells (Nakata *et al.*, 1980), within a very wide temperature range of 4 to 26°C (Wolf, 1966) raise the possibility that this virus could potentially cause serious losses even in warm water fish.

This is especially significant in view of the recent expansion of salmonid culture in the high altitude regions of tropical and sub-tropical countries. This has led to an increased traffic of salmonid eggs from IPN-infected countries to tropical countries for rearing in the upper reaches of rivers which eventually drain into warmer regions where warm water species are farmed. An added hazard in this context is the possibility of transfer of infection via birds. Sonstegard and McDermott (1972) have provided evidence that a wide variety of warm-blooded animals could be mechanical vectors of IPN virus. Since many birds migrate long distances they could also cause IPNV epizootics far from other foci of infection. Birds such as cormorants, kingfishers, fish eagles, herons and pelicans are all important predators of tilapia in their natural and farm environments (Chimits, 1955; Maar *et al.*, 1966), some of these being also predators of salmonid fish.

A number of papers reporting on experimental infections of various warm water fish with IPNV have appeared in the last decade or so. Yu *et al.* (1969) have shown that following injection with IPNV the blue gourami (*Trichogaster trichopterus*) (Pallas) produced antibodies against IPN which were concentrated in the gamma fraction of its serum proteins. Through subsequent splenectomy experiments, these same workers (Yu *et al.*, 1970) showed that in this species the spleen is the major antibody producing organ.

Perlmutter *et al.* (1973) examined the immune response of the blue gourami (*Trichogaster trichopterus*) to IPNV. Under crowded conditions, the fish produced what were described as "water-borne immuno-suppressive factors soluble in methyl chloroform". In a somewhat confused paper they showed that fish in water treated with methylchloroform had slightly higher titres of virus-neutralizing activity than did control fish in untreated water.

Sarot and Perlmutter (1976) showed that intraperitoneal injection of IPNV also resulted in anti-IPN antibody production in the zebra fish *Brachydanio rerio*. Seeley *et al.* (1977) extended this work by injecting zebra fish with IPNV and then spawning them to determine whether the virus is passed on to the eggs. The results showed that transmission of the virus to the eggs did occur and that this transmission was via the female alone. However, if the female was allowed to produce antibodies to the virus, transmission of the virus to the eggs only took place for a short period of time. In addition, when the virus was transmitted to the egg, it remained in the progeny for a period of at least 5 months.

In our laboratories we have carried out a number of experimental infections of *Sarotherodon niloticus* and of *S. niloticus/S. aureus* hybrids with IPNV, Sp strain which had been isolated from farmed rainbow trout. Fry of both *S. niloticus* and the hybrids showed no clinical signs and experienced no mortalities when they were infected by direct immersion and hyperosmotic infiltration. Juvenile *S. niloticus/S. aureus* hybrids orally infected by forced feeding showed no clinical signs of the disease and no mortalities occurred. No virus could be recovered from the kidney of any of the specimens for up to 5 weeks post-infection when experiments were terminated. Moreover, at 5 weeks post-infection, no virus-neutralizing antibodies were detected in the sera.

When juveniles and adults of both *S. niloticus* and the hybrids were infected by intraperitoneal injection of the virus, occasional low level mortalities occurred without any clinical manifestations. From intra-peritoneally injected fish, virus was consistently recovered from the kidney of juvenile fish (only the kidney was examined here) and from the kidney, liver and spleen, but not the gonads, of adult fish for up to 5 weeks post-infection when the experiments were terminated. Five weeks after injection, high levels of virus-neutralizing antibodies could be detected in the sera of all injected fish. Whilst it has to be recognized that intraperitoneal injection may be an unusual mode of establishing infection in natural outbreaks, these observations suggest that IPNV infection can still present a potential hazard to the development of cultures of warm water fish.

Herpesvirus Scophthalmi

Turbot (*Scophthalmus maximus* L.) are nowadays being farmed in warmed sea water from the coolant discharge of nuclear power stations. Some 3 years ago heavy mortalities in one such farm in Scotland led to the discovery of a herpes-type virus (Buchanan *et al.*, 1978) which has provisionally been named *Herpesvirus scophthalmi*. The virus has only been observed under the electron microscope and the evidence for its classification as a herpes-virus include the formation of giant cells, syncytia and giant nuclei, the development of intranuclear inclusions, the assembly of capsids in the nucleus, the envelopment of capsids at the inner nuclear membrane and the architecture of the virus as shown by negative staining (Buchanan and Madeley, 1978). To date, no cell line has been found that will support the growth of this marine virus *in vitro* and until this is achieved, full characterization of this virus will not be possible.

Richards and Buchanan (1978) published a detailed account of the clinical and histopathological manifestations of the disease. Clinical manifestations of the disease involved lethargy, inappetence and the fish often lay in a characteristic position with the head and tail raised when lying on the bottom.

Lesions similar to those observed on the infected farmed fish were observed, even if less frequently, in wild fish providing evidence that this virus may be endemic in wild fish.

Histological examination revealed numerous giant cells in the epithelium of both skin and gills of moribund fish. The nuclei of these cells carried virus-like particles of a roughly hexagonal shape and 100nm in diameter. The cytoplasm also carried virus-like particles but here they were enveloped, covered with spikes and had a diameter of about 200nm. Giant cells in both skin and gill lesions appeared to be in varying stages of maturity even within the same fish.

Virus Diseases of Eels

Like flatfish, eels are also being cultured in heated effluents from power stations. In 1969 a new type of epizootic broke out in eel (*Anguilla japonica*) ponds in Japan and subsequently a new virus designated Eel Virus European (EVE) was isolated. This virus was found to be similar to IPNV in the CPE that it produced on RTG-2 cells. Serologically, EVE was found to be similar to the French strain of IPNV known as d'Honnincthun. However, in infectivity trials, EVE killed Japanese eels (*Anguilla japonica*) but not rainbow trout fry *Salmo gairdneri*. Also IPNV killed rainbow trout fry but not eels. On the basis of these findings, Sano *et al.* (1981) consider

EVE to be either a different agent or possibly a new strain of IPNV. According to Hudson *et al.* (1981), EVE appears to be an Ab serotype of IPN. It is relevant to mention again here that IPNV has been isolated in Japan from cultured European eel *A. anguilla* and Japanese eel *A. japonica* (Sano, 1976), in France (Sp strain) from wild European eels (Castric and Chastel, 1980) and in Britain (Ab strain) from farmed European eel (Hudson *et al.*, 1981). This latter virus did not prove to be pathogenic to European eels following experimental infection.

Recently, two rhabdoviruses have been isolated from eels in Japan by Sano and co-workers (Sano, 1976, 1977; Sano *et al.*, 1977); the first, from young American eels *A. rostrata* was called EVA, the second, from European elvers *A. anguilla* was designated EVEX. The two viruses produce identical CPE in RTG-2 cells (Nishimura *et al.*, 1981) and according to Hill *et al.* (1980) they are related to each other antigenically but show no relationship to the other fish rhabdoviruses in neutralization tests. Hill *et al.* (1980) also reported that EVA and EVEX can infect and cause mortality in rainbow trout fry. Moreover, the diseases produced by these viruses in rainbow trout fry were clinically indistinguishable from VHS. On the other hand, the infectivity trials of Nishimura *et al.* (1981) led them to conclude that the clinical signs and histopathological changes of fish infected with EVA and EVEX were similar to those of IHN.

It is clear that much more work is needed to characterize more fully these three eel viruses.

Golden Shiner Virus (GSV)

A new virus has recently been isolated from the North American cyprinid, the golden shiner *Notemigonus crysoleucas* (Plumb *et al.*, 1979; Schwedler, 1980) from a condition called golden shiner virus (GSV) disease. This virus measures approximately 70nm and is icosahedral and non-enveloped. It has a double-stranded RNA genome and although preliminary investigations indicate that GSV is very similar to the Reoviridae it is as yet uncertain whether the genome consists of 10 separate paired segments as in the Reoviridae or two paired segments as in infectious pancreatic necrosis virus (IPNV). GSV shares many morphological, biochemical and biophysical characteristics with IPNV but the two viruses are serologically unrelated. Moreover, unlike IPNV, GSV is capable of replicating at 30°C (Plumb *et al.*, 1979; Schwedler, 1980; Schwedler and Plumb, 1980). GSV causes a CPE in FHM cells but not BB, RTG-2 or channel catfish ovary cells. CPE in FHM cells is characterized by the formation of focal syncytia with multiple nuclei and cellular vacuolation. Rapid progression of the CPE results in the contraction of the cell sheet and the separation of large rounded particles of cellular debris from the culture surface. Often some degree of cell sheet regeneration follows the development of CPE. Experimentally the virus was successfully transmitted from culture to host and reisolated, but the clinical signs of the disease did not develop suggesting that GSV may have a low pathogenicity. Significantly, there appear to have been no massive mortalities in golden shiner culture ponds as a result of GSV, even on farms from which these initial isolations were made.

Bluegill Virus

A virus isolated from bluegills (*Lepomis macrochirus*) and having single-stranded RNA was originally thought to be either an arenovirus or a paramyxovirus. Recently, however, Beckwith and Malsberger (1979) reported that the virus does not share antigens with prototypes of orthomyxoviruses, paramyxoviruses or arenoviruses. Very little is known about this virus and in fact it has not yet been related to any disease. Indeed, repeated attempts to make another isolation of the virus from bluegills so far seem to have been unsuccessful. Whilst its fish origin needs to be ascertained, the bluegill virus has not been grown in cells of mammals, reptiles or amphibians but only grows in fish cells and seemingly requires fish cells with a fibroblast-like morphology; it achieves highest titres in centrarchid cells. In ultra-thin sections, the virions (80 to 100nm in diameter) are observed to be associated with the cell surface and intra-cellular vacuoles. Beckwith (1974) reported on features of its intracellular replication; at 21°C its replication shows release of new virus at about 10 hours; thereafter it exhibits exponential growth until its maximum titre —about 10^6 tissue culture infectious doses 50% endpoint ($TCID_{50}$) ml^{-1}— is reached.

Concluding Remarks

The foregoing is by no means an exhaustive list of the viruses known to infect warm water fish; a large number of others have been described (see, for example, Edwards *et al.*, 1977; Leibovitz and Riis, 1980), even if some of them only by electron microscopy, but their potential hazards to warm water intensive culture still has to be assessed.

What is amply clear is that great care needs to be exercised when moving fish from one site to another. It cannot be assumed that because two species may have widely differing optimal temperatures for culture, the difference in temperature provides a natural unsurmountable barrier to the transmission of virus from one species to another. This can perhaps be best illustrated by the recent findings of de Kinkelin and his co-workers (1980) that even viral haemorrhagic septicaemia virus, a virus that replicates in fish cell lines at an optimum temperature of 14°C has had a variant selected that replicates at 25°C. This was achieved by serially passaging the virus in the epithelioma papulosum cyprini (EPC) cell line at gradually increasing temperature. After each step of the adaptation process, the new variants were as efficient for inducing *in vitro* cell lysis as they were at 14°C. While the pathogenicity of the virus was attenuated in the process, some of the fish still died after being infected by direct immersion.

References

Ahne, W. (1975). A rhabdovirus isolated from grass carp (*Ctenopharyngodon idella* Val.). *Archives of Virology* **48**, 181–185.

Ahne, W. (1978). Uptake and multiplication of spring viraemia of carp virus in carp, *Cyprinus carpio* L. *Journal of Fish Diseases* **1**, 265–268.

Amin, O. M. (1979). Lymphocystis disease in Wisconsin fishes. *Journal of Fish Diseases* **2**, 207–217.

Bachmann, P. A. and Ahne, W. (1973). Isolation and characterization of agent causing swimbladder inflammation in carp. *Nature, London* **244**, 235–237.

Bachman, P. A. and Ahne, W. (1974). Biological properties and identification of the agent causing swimbladder inflammation in carp. *Archives gessamt Virusforschung* **44**, 261–269.

Bardach, J. E., Ryther, J. H. and McLarney, W. O. (1972). "Aquaculture. The Farming and Husbandry of Freshwater and Marine Organisms." Wiley Interscience, New York, N.Y. 868pp.

Beckwith, D. G. (1974). "Characterization and intracellular replication of the bluegill virus." Ph.D. Thesis, Lehigh University, Bethlehem, Pa. 159pp.

Beckwith, D. G. and Malsberger, R. G. (1979). Characterization and morphology of the bluegill virus. *Journal of General Virology* **43**(3), 489–501.

Bowser, P. R. (1978). "Development and evaluation of a new cell line from the channel catfish *Ictalurus punctatus*." Ph.D. Thesis, Auburn University, Auburn, Ala. 48pp.

Bowser, P. R. and Plumb, J. A. (1980a). Channel catfish virus: Comparative replication and sensitivity of cell lines from channel catfish ovary and the brown bullhead. *Journal of Wildlife Diseases* **16**(3), 451–454.

Bowser, P. R. and Plumb, J. A. (1980b). New cell line—fish cell lines: establishment of a line from ovaries of channel catfish. *In vitro* **16**(5), 365–368.

Braun, F. (1974). The swimbladder inflammation of carp. *Muenchener Beitraege zur Abwasser Fischerei-und Flussbiologie* **25**, 69–74.

Buchanan, J. S. and Madeley, C. R. (1978). Studies on *Herpesvirus scophthalmi* infection of turbot *Scophthalmus maximus* (L.): ultrastructural observations. *Journal of Fish Diseases* **1**, 283–295.

Buchanan, J. S., Richards, R. H., Sommerville, C. and Madeley, C. R. (1978). A herpes-type virus from turbot (*Scophthalmus maximus* L.). *Veterinary Record* **102**, 527–528.

Castric, J. and Chastel, C. (1980). Isolement et essai de caracterisation de trois virus d'anguille (*Anguilla anguilla*): resultats preliminaires. *In* "Virus des Organismes Aquatiques et Marins" pp.15-16. Proceedings Societé Française de microbiologie section de virologie, Jeudi 22 Mai 1980, Institut Pasteur, Paris.

Chimits, P. (1955). Tilapia and its culture: a preliminary bibliography. *FAO Fisheries Bulletin* 10(1), 18-21.

Dobos, P., Hill, B. J., Hallett, R., Kells, D. T . C., Becht, H. and Teninges, D. (1979). Biophysical and biochemical characterisation of five animal viruses with bisegmented double-stranded RNA genomes. *Journal of Virology* 32(2), 593-605.

Edwards, M. R., Samsonoff, W. A. and Kuzia, E. J. (1977). Papilloma-like viruses from catfish. *Fish Health News* 6(2), 94-95.

Fenner, F. (1976). The classification and nomenclature of viruses. Summary of the results of meetings of the International Committee on Taxonomy of viruses in Madrid, September 1976. *Journal of General Virology* 31, 463-470.

Fijan, N., Wellborn, T. L. Jr. and Naftel, J. P. (1970). An acute viral disease of channel catfish. Bureau of Sport Fisheries and Wildlife Technical Paper 43, 11pp.

Fijan, N., Petrinec, Z., Sulimanovic, D., and Zwillenberg, L. O. (1971). Isolation of the viral causative agent from the acute form of infectious dropsy of carp. *Veterinarski Arhiv* 41(5/6), 125-138.

Galla, J. D. and Hartmann, J. X. (1974). Extension of the host range of channel catfish virus CCV to the walking catfish *Clarias batrachus* (Linnaeus). *Florida Scientist* n.v. 31.

Hill, B. J., Underwood, B. O., Smale, C. J. and Brown, C. F. (1975). Physicochemical and serological characterization of five rhabdoviruses infecting fish. *Journal of General Virology* 27, 369-378.

Hill, B. J., Williams, R. F., Smale, C. J., Underwood, B. O. and Brown, F. (1980). Physico-chemical and serological characterization of two rhabdoviruses isolated from eels. *Intervirology* 14, 208-212.

Hudson, E. B., Bucke, D. and Forrest, A. (1981). Isolation of infectious pancreatic necrosis virus from eels, *Anguilla anguilla* L., in the United Kingdom. *Journal of Fish Diseases* 4, 429-431.

Kelly, D. C. and Robertson, J. S. (1973). Icosahedral cytoplasmic deoxyriboviruses. *Journal of General Virology* 20, 17-41.

Kelly, R. K. and Loh, P. C. (1975). Replication of IPN virus: cytochemical and biochemical study in SWT cells. *Proceedings of the Society for Experimental Biology and Medicine* 148, 688-693.

Kelly, R. K., Miller, H. R., Nielsen, O. and Clayton, J. W. (1980). Fish cell culture: Characteristics of a continuous fibroblastic cell line from Walleye (*Stizostedion vitreum vitreum*). *Canadian Journal of Fisheries and Aquatic Sciences* 37, 1070-1075.

de Kinkelin, P., Le Berre, M. B. and Bernard, J. (1980). Viral haemorrhagic septicaemia of rainbow trout: selection of a thermoresistant virus variant and comparison of polypeptide synthesis with the wild-type virus strain. *Journal of Virology* 36(3), 652-658.

Koch, E. A., Dolowy, W. C., Spitzer, R. H., Greenberg, S. and Brown, E. R. (1976). Postulated developmental forms in the life cycle of the lymphocystis virus. *Cancer Biochemistry Biophysics* 1, 163-166.

Krantz, G. E. (1970). Lymphocystis in striped bass *Roccus saxatilis* in Chesapeake Bay. *Chesapeake Science* 11(2), 137-139.

Lawler, A. R., Ogle, J. T. and Donnes, C. (1977). *Dascyllus* spp.: new hosts for lymphocystis, and a list of recent hosts. *Journal of Wildlife Diseases* **13**, 307–312.

Leibovitz, L. and Riis, R. C. (1980). A viral disease of aquarium fish. *Journal of the American Veterinary Medicine Association* **177**, 414–416.

Lidgerding, B. C. and Schultz, C. L. (1979). Fish cell lines: establishment of the first suspension culture (abstr.). *In vitro* **15**, 216.

Liversidge, J. and Munro, A. L. S. (1978). The virology of teleosts. *In* "Fish Pathology" (Ed. R. J. Roberts), x + 318pp. Baillière Tindall, London.

Maar, A., Mortimer, M. A. E. and van der Lingen, I. (1966). Fish culture in Central East Africa. FAO Publication 53608 — 66/E 158pp.

Major, R. D., McCraren, J. P. and Smith, C. E. (1975). Histopathological changes in channel catfish (*Ictalurus punctatus*) experimentally and naturally infected with channel catfish virus disease. *Journal of the Fisheries Research Board of Canada* **32**, 563–567.

Nakata, M., Horiuchi, M. and Kohga, K. (1980). Monolayer culture of ovary cells from eel, *Anguilla japonica*: some characteristics and subcultivation techniques of the cells. *Bulletin of the Japanese Society of Scientific Fisheries* **46**(5), 599–606.

Nicholson, B. L., Thorne, G. W., Janicki, C. and Hanson, A. (1979). Studies on a host range variant from different isolates of infectious pancreatic necrosis virus (IPNV). *Journal of Fish Diseases* **2**, 367–379.

Nishimura, T., Toba, M., Ban, F., Okamoto, N. and Sano, T. (1981). Eel rhabdo-virus, EVA, EVEX and their infectivity to fishes. *Fish Pathology* **15**(3/4), 173–184.

Noga, E. J. and Hartmann, J. X. (1977). Establishment of cell lines from the walking catfish (*Clarias batrachus*) and their infection with channel catfish virus. *In vitro* **13**, 160 (Abstr.)

Paperna, I. (1973). Lymphocystis in fish from East African lakes. *Journal of Wildlife Diseases* **9**, 331–335.

Perlmutter, A., Sarot, D. A., Yu, M., Filazzola, R. and Seeley, R. J. (1973). The effect of crowding on the immune response of the blue gourami (*Trichogaster trichopterus*), to infectious pancreatic necrosis (IPN) virus. *Life Sciences* **13**, 363–375.

Plumb, J. A. (1971). Tissue distribution of channel catfish virus. *Journal of Wildlife Diseases* **7**, 213–216.

Plumb, J. A. (1973). Neutralisation of channel catfish virus by serum of channel catfish. *Journal of Wildlife Diseases* **9**, 324–330.

Plumb, J. A. and Gaines, J. L. Jr. (1975). Channel catfish virus disease. *In* "The Pathology of Fishes" (Eds. W. E. Ribelin and G. Migaki), pp.287–302. University of Wisconsin Press, Madison, Wisconsin.

Plumb, J. A., Wright, L. D. and Jones, V. L. (1973). Survival of channel catfish virus in chilled, frozen, and decomposing channel catfish. *Progressive Fish Culturist* **35**, 170–172.

Plumb, J. A., Bowser, P. R., Grizzle, J. M. and Mitchell, A. J. (1979). Fish virus: a double-stranded RNA icosahedral virus from a North American cyprinid. *Journal of the Fisheries Research Board of Canada* **36**, 1390–1394.

Richards, R. H. and Buchanan, J. S. (1978). Studies on *Herpesvirus scophthalmi* infection of turbot *Scophthalmus maximus* L.: Histopathological observations. *Journal of Fish Diseases* **1**, 251–258.

Sano, T. (1976). Viral diseases of cultured fishes in Japan. *Fish Pathology* **10**, 221–226.

Sano, T. (1977). Viral diseases of cultured salmonids in Japan. *Proceedings of an International Symposium on Diseases of Cultured Salmonids (Tavolek Inc., Seattle)*, pp.120–123.

Sano, T., Nishimura, T., Okamoto, N. and Fukuda, H. (1977). Studies on viral diseases of Japanese fishes. VII. A rhabdovirus isolated from European eel (*Anguilla anguilla*). *Fish Pathology* 43, 491–495.

Sano, T., Okamoto, N. and Nishimura, T. (1981). A new viral epizootic of *Anguilla japonica* Temminck and Schlegel. *Journal of Fish Diseases* 4(2), 127–139.

Sarig, S. (1971). Diseases of Fishes. The prevention and treatment of diseases of warmwater fishes under subtropical conditions, with special emphasis on intensive fish farming. *In* "Diseases of Fish, Book 3" (Eds. S. F. Snieszko and H. R. Axelrod), 127pp. TFH Publications, Reigate, Surrey.

Sarot, D. A. and Perlmutter, A. (1976). The toxicity of zinc to the immune response of the Zebra fish, *Brachydanio rerio* injected with viral and bacterial antigens. *Transactions of the American Fisheries Society* 3, 456–459.

Schwedler, T. E. (1980). "Characteristics of a new virus of golden shiners *Notemigonus crysoleucas*." Ph.D. Thesis, Auburn University. 70pp.

Schwedler, T. E. and Plumb, J. A. (1980). Fish viruses: Serologic comparison of the Golden Shiner and Infectious Pancreatic Necrosis Viruses. *Journal of Wildlife Diseases* 16(4), 597–599.

Seeley, R. J., Perlmutter, A. and Seeley, V. A. (1977). Inheritance and longevity of infectious pancreatic necrosis virus in the zebra fish *Brachydanio rerio* (Hamilton-Buchanan). *Applied Environmental Microbiology* 34(1), 50–55.

Sonstegard, R. A. and McDermott, L. A. (1972). Epidemiological model for passive transfer of IPNV by homeotherms. *Nature, London* 237, 104–105.

Stephens, E. B., Newman, M. W., Zachary, A. L. and Hetrick, F. M. (1980). A viral aetiology for the annual spring epizootics of Atlantic menhaden *Brevoortia tyrannus* (Latrobe) in Chesapeake Bay. *Journal of Fish Diseases* 3, 387–398.

Templeman, W. (1965). Lymphocystis disease in American plaice of the Eastern Grand Bank. *Journal of the Fisheries Research Board of Canada* 22, 1345–1355.

Thakur, N. K. and Nasar, S. A. K. (1977). On the occurrence of lymphocystis in *Anabas testudineus* (Bloch). *Current Science* 46(5), 150–151.

Uchida, R. N. and King, J. E. (1962). Tank culture of tilapia. *United States Fisheries and Wildlife Service, Fisheries Bulletin* 62, 21–52.

Underwood, B. O., Smale, C. J., Brown, F. and Hill, B. J. (1977). Relationship of a virus from *Tellina tenuis* to infectious pancreatic necrosis virus. *Journal of General Virology* 36, 93–102.

Vaughan, G. E. (1979). Comparative vulnerability of bluegills with and without lymphocystis disease to predation by largemouth bass. *Progressive Fish Culturist* 41(3), 163–164.

Walker, D. P. and Hill, B. J. (1980). Studies on the culture, assay of infectivity and some *in vitro* properties of lymphocystis disease. *Journal of General Virology* 51, 385–395.

Watanabe, Y., Hanada, H. and Ushiyama, M. (1981). Monolayer cell cultures from marine fishes. *Fish Pathology* 15(3/4), 201–205.

Weissenberg, R. (1965). Morphological studies on lymphocystis tumour cells of a cichlid from Guatemala, *Cichlasoma synspilum* Hubbs. *Annals of the New York Academy of Science* 126, 396–413.

Wolf, K. (1966). Infectious pancreatic necrosis (IPN) of salmonid fishes. United

States Fisheries and Wildlife Service Bureau, Sport Fisheries and Wildlife, Fisheries Leaflet No. 1.

Wolf, K. (1976). Fish viral diseases in North America, 1971–1975, and recent research of the Eastern Fish Disease Laboratory, U.S.A. *Fish Pathology* **10**(2), 135–154.

Wolf, K. and Carlson, C. P. (1965). Multiplication of lymphocystis virus in the bluegill (*Lepomis macrochirus*). *Proceedings of the National Academy of Science, U.S.A.* **216**, 414–419.

Wolf, K. and Mann, J. A. (1980). Poikilothermic vertebrate cell lines and viruses: A current listing for fishes. *In vitro* **16**, 168–179.

Wolf, K., Snieszko, S. F., Dunbar, C. E. and Pyle, E. (1960). Virus of infectious pancreatic necrosis in trout. *Proceedings of the Society for Experimental Biology and Medicine* **104**, 105–108.

Wolf, K., Herman, R. L. and Carlson, C. P. (1972). Fish viruses: Histopathologic changes associated with experimental channel catfish virus disease. *Journal of the Fisheries Research Board of Canada* **29**, 149–150.

Yamamoto, T., MacDonald, R. D., Gillespie, D. C. and Kelly, R. K. (1976). Viruses associated with lymphocystis disease and dermal sarcoma of walleye (*Stizostedion vitreum vitreum*). *Journal of the Fisheries Research Board of Canada* **33**, 2408–2419.

Yu, M., Sarot, D. A., Filazzola, R. J. and Perlmutter, A. (1969). Immune response of the blue gourami *Trichogaster trichopterus* to infectious pancreatic necrosis (IPN) virus. *Life Sciences* **8**(2), 1207–1213.

Yu, M., Sarot, D. A., Filazzola, R. J. and Perlmutter, A. (1970). Effects of splenectomy on the immune response of the blue gourami (*Trichogaster trichopterus*) to infectious pancreatic necrosis (IPN) virus. *Life Sciences* **9**, 749–755.

7

The Pathogenesis of
Bacterial Diseases of Fishes

A. L. S. MUNRO

DAFS Marine Laboratory
Victoria Road, Aberdeen, Scotland, U.K.

The pathogenesis or progressive development of bacterial diseases in fishes from initiating events to some subsequent stage in the host pathogen relationship is the subject of this review. The division of the subject by the following headings is more derived by analogy with disease in mammals than actual information on events in fish. Although such division is useful, it is a form of generalization which may not be applicable necessarily to all diseases. That concepts of pathogenesis and pathogenicity (Smith, 1978; Mims, 1976) in higher animals have parallels in fish should come as no surprise as we learn how comparable are the fishes defence mechanisms (Ellis, 1977). However, the list of known bacterial disease agents (Table 1) is not long when the number of fish species, their diversity and their abundance in global terms is considered. This might imply that fish are very efficient in dealing with bacterial invaders or that many more bacterial diseases have yet to be described.

Initial Events

Attachment of the potential bacterial pathogen to host surfaces is of critical importance for initiation of infection (Smith, 1977; Costerton *et al.*, 1978). The bacteria meet their potential host by carriage in water, association with particles in water such as silt and faeces, by direct contact between other fish or animals, or by their presence in the fishes' food. Attachment of pathogens in mammals is commonly a prelude to entry of the tissues by killing the epithelial cells, by passage through or between them or perhaps by-passing the surface and gaining attachment and entry through a site of damage. The diphtheria bacillus and *Vibrio cholera* are examples where attachment and elaboration of toxin at that site are sufficient in themselves to cause systemic disease.

Table 1. Taxonomy of bacterial pathogens of fishes (after Roberts, 1978)

Family	Genus	Species	Main pathological feature
Cytophagaceae (gliding bacteria)	*Flexibacter*	*F. columaris*[b] *F. psychrophila*[a,b] *F. marinus*[a,b]	Gill and skin lesions
Pseudo-monadaceae	*Pseudomonas*	*Ps. fluorescens*	Septicaemias, haemor-rhage
		Ps. anguilliseptica[a]	Septicaemias and haem-orrhage in eels
Enterobacteriaceae	*Edwardsiella*	*E. tarda*	Septicaemias, haemor-rhage and skin lesions
	Yersinia	*Y. ruckerii*[a]	
Vibrionaceae	*Vibrio*	*V. anguillarum* *V. spp.*	Septicaemias, haemor-rhage and skin lesions
	Aeromonas	*A. hydrophila* *A. salmonicida*	
Uncertain but Gram-negative	*Flavobacterium*	*F. sp.*	Skin lesions, haemor-rhage, septicaemias
	Pasteurella	*Past. piscicida*[a,b]	Granulomas
	Haemophilus	*H. piscium*	Skin lesions, septi-caemias and haemor-rhage
Streptococcaceae	*Streptococcus*	*Str. faecalis* *Str. sp.*	Granulomas, haemorrhage
Norcardiaceae	*Nocardia*	*N. asteroides* *N. kampachi*[a,b]	Granulomas esp. tubercles
Uncertain but Gram-positive	Uncertain	Bacterial kidney disease or *Renibacterium salmoninarum*[a,b]	Granulomas in salmonids, haemor-rhage
Bacillaceae	*Clostridium*	*Cl. botulinum*	Intoxication
Mycobacteria-ceae	*Mycobacterium*	*M. fortuitum* *M. marinum*	Granulomas esp. tubercles
Chlamydiaceae	Uncertain	Uncertain	Epithelial cysts

[a]Not listed in Bergey's, 8th edition
[b]Not listed in "Approved Lists of Bacterial Names"

The surfaces for primary attachment and entry of pathogens into the fish are shown in Fig. 1. The integument of the outer surfaces is covered by a variably thick layer of mucus, the cuticle, which may inhibit bacterial growth (Sieburth, 1975). Bacterial penetration of the cuticle is probably highly significant in the establishment of infection and can be achieved by mechanical abrasion, by parasite abrasion and by eruptions in the epidermis, for example sloughing of epidermal papillomata (Carlisle, 1977). Gill and other internal epithelial surfaces do not have this thick layer of mucus covering them although mucus is shed continuously. In the author's experience, infectious disease of even the remoter surfaces such as the pneumatic duct, the gall bladder, the abdominal pores (Bles, 1898; George *et al.*, 1981) and the eye (Hendricks and Leek, 1975) is possible. The presence of numerous bacteria in close proximity to fish surfaces is well attested (Shewan, 1961; Colwell, 1962; Trust and Sparrow, 1973).

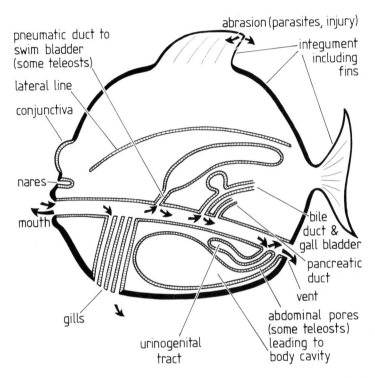

Fig. 1. Diagrammatic representation of fish body surfaces as sites of microbial infection and shedding.

Of the bacterial pathogens of fishes *Aeromonas salmonicida* has received most attention. It commonly causes a systemic disease, called furunculosis in salmonids, in several freshwater species of fish. It may also cause skin diseases only in all these fishes. In studies of fin rot at two salmon hatcheries, Schneider and Nicholson (1980) described healthy fish skin surfaces as almost devoid of bacteria. However, when fin rot was prevalent *A. salmonicida* dominated the flora of the lesion at one hatchery and *Flexibacter* sp. at the other. When *A. salmonicida* dominated the lesion, glycocalyx fibres extended from bacteria on the surface of the lesion to the host surface. Such fibres are known to mediate adhesion and concentrate virulence factors such as toxins and enzymes (Costerton *et al.*, 1978). Smith

(1977) has described this phase as a major determinant in the initiation of disease. In studies of furunculosis, virulence has been associated with self-agglutinating isolates since the early work of the 1930s but only recently has this property been associated with a newly identified additional cell wall layer, called the A layer, first described by Udey and Fryer (1978). The A layer is also common to virulent isolates from non-salmonids and to achromogenic isolates (Hamilton *et al.*, 1981). Characterization of the A layer by Trust *et al.* (1980a) has shown a molecular weight component of 49,000 and, using the electron microscope, negative staining has revealed a patterned surface similar to that of bacterial pathogens of homoeotherms where it is associated with antiphagocytic properties and sometimes adhesion. Hubbert and Brain (1980) have reported that the A layer of an achromogenic isolate from roach (*Rutilus rutilus*) has regularly arranged tetragonal subunits both in culture and in diseased fish. They reported a second layer of hexagonal subunits was also present. These differences in the findings of workers studying the outer surfaces of *A. salmonicida*, namely glycocalyx structures and more than one A layer, may reflect strain or cultural differences or, more accurately, reflect the immediate past history of the cells which were visualized. Costerton *et al.* (1981) and Smith (1981) emphasize *in vivo* study of the pathogen in the process of producing disease in the host as the way to resolve questions of presence or absence of structural components and their probable function. Both *A. salmonicida* and *A. hydrophila*, another fish pathogen, have adhesins which allow them to attach to selected eucaryotic cells, including trout red blood cells (Trust *et al.*, 1980b). The selectivity of the adhesins was shown to be based on recognition of D-mannose and L-fucose side chains on polymers on the surface of the eucaryotic cells.

Zobell and Wells (1934) described a condition they named infectious dermatosis, common in recently caught fish from the Pacific Ocean and held in the Scripps Institute aquarium. Caused by *V. anguillarum* they described *in vivo* bacteria as possessing a large capsule, another type of glycocalyx structure. Capsules have not been described subsequently in other cases of vibriosis, but they are often associated with virulence in pathogens of homoeotherms.

The myxobacterioses are another significant and widespread group of bacterial fish skin diseases including columnaris disease, gill disease, cold water and peduncle diseases (Bullock *et al.*, 1971) and saddleback disease (Morrison *et al.*, 1981). Their taxonomic position is an evolving subject and the inter-relationships between isolates are often difficult to determine. However, there is little doubt they are often commensals on gill epithelium and also on outer integument epithelium if given the opportunity. Serological comparisons have indicated differences between pathogenic and non-pathogenic strains (Pacha and Porter, 1968). Many strains causing skin disease appear to have a tropism for dermal tissue but the chemical basis for this is obscure.

Beneath the Epithelial Barrier

Examination of the tissues commonly coming into contact with bacteria, viz — gill, gut and outer integument, is instructive in giving insights into the arrangement of the fishes' defences in areas where we might infer that invaders are common.

Gill

The secondary lamellae of the gills have little mucus, a single cell epithelial layer (Roberts, 1978) and the blood capillaries are lined with alternating pillar and macrophage cells (Chilmonczyk, 1980). The primary lamellae and gill arches housing the blood supply to and from the gill area are well endowed with lymphocytes and eosinophilic granulocytes (EGCs).

Of the many reports of bacterial gill diseases an account by Wakabayashi and Egusa (1980) is instructive. They reported a gill disease of cultured salmonids caused by a *Flavobacterium* sp. which extensively colonized gill surfaces in experimental studies but did not reproduce the original disease. Colonization was followed by host gill epithelial hyperplasia and subsequent shedding of most of the bacteria from the surface.

In more severe cases of gill disease, mucus accumulation, epithelial hyperplasia followed by death of epithelial cells, embolisms and mobilization of EGCs and lymphocytes to the secondary lamellae may occur.

Gut

Another area much exposed to microbes is the intestinal tract. Beneath the columnar epithelium there are a variety of fixed and wandering leucocytes, in addition to which the spongy nature of the tissue suggests copious quantities of fluid which, in the plaice (*Pleuronectes platessa*), has been shown to be rich in antibody (Ellis, 1974). Fletcher and Grant (1969) have demonstrated antibody in gut mucus and Lobb and Clem (1981b) have shown that bile mucus contains secretory type antibody.

Several diseases are reported to start from initial events in the gut, thus Egusa (1982) reports that vibriosis may start from an enteritis as may streptococcosis (Kusuda and Kimura, 1978), enteric redmouth disease (Dulin *et al.*, 1976) and furunculosis (Sakai, 1979). Other descriptions of the pathology of vibriosis outbreaks (Anderson and Conroy, in Bullock *et al.*, 1971) indicate a primary intestinal lesion suggesting parallels with *V. cholera* and *V. parahaemolyticus* and their attachment to gut epithelial cells and toxin elaboration there.

Skin

A mucus cuticle and non-vascularized epidermis, often several cells thick and within which scales may be embedded, covers the body surface. Fletcher and Grant (1969) have shown antibody in this mucus and Lobb and Clem (1981a) have demonstrated a secretory antibody in one species. Lymphocyte-like cells whose function is uncertain can be seen in this epidermal layer. Below this is a basement membrane and a weakly vascularized dermis. In wild fish, damage to the mucus cuticle and epidermis is perhaps uncommon, the intact surface continuously shedding mucus and thus giving considerable protection from invasive bacteria. However, in fish culture conditions, crowding and abrasion of surfaces may greatly increase the risk of damage with the consequence that a portal of entry is available. Parasites of the integument, which are often more numerous in culture conditions, are another factor likely to cause damage sufficient to allow entry and attachment of bacteria beneath the epithelial surface. When entry occurs by the skin route there is often direct visual evidence of localized entry because of lesions and inflammatory responses. The furuncle caused by *A. salmonicida* is most often a single lesion which may represent a point source of entry in the skin. Vibrio, aeromonad, myxobacter and possibly many other pathogens may gain entry from this route. A demonstration that bacterial pathogens may enter the host by more than one route was given by Sakai (1979), who showed that healthy fish bathed in water rich in *A. salmonicida* did not succumb to disease whereas intubation of bacteria into stomach or rectum resulted in 50% and 10% diseased fish respectively. Additionally, when caudal or dorsal fin clipped fish were bathed in pathogen-rich water, 80% and 60% respectively became diseased.

The Spread of Infection

Once a bacterium has penetrated the epithelium of gill or gut and passed the leucocyte defences of those organs, or has passed through the integument of outer fish surfaces, it may be assumed it has penetrated one or other or both of the fluid conduits of the fish, namely the blood and lymph. Inflammatory responses, if ineffective, may well spread the infection by allowing faster penetration of the blood and lymph. Serum anti-bacterial factors including antibody, complement (Nonaka *et al.*, 1981a, b) and opsonization are all part of the fishes' defensive system as are circulating phagocytes.

Both lymphatic and blood circulation systems pass through the spleen and kidney which should be viewed as functioning, amongst other activities, as organs of filtration (Ellis *et al.*, 1976). Study of the fate of injected colloidal carbon particles, which is analogous to bacterial septicaemia, has shown that in the plaice almost all the carbon is accumulated in the macrophages of kidney and spleen with very small amounts seen in other places such as the serosal epithelia of the organs of the body cavity, in blood and heart macrophages and in gill leucocytes (Ellis *et al.*, 1976). Of course, carbon is inert and, when substituted by a pathogen, interactive and highly specific changes can be anticipated. In the pathogenesis of experimentally induced furunculosis in rainbow trout (*Salmo gairdneri*), Klontz *et al.* (1966) found a series of sequential changes; at 8 hours after intramuscular (i.m.) inoculation a transient bacteraemia occurred while at the site of injection there was a marked inflammatory response consisting of lymphocytes, neutrophilic granulocytes, macrophages and fibroblasts; after 40 hours there was significant diminution of the inflammatory response at the site of injection, while in the anterior kidney and spleen degenerative changes showed; by 56 hours the bacteraemia had recurred; after 72 hours the kidney, spleen and site of injection were devoid of granulocytes and macrophages, the tissues were undergoing liquefactive necrosis and blood leucocyte levels dropped to 33–0% of normal; by 96 hours fish were dying with massive bacteraemia. Wolke (1975), reviewing the disease, noted a prominent feature was the lack of an inflammatory response, while the destruction of the ellipsoids of the spleen is the most consistent feature noted by histopathologists (Ferguson and McCarthy, 1978; Bach *et al.*, 1978; McCarthy and Roberts, 1980) in cases of naturally occurring disease. The overwhelming of the leucocytic response and their subsequent death and liquefaction both in their reservoir bases and in the blood indicate how *A. salmonicida* achieves its spread and dominance in the fish. A toxin (or toxins) perhaps acting as a leucocytolysin was postulated by Klontz *et al.* (1966) to explain this observation.

In contrast to the last example of an acute and virulent disease, mycobacteriosis represents an example of a chronic disease with focal lesions, the outcome of which may not be fatal. Timur and Roberts (1977) studied the pathogenesis of an experimentally induced focal lesion following i.m. injection of *Mycobacterium marinum* in the plaice. Within a few days muscle damage at the site of injection was observed as were small numbers of infiltrating polymorphs, lymphocytes and acid-fast bacilli both extracellularly and intracellularly within macrophages. By day 18 all bacilli were located intracellularly in phagocytes and from then to day 35 tubercle formation typical of higher animals occurred, with clear signs of multi-nucleated giant cells occurring during this period. After day 35 the tubercle was a fully formed epithelioid granuloma with a central focus of caseation in which numerous acid-fast bacilli occurred. The presence of numerous acid-fast bacilli inside the tubercle is evidence that the defensive mechanisms of the plaice failed to kill all the mycobacteria and that, although they were apparently contained in the tubercle, their escape and further tubercle formation was probable. Naturally occurring myco-bacterial infections of fish result in widespread tubercle formation especially in the kidney and spleen (Nigrelli and Vogel, 1963). In this example it is clear that the bacilli do not elaborate powerful toxins but are strongly resistant to host killing mechanisms.

The pathogenesis of vibriosis caused by *V. anguillarum* is not as well studied as is furunculosis, but the clinical and histopathological evidence also suggests toxin elaboration with immobilization and destruction of leucocytes and red blood cells followed by overwhelming bacteraemia. The pathogenesis of bacterial kidney disease (BKD) is also not well documented, but it is clear that intracellular survival and multiplication of bacteria in macrophages in the kidney and spleen figure prominently (Young and Chapman, 1978) suggesting that the bacilli are transported there. Although BKD shares in common with mycobacteriosis a chronic course, giant cell formation and intracellular presence and survival in macrophages, it differs in producing a diffuse rather than a focal granuloma and a degree of widespread organ damage suggestive of some toxin formation. Two diseases of yellow-tail (*Seriola* sp.), pseudotuberculosis caused by *Pasteurella piscicida* (Kubota *et al.*, 1970a, b, 1972), and nocardiosis caused by *Nocardia kampachi* (Kusuda, 1975), produce tubercle-like conditions although the pathology of each disease is rather different. From Table 1, as a broad generalization, the Gram-positive (including acid-fast) bacterial diseases are chronic, produce granulomas and have a tropism for phagocytes. It is not possible to group the Gram-negative caused diseases together but there is a strong suggestion that toxin production plays a significant role in some as will be shown in the next section.

Mechanisms of Cell and Tissue Damage

Exotoxins

Although it has long been suspected that bacterial fish pathogens produce toxic factors important in the pathogenesis of disease, only recently has evidence been presented on the *in vivo* effects of crude and partially purified preparations.

Thus for *A. salmonicida*, where it has been suspected for some time that toxin production was significant in the pathogenesis of disease, there were accounts of *in vitro* production of haemolysin (Karlsson, 1962; Titball and Munn, 1981), leucocytolysin (Klontz *et al.*, 1966) and protease (Dahle, 1971; Shieh and McLean, 1975). Sakai (1977) has shown that extracellular protease is a major causative factor in the pathology of furunculosis. Munro *et al.* (1980) have since shown that *in vitro* prepared extracellular products (ECP) of *A. salmonicida* grown on cellophane are cytolytic and at lower concentrations toxic for a variety of fish cells including red blood cells, macrophages and tissue culture cells, that ECP has lipase and protease activity, is fatal for fish when introduced by i.m. and i.p. routes and that i.m. injections produce swellings histologically similar to the furuncle seen in diseased fish. Ellis *et al.* (1981) have further extended this work to show that i.p. and i.m. injections of ECP collectively produce most of the pathological and histopathological changes reported in cases of furunculosis, whilst Ellis (1981a) has separately shown that ECP introduced by the i.p. route causes significant histamine release in gut tissues of rainbow trout, probably from degranulating eosinophilic granulocytes which are most prevalent in this tissue. Sheeran and Smith (1981) have shown that *A. salmonicida* produces two protease enzymes which differ in both their susceptibility to inhibitors and in their substrate specificity. The caseinolytic protease corresponds to that of Shieh and McLean (1975) while the other, unable to hydrolyse casein, is gelatinolytic and possibly a metallo-enzyme.

The closely related *A. hydrophila* produces a multiplicity of enzymes and toxins (Wadstrom *et al.*, 1976). One isolate from fish produces an enterotoxin (Baulanger *et al.*, 1977). Stevenson and Allen (1981) have shown that ECP from *A. hydrophila* is toxic for fish and contains at least haemolysis and protease activity which could be separated by chromatography. Allen and Stevenson (1981) have further shown that a protease-deficient mutant retains most of the toxic ECP activity implicating the haemolytic component as the significant toxic factor. In contrast to the significance that Allen and Stevenson's (1981) results place on the haemolysin of *A. hydrophila*, Sakai's (1977) findings with a protease deficient mutant of *A. salmonicida* indicate the importance of protease in furunculosis pathology.

The electron micrographs of Schneider and Nicholson (1980) give visual evidence of the action of *A. salmonicida* proteases when a bacterial cell is lodged on the integument of a fin. They also illustrate how the glycocalyx may not only act as an attachment mechanism but also prevent the loss of aggressive factors by concentrating them at the host–pathogen interface. In this context, it is interesting to recall that *Haemophilus*, *Streptococcus* (Male, 1979) and *Gonococcus* (Blake and Swanson, 1978) produce immunoglobulin A proteases, the action of which is important in allowing colonization of mucus surfaces in mammals. The destruction of the splenic ellipsoids in the presence of microcolonies of *A. salmonicida* in cases of clinical furunculosis (Ferguson and McCarthy, 1978) is probably another example of pathogen protease in action. This destruction of the splenic architecture where the association of melanomacrophage, antigen trapping ellipsoidal sheath and lymphocytes may act to prime uncommitted lymphocytes is perhaps one reason for the early failure of lymphocyte responses to systemic infection by *A. salmonicida*.

The antiprotease activity reported in trout serum by Munro *et al.* (1980) has been shown by Grisley *et al.* (1982) to be analogous to the α-macroglobulin antiproteases in the serum of many mammals. A characteristic feature of these antiproteases is that the protease–antiprotease complex retains proteolytic activity for small peptides.

Anaemia characterized by low haematocrit values is a typical finding in many bacterial fish diseases. Whether this is due to specific haemolysins, non-specific cytolysins or to other factors, for example haemorrhage or haemodilation, is not always clear. However, in vibriosis caused by *V. anguillarum*, the concurrent accumulation of considerable deposits of iron in the spleen and kidney is presumptive evidence (Richards, 1980) for haemolytic activity. Munn (1978) has partially purified preparations of extracellularly produced material from *V. anguillarum* cultures which are both haemolytic for eel red blood cells and toxic for eels (*Anguilla anguilla*). In common with *V. cholera* and *V. parahaemolyticus*, the *V. anguillarum* haemolysin is inhibited by the presence of certain gangliosides, the probable membrane receptor components for the cytolysin (Munn, 1980).

The ability of a host to deny a bacterium iron, or of the invader to acquire this essential element, may be of importance for microbial growth *in vivo* or for the elaboration of specific virulence factors (Weinberg, 1978). An example of a plasmid-coded iron-chelating compound with the ability to determine virulence has been shown in several isolates of serotype I of *V. anguillarum* (Crosa, 1980; Crosa and Hodges, 1981). In this example, new outer-membrane proteins are induced under conditions of iron limitation. Transferrin genotype of host fish has been implicated in determining resistance to experimentally induced BKD in Pacific salmon (*Oncorhynchus* spp.) (Suzumoto *et al.*, 1977; Winter *et al.*, 1980).

In experimental streptococcosis of yellowtail, Kimura and Kusuda (1979) prepared a cell-free culture filtrate from a virulent strain of *Streptococcus* sp. and injected it in fish shortly before injection of a virulent or low virulence culture. The supernatant speeded the onset of disease with the virulent culture and caused disease when introduced with the low virulence culture, whereas the latter did not produce disease when injected alone. The authors concluded that this was direct evidence for exotoxin formation by virulent strains of the bacterium.

Clostridium botulinum toxin has been found to cause death in farmed trout in Denmark (Huss and Eskildsen, 1974). The very high levels sometimes found in dead or dying trout cannot always be ascribed to the levels of toxin found in their food. Although the bacillus is non-invasive, some vegetative multiplication and toxin production may possibly occur in the intestine of fish.

Endotoxin

The endotoxin or lipopolysaccharide (LPS) of Gram-negative bacteria is toxic for most homoeotherms inducing a variety of pathological conditions including shock, haemorrhage, fever and death but, despite considerable research, the mechanisms remain obscure. In fish no evidence has been found that LPS is toxic (Bercz *et al.*, 1966; Wedemeyer *et al.*, 1969; Paterson and Fryer, 1974). However, Reynolds *et al.* (1978) have shown febrile responses in the goldfish (*Carassius auratus*) injected with LPS from *A. salmonicida* and *Escherichia coli*. At high concentrations, LPS is mitogenic for B cells, macrophages and granulocytes in homoeotherms and consequently induces polyclonal stimulation of B cells (Moller, 1972). At lower concentrations it induces an antigen specific T-cell—and macrophage-independent response from the "correct" B-cell population. In rainbow trout Etlinger *et al.* (1976) showed that LPS is mitogenic for some lymphocytes while many reports show LPS is antigenic at lower than mitogenic concentrations in fish.

Persistence of Infection

Most pathogens must persist and proliferate to produce enough toxins/aggressins to be effective or to develop sufficient numbers for tissue invasion and/or septicaemia. There are significant advantages for the bacterial pathogen if it can establish a persistent or carrier state infection of the host. Persistence coupled with shedding confers other advantages, namely lateral transmission to new hosts (Mims, 1976). For most bacterial pathogens of fish it is not known whether or for how long they may infect a host. However, within fish populations it is probable that many pathogens may establish a near permanent relationship. Persistent infection of wild and farmed Pacific and Atlantic salmon (*Salmo salar*) and other salmonids by the kidney disease bacterium (*Renibacterium salmonis*) often without pathology, has been recorded (Bell, 1961; Mitchum and Sherman, 1979; Paterson *et al.*, 1979). The long held suspicion of persistent infection of salmonids by *A. salmonicida* was substantiated by the finding of Bullock and Stuckey (1975) that corticosteroid injections activated latent infection (not detectable by culture methods) to produce clinical disease. Using this method, McCarthy (1977) demonstrated that farmed brown trout (*Salmo trutta*) populations had a high carrier rate of *A. salmonicida* (<80%) while farmed rainbow trout had a low prevalence (0–5%). He also showed that latent infection could occur without any prior record of clinical disease. Jensen and Larsen (1980) also used similar methods to study the seasonal occurrence of both *A. salmonicida* and *A. hydrophila* in farmed brown and rainbow trout. They recorded a high prevalence of *A. salmonicida* in summer in both species (90 and 66% respectively) but no infection in either in winter. However, *A. hydrophila* infection was detected in winter and summer in both fish species at intermediate levels (5–34%).

Kusuda and Kimura (1978) record that the streptococcal infection of yellowtail persists in the intestine in the fish. Egusa (1982) discussing this disease records that it has a chronic course and surviving fish may have further episodes of disease. Busch and Lingg (1975) recorded an asymptomatic carrier-state of infection for the enteric redmouth bacterium (*Yersinia ruckeri*) in farmed rainbow trout.

There is an urgent need to identify the sites of persistence with individual infections. Are some intracellular, or is persistence at tissue surfaces the site of infection (Costerton *et al.*, 1981)? From the foregoing observations we can conclude the fish, like higher animals, may regularly harbour pathogens without clinically significant disease. This suggests that factors other than simply the presence of the pathogen are important in pathogenesis. Some stressful influences, for example handling and crowding, induce elevated levels of cortisol resulting in depression of one or several defensive mechanisms (Ellis, 1981b). The presence of the *Renibacterium salmonis* in faeces suggests colonization of an epithelial surface or a site which allows discharge into the intestine (Bullock *et al.*, 1980; Mitchum and Sherman, 1981). However, the bacterium is found also in internal organs, especially the kidney, without any clear indication if these are preferred or protected sites.

Another aspect of persistence is the degree of virulence possessed by the strain of the pathogen. Thus McCarthy and Roberts (1980) reported that freshly isolated strains from acute furunculosis may show a minimum lethal dose as low as 10^{-2}–10^{-3} viable cells whereas an isolate obtained from a carrier fish artificially stressed by injection with prednisolone acetate requires the injection of 10^{-5} viable cells to kill non-carrier fish. Therefore it may be that persistent infections are due to strains of lesser or intermediate virulence and that strains associated with epidemics are of greater virulence. How readily strains of lesser virulence may be transformed into strains of greater virulence and *vice versa* and to what extent host factors might influence these events is not known, but the example of gonorrhoea in humans is evidence of such complex events (Swanson, 1980). We should also consider that if the phenotypic characteristics of an established bacterial population reflect the selection pressures of the host environment a comparison of such bacteria *in situ* with laboratory cultures used for the study of pathogenesis may be rewarding. The role of the distal surface structures of the bacterial wall, e.g. the glycocalyx polysaccharides (Costerton *et al.*, 1981), which maintain contact between host and pathogen, is one such aspect that deserves greater attention.

Persistent shedding of the pathogen may put at risk other fish in a population and may, in some cases, cause transmission to the fish's progeny. The use of vaccines in fish may give some cause for concern if increases in existing disease reservoirs result. In studies of the experimental vaccination of Atlantic salmon against bacterial kidney disease, Paterson *et al.* (1981) have shown a protective effect from their use of a killed bacterial cell suspension in Freund's adjuvant. However, they also recorded that all of the protected and surviving salmon carried detectable levels of the KD bacterium and it can probably be concluded that these fish were shedding bacteria. If such a result is common to many fish vaccines, *viz* that vaccinated fish become persistently infected and shed the disease agent, there are some general implications for the use of vaccines in fish:

(1) at a fish farm where vaccinated fish are present no susceptible stocks should be introduced;
(2) the risks of vertical transmission via ova must be evaluated;
(3) shedding of the pathogen if it is sufficiently extensive may contribute to loss of population protection. The significance of shedding, e.g. numbers shed, seasonality of shedding, virulence of bacteria, requires further study.

Conclusions

Many of the reports previously referred to either demonstrate or imply that strains of pathogen vary with regard to their properties of virulence. Only by describing the molecular basis of virulence and defining phenotypic and genotypic controls regulating the production of virulence factors can we begin to understand the complex interplay between host and pathogen. In such a scenario we should anticipate that host defensive systems influence the expression of bacterial virulence in many subtle ways. Only at this molecular level will be understand how stressful events on the host play their part in initiating the infectious disease process (Pickering, 1981).

The study of bacterial fish diseases is now moving from the descriptive stage towards defining the molecular basis of pathogenicity. We can expect many more accounts of the isolation and characterization of toxic factors and of virulence mechanisms including those mediating attachment.

Emphasis on persistent bacterial infection should be an important part of future studies. This is necessary if we are to achieve greater control of disease in farmed fish because there is much to learn about reservoirs of infection in farmed and wild fish, how fish behave in terms of shedding pathogen, the properties of the bacteria shed, and how vaccines may influence persistence patterns.

The studies reviewed here show that the fish is likely to be challenged simultaneously at the gut, gill and skin as well as at other less important sites. It may therefore be asked if vaccination by one method is sufficient to protect the host sufficiently at all the major sites of invasion. In testing the efficacy of experimental vaccines challenge by all these routes of invasion should be compared.

References

Allen, B. J. and Stevenson, R. M. V. (1981). Extracellular virulence factors of *Aeronomonas hydrophila* in fish infections. *Canadian Journal of Microbiology* (in press).

Bach, R., Chen, P. K. and Chapman, G. B. (1978). Changes in the spleen of the channel catfish *Ictalurus punctatus* (Rafinesque) induced by infection with *Aeromonas hydrophila*. *Journal of Fish Diseases* 1, 205–217.

Baulanger, Y., Lallier, R. and Cansineau, G. (1977). Isolation of enterotoxigenic *Aeromonas* from fish. *Canadian Journal of Microbiology* 23, 1161–1164.

Bell, G. R. (1961). Two epidemics of apparent kidney disease in cultured pink salmon *Oncorhynchus gorbuscha*. *Journal of the Fisheries Research Board of Canada* 18, 559–569.

Bercz, I., Bertok, I. and Bereznai, D. (1966). Comparative studies of the toxicology of *Escherichia coli* lipopolysaccharide endotoxin in various animal species. *Canadian Journal of Microbiology* 12, 1070–1071.

Blake, M. S. and Swanson, J. (1978). Studies of gonococcus infection. XVI. Purification of *Neisseria gonorrhoeae* immunoglobulin A1 protease. *Infection and Immunology* 22, 350–358.

Bles, E. J. (1898). The correlated distribution of abdominal pores and nephrostomes in fishes. *Journal of Anatomy and Physiology* 32, 484–512.

Bullock, G. L. and Stuckey, H. M. (1975). *Aeromonas salmonicida* detection in asymptomatically infected trout. *Progressive Fish-Culturist* 37, 237–239.

Bullock, G. L., Conroy, D. A . and Snieszko, S. F. (1971). Bacterial diseases of fishes. *In* "Diseases of Fishes" (Eds. S. F. Snieszko and H. R. Axelrod). TFH Publications, Neptune City, New Jersey.

Bullock, G. L., Griffin, B. R. and Stuckey, H. M. (1980). Detection of *Corynebacterium salmonis* by direct fluorescent antibody test. *Canadian Journal of Fisheries and Aquatic Sciences* **37**, 719–721.

Busch, R. A. and Lingg, A. (1975). Establishment of an asymptomatic carrier state infection of enteric redmouth disease in rainbow trout (*Salmo gairdneri*). *Journal of the Fisheries Research Board of Canada* **32**, 2429–2432.

Carlisle, J. C. (1977). An epidermal papilloma of the Atlantic salmon (*S. salar*). II. Ultrastructure and etiology. *Journal of Wildlife Diseases* **13**, 235–239.

Chilmonczyk, S. (1980). Some aspects of trout gill structure in relation to egtved virus infection and defence mechanisms. *In* "Fish Diseases. Third COPRAQ— Session" (Ed. W. Ahne), pp.18–22. Springer Verlag, Berlin.

Colwell, R. (1962). The bacterial flora of Puget Sound fish. *Journal of Applied Bacteriology* **25**, 147–158.

Costerton, J. W., Geesey, G. G. and Cheng, K. S. (1978). How bacteria stick. *Scientific American* **238**, 86–95.

Costerton, J. W., Irven, R. J. and Cheng, K-J. (1981). The role of bacterial surface structures in pathogenesis. *Critical Reviews in Microbiology* **8**, 303–338.

Crosa, J. H. (1980). A plasmid associated with virulence in the marine fish pathogen *Vibrio anguillarum* specifies an iron-sequestering system. *Nature, London* **284**, 566–568.

Crosa, J. H. and Hodges, L. L. (1981). Outer membrane proteins induced under conditions of iron limitation in the marine fish pathogen *Vibrio anguillarum*. *Infection and Immunity* **31**, 223–227.

Dahle, H. K. (1971). The purification and some properties of two *Aeromonas* proteinases. *Acta Pathologica Scandanavia, Section B* **79**, 726–738.

Dulin, M. D., Huddleston, T., Larson, R. E. and Klontz, G. W. (1976). "Enteric Redmouth Disease". Bulletin No. 8. College of Forestry, Wildlife and Range Sciences, University of Idaho, Moscow.

Egusa, S. (1982). Disease problems in Japanese yellowtail (*Seriola quinqueradiata*) culture: a review. *In* "Special Meeting on Diseases of Commercially Important Marine Fish and Shellfish", Copenhagen, 1–3 October 1980 (Ed. J. Stewart). *Rapports et Procès-Verbaux des Reunions Council International pour l'Exploration de la Mer* (in press).

Ellis, A. E. (1974). "Aspects of the lymphoid and reticulo-endothelial systems in the plaice, *Pleuronectes platessa* L." PhD Thesis, University of Aberdeen.

Ellis, A. E. (1977). The leucocytes of fish: a review. *Journal of Fish Biology* **11**, 453–491.

Ellis, A. E. (1981a). Histamine, mast cells and hypersensitivity responses in fish. *Developmental and Comparative Immunology* (in press).

Ellis, A. E. (1981b). Stress and modulation of the immune response in fish. *In* "Stress and Fish" (Ed. A. D. Pickering), pp.147–169. Academic Press, London.

Ellis, A. E., Munro, A. L. S. and Roberts, R. J. (1976). Defence mechanisms in fish 1. A study of the phagocytic system and the fate of intraperitoneally injected particulate material in the plaice (*Pleuronectes platessa*). *Journal of Fish Biology* **8**, 67–78.

Ellis, A. E., Hastings, T. S. and Munro, A. L. S. (1981). The role of *Aeromonas salmonicida* extracellular products in the pathology of furunculosis. *Journal of Fish Diseases* **4**, 41–51.

Etlinger, H. M., Hodgins, H. O. and Chiller, J. M. (1976). Evolution of the lymphoid system. I. Evidence for lymphocyte heterogeneity in rainbow trout revealed by the organ distribution of mitogenic response. *Journal of Immunology* **116**, 1547–1553.

Ferguson, H. and McCarthy, D. H. (1978). Histopathology of furunculosis in brown trout *Salmo trutta* L. *Journal of Fish Diseases* **1**, 165–174.

Fletcher, T. C. and Grant, P. T. (1969). Immunoglobulins in the serum and mucus of the plaice (*Pleuronectes platessa*). *Biochemical Journal* **115**, 65D.

George, C. J., Ellis, A. E. and Bruno, D. W. (1981). On remembrance of the abdominal pores in rainbow trout. *Journal of Fish Biology* (in press).

Grisley, M. S., Ellis, A. E., Hastings, T. S. and Munro, A. L. S. (1982). An alpha-migrating anti-protease in normal salmonid plasma and its relationship to the neutralisation of *Aeromonas salmonicida* toxins. *In* "Fish Diseases. Fourth COPRAQ Session" (in press).

Hamilton, R. C., Kalnins, H., Ackland, N. R. and Ashburner, N. D. (1981). An extra layer in the surface layer on an atypical *Aeromonas salmonicida* isolated from Australian goldfish. *Journal of General Microbiology* **122**, 363–366.

Hendricks, J. D. and Leek, S. L. (1975). Kidney disease postorbital lesions in spring chinook salmon (*Oncorhyncus tshawytscha*). *Transactions of the American Fisheries Society* **104**, 805–807.

Hubbert, R. M. and Brain, A. P. R. (1980). Studies on the ultrastructure of *Aeromonas salmonicida* subsp. *achromogenes*. *Bamidgeh* **32**, 101–107.

Huss, H. H. and Eskildsen, U. (1974). Botulism in farmed trout caused by *Clostridium botulinum* type E. *Nordic Journal of Veterinary Medicine* **26**, 733–738.

Jensen, N. J. and Larsen, J. L. (1980). Seasonal occurrence of *Aeromonas salmonicida* carriers. *In* "Fish Diseases. Third COPRAQ—Session" (Ed. W. Ahne), pp.87–89. Springer Verlag, Berlin.

Karlsson, K. A. (1962). The haemolysin of *Aeromonas salmonicida*. *Nord. Veterinaermoede, Beretn, Copenhagen* **9**, **2**, 793–797.

Kimura, H. and Kusuda, R. (1979). Studies on the pathogenesis of streptococcal infection in cultured yellowtails *Seriola* spp.: effect of cell free culture on experimental streptococcal infection. *Journal of Fish Diseases* **2**, 501–510.

Klontz, G. W., Yasutake, W. T. and Ross, A. J. (1966). Bacterial diseases of the Salmonidae in the western United States. Pathogenesis of furunculosis in rainbow trout. *American Journal of Veterinary Research* **27**, 1455–1460.

Kubota, S., Kimura, M. and Egusa, S. (1970a). Studies of a bacterial tuberculoidosis of the yellowtail I. Symptomatology and histopathology. *Fish Pathology* **4**, 103–110.

Kubota, S., Kimura, M. and Egusa, S. (1970b). Studies of bacterial tuberculoidosis of the yellowtail II. Mechanisms of nodule formation. *Fish Pathology* **5**, 31–34.

Kubota, S., Kimura, M. and Egusa, S. (1972). Studies of a bacterial tuberculoidosis of the yellowtail III. Findings on nodules and bacterial colonies in tissues. *Fish Pathology* **6**, 69–72.

Kusuda, R. (1975). Nocardial infection in cultured yellowtail. Proceedings of 3rd U.S.–Japan Meeting on Aquaculture, Tokyo, Japan, pp.63–66.

Kusuda, R. and Kimura, H. (1978). Studies of the pathogenesis of streptococcal infection in cultured yellowtails *Seriola* spp.: the fate of *Streptococcus* sp. bacteria after inoculation. *Journal of Fish Diseases* **1**, 109–114.

Lobb, C. J. and Clem, L. W. (1981a). Phylogeny of immunoglobulin structure and function. XI Secretory immunoglobulins in the cutaneous mucus of the sheepshead *Archosargus probatocephalus*. *Developmental and Comparative Immunology* **5**(2), 271–282.

Lobb, C. J. and Clem, W. (1981b). Phylogeny of immunoglobulin structure and function. XII Secretory immunoglobulins in the bile of the marine teleost *Archosargus probatocephalus*. *Molecular Immunology* **18**, 615–619.

McCarthy, D. H. (1977). Some ecological aspects of the bacterial fish pathogen, *Aeromonas salmonicida*. In *"Aquatic Microbiology"*. *Society for Applied Bacteriology Symposia* **6**, 299–324.

McCarthy, D. H. and Roberts, R. J. (1980). Furunculosis of fish—the present state of our knowledge. *Advances in Aquatic Microbiology* **2**, 293–341.

Male, C. J. (1979). Immunoglobulin A1 protease production by *Haemophilus influenzae* and *Streptococcus pneumoniae*. *Infection and Immunity* **26**, 254–260.

Mims, C. A. (1976). "The Pathogenesis of Infectious Disease". Academic Press, London.

Mitchum, D. L. and Sherman, L. E. (1979). Bacterial kidney disease in feral populations of brook trout (*Salvelinus fontinalis*), brown trout (*Salmo trutta*) and rainbow trout (*Salmo gairdneri*). *Journal of the Fisheries Research Board of Canada* **36**, 1370–1376.

Mitchum, D. L. and Sherman, L. E. (1981). Transmission of bacterial kidney disease from wild to stocked hatchery trout. *Canadian Journal of Fisheries and Aquatic Sciences* **38**, 547–551.

Moller, G. (1972). Lymphocyte activation by mitogens. *Transplantation Review* **11**, 53–75.

Morrison, C., Cornick, J., Shum, G. and Zwicker, B. (1981). Microbiology and histopathology of saddleback disease of underyearling Atlantic salmon, *Salmo salar* L. *Journal of Fish Diseases* **4**, 243–258.

Munn, C. B. (1978). Haemolysin production by *Vibrio anguillarum*. *Federation of European Microbiological Societies, Microbiology Letters* **3**, 265–268.

Munn, C. B. (1980). Production and properties of a haemolytic toxin by *Vibrio anguillarum*. In "Fish Diseases. Third COPRAQ—Session" (Ed. W. Ahne), pp.69–74. Springer Verlag, Berlin.

Munro, A. L. S., Hastings, T. S., Ellis, A. E. and Liversidge, J. (1980). Studies on an ichthyotoxic material produced extracellularly by the furunculosis bacterium, *Aeromonas salmonicida*. In "Fish Diseases. Third COPRAQ—Session" (Ed. W. Ahne), pp.98–106. Springer Verlag, Berlin.

Nigrelli, R. G. and Vogel, H. (1963). Spontaneous tuberculosis in fish and in other cold-blooded vertebrates with special reference to *Mycobacterium fortuitum* from fish and human lesions. *Zoologica, New York* **48**, 131–144.

Nonaka, M., Yamaguchi, N., Natsuume-Sakai, S. and Takahashi, M. (1981a). The complement system of rainbow trout (*Salmo gairdneri*). I. Identification of the serum lytic system homologous to mammalian complement. *Journal of Immunology* **126**, 1489–1491.

Nonaka, M., Natsuume-Sakai, S. and Takahashi, M. (1981b). The complement system in rainbow trout (*Salmo gairdneri*). II. Purification and characterisation of the fifth component (C5). *Journal of Immunology* **126**, 1495–1498.

Pacha, R. E. and Porter, S. (1968). Characteristics of myxobacteria isolated from the surface of freshwater fish. *Applied Microbiology* **16**, 1901–1906.

Paterson, W. D. and Fryer, J. L. (1974). Effect of temperature and antigen dose on the antibody response of juvenile coho salmon (*Oncorhynchus kisutch*) to *Aeromonas salmonicida* endotoxin. *Journal of the Fisheries Research Board of Canada* **31**, 1743-1749.

Paterson, W. D., Gallant, C., Desautels, D. and Marshall, L. (1979). Detection of bacterial kidney disease in wild salmonids in the Margaree River system, and adjacent waters using an indirect fluorescent antibody technique. *Journal of the Fisheries Research Board of Canada* **36**, 1464-1468.

Paterson, W. D., Desautels, D. and Weber, J. M. (1981). The immune response of Atlantic salmon, *Salmo salar* L., to the causative agent of bacterial kidney disease, *Renibacterium salmoninarum*. *Journal of Fish Diseases* **4**, 99-111.

Pickering, A. D. (1981). "Stress and Fish". Academic Press, London.

Reynolds, W. W., Covert, J. B. and Casterlin, M. E. (1978). Febrile response of goldfish *Carassium auratus* (L.) to *Aeromonas hydrophila* and to *Escherichia coli* endotoxin. *Journal of Fish Diseases* **1**, 271-273.

Richards, R. H. (1980). Observations on vibriosis in cultured flatfish. In "Fish Diseases. Third COPRAQ—Session" (Ed. W. Ahne), pp.75-81. Springer Verlag, Berlin.

Roberts, R. J. (1978). The pathophysiology and systematic pathology of teleosts. *In* "Fish Pathology" (Ed. R. J. Roberts), pp.55-91. Bailliere Tindall, London.

Sakai, D. K. (1977). Causative factor of *Aeromonas salmonicida* in salmonid furunculosis: extracellular protease. *Scientific Reports of Hokkaido Fish Hatchery* **32**, 61-89.

Sakai, D. K. (1979). Invasive routes of *Aeromonas salmonicida* subsp. *salmonicidae*. *Scientific Reports of the Hokkaido Fish Hatchery* **34**, 1-6.

Schneider, R. and Nicholson, B. L. (1980). Bacteria associated with fin rot disease in hatchery-reared Atlantic salmon (*Salmo salar*). *Canadian Journal of Fisheries and Aquatic Sciences* **37**, 1505-1513.

Sheeran, B. and Smith, P. R. (1981). A second extracellular proteolytic activity associated with the fish pathogen *Aeromonas salmonicida*. *Federation of European Microbiological Societies Microbiology Letters* **11**, 73-76.

Sheeran, B., Drinan, E. and Smith, P. R. (1982). Preliminary studies on the role of extracellular proteolytic enzymes in the pathogenesis of furunculosis. *In* "Fish Diseases. Fourth COPRAQ Session" (in press).

Shewan, J. M. (1961). The microbiology of seawater fish. *In* "Fish as Food" (Ed. G. Bergstrom), Vol. 1, pp.487-560. Academic Press, London.

Shieh, H. S. and McLean, J. R. (1975). Purification and properties of an extracellular protease of *Aeromonas salmonicida*, the causative agent of furunculosis. *International Journal of Biochemistry* **6**, 653-656.

Sieburth, J. M. (1975). "Microbial Seascapes". University Park Press, Baltimore, London and Tokyo.

Smith, H. (1977). Microbial surfaces in relation to pathogenicity. *Bacteriological Reviews* **41**, 475-500.

Smith, H. (1978). The determinants of pathogenicity. *In* "Essays in Microbiology" (Eds. M. H. Richmond and J. Norris), 13/1-13/32. John Wiley and Sons, Chichester.

Smith, H. W. (1981). Introduction. *In* "The Molecular Basis of Microbial Pathogenicity" (Eds. H. Smith, B. Skehel and C. Turner), pp.11-16. Verlaz Chemie.

Stevenson, R. M. W. and Allen, B. J. (1981). Extracellular virulence products in *Aeromonas hydrophila* disease processes in salmonids. *In* "Symposium on Fish Biologics: Serodiagnostics and Vaccines" (in press).

Suzumoto, B. K., Schreck, C. B. and McIntyre, J. D. (1977). Relative resistances of three transferrin genotypes of coho salmon (*Oncorhynchus kisutch*) and their hematological responses to bacterial kidney disease. *Journal of the Fisheries Research Board of Canada* **34**, 1–8.

Swanson, J. (1980). Adhesion and entry of bacteria into cells: a model of the pathogenesis of gonorrhea. *In* "The Molecular Basis of Microbial Pathogenicity" (Eds. H. Smith, B. Skehel and C. Turner), pp.17–37. Verlag Chemie.

Timur, G. and Roberts, R. J. (1977). The experimental pathogenesis of focal tuberculosis in the plaice (*Pleuronectes platessa* L.). *Journal of Comparative Pathology* **87**, 83–87.

Titball, R. and Munn, C. B. (1981). Evidence for two haemolytic activities from *Aeromonas salmonicida*. *Federation of European Microbiological Societies, Microbiology Letters* **12**, 27–30.

Trust, T. J. and Sparrow, R. A. H. (1973). The bacterial flora in the alimentary tract of freshwater salmonid fishes. *Canadian Journal of Microbiology* **19**, 1219–1228.

Trust, T. J., Howard, P. S., Chamberlain, J. B., Ishiguro, E. E. and Buckley, J. T. (1980a). Additional surface protein in autoaggregating strains of atypical *Aeromonas salmonicida*. *Federation of European Microbiological Societies, Microbiology Letters* **9**, 35–38.

Trust, T. J., Canotice, I. D. and Atkinson, H. M. (1980b). Haemagglutination properties of *Aeromonas*. *In* "Fish Diseases. Third COPRAQ—Session" (Ed. W. Ahne), pp.218–223. Springer Verlag, Berlin.

Udey, L. R. and Fryer, J. F. (1978). Immunization of fish with bacterium of *Aeromonas salmonicida*. *Marine Fisheries Review* **40**, 12–17.

Wadstrom, T., Lungh, A. and Waetlend, B. (1976). Enterotoxin, haemolysin and cytotoxic protein in *Aeromonas hydrophila* from human infections. *Acta pathologica et microbiologica, Scandinavica* **B 84**, 112–114.

Wakabayashi, H. and Egusa, S. (1980). Characteristics of filamentous bacteria isolated from a gill disease of salmonids. *Canadian Journal of Fisheries and Aquatic Sciences* **37**, 1499–1504.

Wedemeyer, G., Ross, A. J. and Smith, L. (1969). Some metabolic effects of bacterial endotoxins in salmonid fishes. *Journal of the Fisheries Research Board of Canada* **26**, 115–122.

Weinberg, E. D. (1978). Iron and infection. *Microbiology Reviews* **42**, 45–86.

Winter, G. W., Schreck, C. B. and McIntyre, J. D. (1980). Resistance of different stocks and transferrin genotypes of coho salmon (*Oncorhynchus kisutch*) and steelhead trout (*Salmo gairdneri*) to bacterial kidney disease and vibriosis. *Fishery Bulletin* **77**, 795–802.

Wolke, R. E. (1975). Pathology of bacterial and fungal diseases affecting fish. *In* "Pathology of Fishes" (Eds. W. E. Ribelin and G. Migaki), pp.33–116. University of Wisconsin Press, Madison.

Young, C. L. and Chapman, G. B. (1978). Ultrastructural aspects of the causative agent and renal histopathology of bacterial kidney disease in brook trout (*Salvelinus fontinalis*). *Journal of the Fisheries Research Board of Canada* **35**, 1234–1248.

Zobell, C. E. and Wells, N. A. (1934). An infectious dermatitis of certain marine fishes. *Journal of Infectious Disease* **55**, 299–305.

8

Progress Towards Furunculosis Vaccination

C. MICHEL

Laboratoire d'Ichtyopathologie, I.N.R.A.
Route de Thiverval, 78850 Thiverval-Grignon, France

Introduction

Although furunculosis of salmonids was the first bacterial disease of fish to be fully recognized (Emmerich and Weibel, 1894), and although it was also the first to stimulate a vaccination attempt in fish (Duff, 1942), more than 80 years of intensive research have failed to provide the solution for the control of this disease. Owing to its economic significance both for cultivated species and wild populations of salmonids, furunculosis remains one of the most intensively studied of the teleost infections and a digest of the significant information presently available can be found in recent reviews (McCraw, 1952; Hermann, 1968; McCarthy and Roberts, 1980).

The causative organism, *Aeromonas salmonicida* was very early characterized and finally classified in the family of Vibrionaceae, but since Kimura described a new sub-species in 1970, an increasing number of reports have been made concerning atypical strains which resemble the initial isolates less and less. Thus furunculosis appears no longer as a disease confined to the salmonids, but as a large group of infections of worldwide distribution, affecting almost every species of freshwater fish, and caused by non-motile Gram-negative microorganisms displaying various morphological, physiological and biochemical properties. This heterogeneity in the phenotypical characters is compensated by a striking homogeneity of the genotypes (McCarthy, 1978; McInnes *et al.*, 1979; Paterson *et al.*, 1980). It must be noted, however, that although they are susceptible to atypical strains of *A. salmonicida*, salmonids more often exhibit the classical signs of the disease, and the most serious threat for fish-culture still stems from the typical pigmented strains. Moreover, the major part of the work concerning the vaccination procedures for the control of furunculosis has been undertaken in salmonids with typical strains. For these reasons, and to avoid an excessive complication of this report, non-typical strains will not be considered.

151

The history of furunculosis vaccination can be roughly divided into two phases. The first ran from 1942 to the middle 1970s, with a 10 years interruption just after the Second World War, corresponding to an extensive and temporarily conclusive use of antimicrobial drugs. During this time, the workers adopted a pragmatic approach and tried to induce the protection of fish through the administration of crude bacterins, using different methods of immunization. The results were uniformly unsuccessful and since 1975 new directions of research have been developed, which aim to a more comprehensive knowledge of the interactions between the pathogen and its host. Such investigations, dealing with the mechanisms of the virulence and the specific or non-specific defences of the host, are expected to allow the design of a reliable vaccine and have already provided very interesting data. This paper will sequentially document the major progress of the last 40 years, and will try to define the main problems which require to be solved before a feasible vaccine is likely to become available.

Immunization of Fish with Crude Bacterial Preparations

Having assessed the frequency and economic importance of furunculosis, first investigators had to promote some control measures in order to limit the losses in trout hatcheries. No drugs were available at that time and, apart from sanitary precautions and technological improvements, the best solution looked to be the active immunization of trout. The ability of fish to elicit an immune response was known since the early work of first immunologists (see Corbel, 1975), but it was not until 1942 that a vaccination trial was carried out by Duff in cutthroat trout (*Salmo clarki*), using an orally administered chloroform-killed vaccine. This attempt provided a fair result with 25% mortality in treated fish compared with the 75% of the control group. There were two reasons for satisfaction with such a result since the preparation of the bacterin was easy, and the oral route of administration of practical interest in the field situation. Unfortunately, Snieszko and Friddle (1949) failed to confirm this work and to detect any protection.

During the following decade, the increasing use of antimicrobial drugs for the control of furunculosis led to the abandonment of vaccination development programmes. However, a new interest arose when it became evident that the extensive use of antibiotics was not devoid of hazards both for the natural environment and for human health. Many projects were instigated but as can be seen from Tables 1 and 2, vaccination attempts between 1960 and 1980 provided rather inconsistent results. The discrepancies between the observations of different authors may be partially explained by variables in experimental conditions such as fish species, temperature of water during the immunization programmes and during the challenge infections and preparation procedure of the bacterins. Two factors must be stressed for their special importance: the route of administration of the vaccine and the challenge procedure. The last point will be discussed further, but the current use of field testing as a challenge procedure must be immediately pointed out, since this seemingly realistic procedure can fail if the expected natural disease outbreak does not occur (Frost, 1968; Antipa and Amend, 1977) or proves insufficient (Udey and Fryer, 1978; Palmer and Smith, 1980). What is worse, other diseases can produce mortalities in experimental groups and add their effect to those of furunculosis (or even alter the course of the infection) as was the case in the trials by Hara and Inoue, in 1976.

The possibility of immunizing fish with a bacterin in the food was not confirmed by Snieszko and Friddle in 1949. At different times, investigations were carried out to resolve this question, without any more success (Table 1). Some workers were unable to observe any protection (Spence *et al.*, 1965; Udey and Fryer, 1978; Michel, 1979), but recently, Smith *et al.* (1980) stated a positive result after feeding brown trout (*Salmo trutta*) with a formalin-killed vaccine. Large-scale field trials, conducted from 1965 to 1968 in hatcheries and summarized by Klontz and Anderson (1970) were of peculiar importance, as they used a sonicated and alum-precipitated crude antigen. Even in such conditions, results were conflicting, and the commercial production of the vaccine was not developed and an oral vaccine to combat furunculosis is still far from being available.

Administration by bath treatment is another method quite well adapted for treating large numbers of fish. As the size of intact bacterial cells appeared to preclude good penetration of the bacterin into the fish tissues, there were no trials by this route until a hyperosmotic infiltration procedure (HI) was developed by Amend and Fender (1976). Three studies on this technique have been published of which two (Antipa and Amend, 1977; Palmer and Smith, 1980) remained inconclusive for want of challenge. Smith *et al.* (1980) observed slight protection. Although Duff had detected low titres of agglutinins in vaccinated trout, all subsequent studies have demonstrated that circulating antibodies are not found following oral or bath immunization. Smith, using a leucocyte migration inhibition test, could assess that the cells of vaccinated fish were sensitized to *A. salmonicida* indicating the likelihood that the immune response to local administration of anti-furunculosis bacterins could involve local or cellular mechanisms.

Parenteral methods of immunization (Table 2) have not provided any more conclusive data than the other methods, although the protection of

Table 1. Vaccination trials against furunculosis, using a local administration of bacterin

References	Species	Inactivating agents	Route of vaccination	Route of challenge	Protection	Observations
Duff (1942)	S. clarki	Chloroform	Oral	Bath	+	
Snieszko and Friddle (1949)	S. fontinalis	Heat	Oral	Intraperitoneal	−	
Spence et al. (1965)	O. kisutch	Formalin	Oral	Scrape + bath	−	Variable results
Klontz and Anderson (1970)	S. fontinalis, Oncorhynchus	Sonication + alum (FSA)	Oral	Field	±	
Hara and Inoué (1976)	Varied	FSA	Oral	Field	+ slight (?)	Interfering diseases
Udey and Fryer (1978)	O. kisutch	Formalin FSA	Oral	Field	−	
Michel (1979)	S. gairdneri	Formalin	Oral	Intramuscular	−	
Palmer and Smith (1980)	S. salar	Formalin	Hyperosmotic infiltration (HI)	Field	−	Insufficient challenge
Smith et al. (1980)	S. trutta	Formalin Sonication or SDS.	Oral HI	Field	+ + slight	Cellular response

Table 2. Vaccination trials using parenteral injections of furunculosis bacterin

Authors	Species	Vaccine preparation	Vaccination	Route of challenge	Protection	Observations
Krantz et al. (1963)	S. trutta and S. fontinalis	Formalin	Intraperitoneal (i.p.)		−	
			i.p. + FCA	i.p.	+	
Spence et al. (1965)	O. kisutch	Hyperimmune serum	i.p.	Scrape + bath	+	Passive protection
Paterson and Fryer (1974)	O. kisutch	Formalin	i.p. + FCA	i.p.	+	
Hara and Inoue (1976)	Varied	Formalin	i.p., i.p. + FCA i.m.	Field	+ slight	Interfering infections
Udey and Fryer (1978)	O. kisutch	Formalin	i.p. + FCA	Field	+ slight	Insufficient challenge
Michel (1979)	S. gairdneri	Formalin	i.p.	Intramuscular	−	
Palmer and Smith (1980)	S. salar	Formalin	i.p. + FCA	Field	−	Insufficient challenge
W. D. Paterson (unpublished observations)	S. salar S. fontinalis	?	i.p.	Bath	+	

fish was more often asserted, mainly when an adjuvant was associated to the bacterin (Krantz *et al.*, 1963; Paterson and Fryer, 1974b). Without adjuvant, and using a parenteral injection of *A. salmonicida* as a challenge, Krantz *et al.* (1963) and Michel (1979) failed to detect a protective immunity. Whatever the significance of their results for protective purposes, these experiments stimulated the advance of our knowledge concerning the humoral response of fish to furunculosis infection. In all cases of parenteral immunization, such a response was initiated, demonstrating the immunogenic properties of the bacteria. Agglutinins were the most studied of the resultant antibodies, and the easier to detect, but precipitins (Anderson and Klontz, 1970) and complement fixing antibodies (Dorson *et al.*, 1979) were also described. It seems that the aggregating or non-aggregating nature of the injected bacteria does not change the resulting titres of agglutinins. Although Klontz and Anderson (1968) considered that several serotypes were distinguishable using fluorescent antibody techniques, the majority of authors have failed to obtain confirmatory results, and the serological homogeneity of *A. salmonicida* is generally accepted. In fact, some variations between the strains can be observed, but it is difficult to assess their systematic character, since fish themselves display a great variability of individual responses. Antibody production can be enhanced by the use of adjuvants, and response also depends upon the temperature of water, as indicated by Paterson and Fryer (1974a, b).

For many years the occurrence and persistence of agglutinating antibodies was considered to indicate protection against furunculosis. This was substantiated by Spence *et al.* (1965) in experiments in which coho salmon (*Oncorhynchus kisutch*) had proven protected after intraperitoneal (i.p.) injection of vaccinated trout serum. However, researchers who had observed a protection after oral immunization of fish emphasized that presence of humoral antibodies was not necessary to protection (Klontz and Anderson, 1970). Conversely, Table 2 shows that in spite of high agglutinin titres, some protection experiments remained unsuccessful. It is now well established that while circulating agglutinins may be of interest to allow study of the immune response of salmonids, they do not necessarily directly play a part in the protection mechanism.

Recent Progress Toward the Virulence Mechanisms in Furunculosis

Thirty years after the first attempt at vaccination by Duff, the question of specific protection of fish against furunculosis had not been definitively cleared up, and it became evident that further understanding of the biology of the microorganism and of its relations with the fish were necessary if any further progress was to be achieved. The morphological heterogeneity of *A. salmonicida* had been recognized as early as 1937 when Duff described three types of colonies, of which two at least were regularly observed and called rough (R) and smooth (S), for they strongly resembled the so-called *Salmonella* forms. But the real importance and meaning of this dissociation were not immediately perceived, and most authors seldom specified the kind of strain that they used, until Udey and Fryer (1978) positively demonstrated that the aggregating "R" strains were more virulent than the non-aggregating "S" strains. In contrast with the *Salmonella* for which pathogenicity is related to the lipopolysaccharide (LPS) conformation, a different mechanism was suspected to occur in the case of *A. salmonicida*. In the same publication, Udey and Fryer produced electron micrographs showing the presence of an additional layer at the surface of the aggregating cells. Subsequent studies have confirmed the aggregating character of the virulent strains, and it seems that all the strains isolated from clinical cases belong to this same type.

These findings had a stimulating action on furunculosis research, and during the last few years, a range of new initiatives into the biochemical and structural properties of *A. salmonicida*, and their possible effect on virulence and immunogenicity have been made. Anderson (1973) had tried to extract and compare the LPS production of aggregating and non-aggregating strains. Production was generally better with the non-aggregating forms, for which a carbohydrate analysis revealed a higher number of constituent sugars. But it is difficult to be sure that the extraction method was really convenient for these "R" strains. In any case, the *A. salmonicida* LPS appeared comparable to those of other Gram-negative bacteria. Later, Paterson and Fryer (1974a) studying some biological properties of these components did not find significant differences between *A. salmonicida* and *Escherichia coli* endotoxins. Both exhibited a great toxicity for mice while the fish were more resistant. The *A. salmonicida* LPS was strongly antigenic, and a fair immune response could be observed in fish inoculated with a culture supernatant, demonstrating the release of free endotoxin into the medium. It seems likely that the agglutinating antibodies synthesized by fish during a conventional immunization are principally induced by the antigenic determinants of the endotoxin.

Proteolytic enzymes are widespread among Vibrionaceae. Moreover almost all cases of fish infections involving members of this family are characterized by necrotic lesions of the fins, of the skin and sometimes of the underlying musculature. Then, several authors have suspected that the proteases had a significant role in such pathogenic processes, and there were some trials to isolate and purify these products. With regard to *A. salmonicida*, the first protease study was by Dahle (1971a, b) who described an enzyme synthesized *in vitro* by a non-virulent strain. The molecular weight of this proteinase B was estimated at about 43000 and its production was demonstrated to depend on the medium composition and Shieh and McLean (1975) managed to purify, concentrate and chemically study a specific 11000 molecular weight component, but the biological properties of these products were not reported.

The already indicated additional layer possessed by virulent *A. salmonicida* strains has been named A-layer by Udey and Fryer (1978). These authors assumed that this A-layer was directly correlated to the pathogenic properties of the strains, and established that it was responsible for the attachment of the bacteria to various cells and tissues of the host. The electron-microscopic observation of negatively-stained bacteria has revealed a regular tetrameric arrangement of material surrounding the cells, which does not exist in non-aggregating strains and probably represents the A-layer. Trust *et al.* (1980b) undertook the purification of this material and concluded it was a protein with a molecular weight of 49000, conferring the properties of clumping and cell-adherence. It would be of interest to attempt to establish a relationship between this material and the haem-agglutinating properties exhibited by *A. salmonicida* against several types of red blood cell. The haemagglutinin was destroyed by heating for 5 minutes at 55°C and had a specific affinity for L-fucose and D-mannose (Trust *et al.*, 1980a). Among the biological characters correlated to the additional layer, the susceptibility to different phages has provided a good means for differentiation of virulent and non-virulent strains (Udey and Guzman, 1980). A lysogenic condition could be induced when lytic phages penetrated bacteria having the A-layer.

Another important step was made in the understanding of furunculosis pathogenesis when Fuller *et al.* (1977) claimed that a leucocytolytic factor (LF) had been isolated from a virulent strain. Former investigations had led several workers to postulate the existence of such a factor, and Klontz *et al.* (1966) had given a good description of the leucocyte depletion induced during the course of an experimental disease: after an initial inflammatory response at the site of injection, a gradual diminution of the process, associated with the disappearance of the leucocytes and the necrosis of the leucocytopoietic tissues occurred within 50 hours post-infection. Fuller *et al.* (1977) characterized the LF as a glycoprotein of 100,000 to 300,000 molecular weight, and studied its leucocytic activity in rainbow trout. It was found that this extract, simultaneously injected into fish with a non-virulent strain, greatly enhanced the pathogenicity of the bacteria. Precipitins could be detected using gel-diffusion tests, after immunization of rabbits or trout with this substance.

Munro *et al.* (1980) used the cellophane overlay technique to grow a virulent strain of *A. salmonicida* and harvest its soluble extracellular products (ECP). This preparation had several biological effects, including proteolytic activity, lecithinase activity, haemolysis of rabbit and trout erythrocytes and cytolytic action for RTG cells or leucocytes of fish. Parenteral injection of the product to rainbow trout produced a lethal condition, with the general signs of furunculosis, including furuncle formation at the site of injection when the intramuscular (i.m.) route was used. Ellis *et al.* (1981) have given a histopathological description of the induced lesions and concluded that ECP could account for almost all of the clinico-pathological features of furunculosis. A neutralizing activity was detected in normal trout serum, and the authors have suggested that in cases of fatal furunculosis, some mechanisms, perhaps involving histamine release by activated eosinophilic cells, could paralyse the host defences. It is probable that ECP contains several components, including a protease and a leucocytolytic factor.

A recent thesis (Cipriano, 1980) also reports the production of extracellular factors (ECF) which were fractionated and studied for their properties. Two of these fractions could reproduce the furuncle lesions, and one was considered similar to the leucocytolytic factor of Fuller. The presently known extracellular substances are listed in Table 3, with their main characteristics. It must be kept in mind that in most cases, these substances have not been chemically analysed, and many effects may be produced by one substance.

Some very recent vaccination attempts are worth reporting. W. D. Paterson (unpublished observations) compared the respective efficacy of virulent and non-virulent strains of *A. salmonicida* in immunizing and, using a bath challenge, found a better protection when the bacterin was prepared from virulent bacteria. Cipriano (1980) could confer some protection with a fraction of his extracellular factor. B. Austin (unpublished observations) obtained an interesting result during a field experiment. The vaccine consisted of killed bacteria associated to a toxoid prepared from the ECP defined by Munro *et al.* (1980). The oral administration of this complex afforded significant protection against natural furunculosis outbreaks.

Further Investigations: The Questions to be Solved

Forty years of attempts to immunize fish populations against furunculosis have not resulted in the launching of a commercial bacterin, and though many data have been gathered, authors have obtained variable success in vaccination experiments. In such a situation, certain questions can be

Table 3. Properties of the soluble factors presently identified from *Aeromonas salmonicida* cultures

Factors	Chemical nature	Molecular weight	Type of strains	Role in virulence	Immuno-genicity	Possibility for protection
Free-endotoxin	Lipopoly-saccharide		All strains	Toxic (mammals) Slightly toxic (fish)	+	+
Protease Proteinase B	Proteins	11000 43000	? Non-virulent	Proteolytic	?	?
A-layer	Protein	49000	Virulent	Attachment hemagglutination (?)	Slight	?
Leucocytolytic factor (LF)	Glycoprotein	100–300000	Virulent	Leucocytic	+	?
Extracellular product (ECP)	Complex		All strains	Cytolytic Proteolytic Lipolytic Toxic	+	+
Extracellular factor (ECF)	Complex (3 fractions)		All strains	Toxic (Virulent strains)	+	+

asked, from which three seem to be of particular consequence. Is there really a protective immune response in furunculosis? If so, how to detect it in fish? And what kind of vaccine could be the best, both for its efficacy and its practical interest?

Protective Immunity in Furunculosis

The heterogeneity of the results obtained in furunculosis vaccination experiments has been emphasized. It is difficult to compare and explain the discrepancies in Tables 1 and 2, because the experimental conditions always differed. Salmonid species, administration routes, use of adjuvants, experimental facilities and water quality could vary, as well as the challenge method. Some workers have tried to explain the great diversity of experimental results by supposing that in furunculosis the induced protection is very weak, and that a "subtle" challenge technique is needed to detect it. According to this opinion, the protective immunity would be real, but slight. The question of the challenge technique will be discussed later. It can be noted that the high amounts of agglutinins observed when fish are intraperitoneally (i.p.) or intramuscularly (i.m.) injected reveal a strong stimulation of the general defence mechanisms, and that if such general defences were involved in furunculosis protection, it would be easily detected. The immune status of fish surviving natural outbreaks of furunculosis could provide some interesting data concerning this problem.

It has been known for a long time that fish which recover from a furunculosis infection generally reach a carrier status (McCraw, 1952). The location of the bacteria in the fish tissues remains enigmatic, but their persistence can be demonstrated using a stress technique described by Bullock and Stuckey (1975). Direct isolation of the bacteria is very uncertain, and a noticeable feature is the low level or absence of agglutinating antibodies, which restricts the value of serological diagnosis. Experimental work conducted in our laboratory (unpublished observations) has shown that when rainbow trout (*Salmo gairdneri*) were injected i.m. with a virulent strain of *A. salmonicida*, it was not possible to observe high titres of agglutinins in the surviving fish. Even when low doses were used in repeated infections, fish did not exhibit antibodies (Table 4). However, fish which had been treated with an antimicrobial drug during the course of the disease exhibited agglutinating antibodies. It seems that the ability of fish to elicit a general immune response to furunculosis requires very large amounts of bacteria, as when fatal septicaemia occurs or when a bacterin is parenterally injected. Conversely, a limited infection developing in a local area of the body could be overcome, but without stimulation of the systemic defences.

Table 4. Failure in detection of agglutinins in 70g rainbow trout fingerlings repeatedly infected with mild doses of a virulent *Aeromonas salmonicida* strain

Serology			Experimental infections		
Number of positive sera	Maximum agglutinating titre	Time (days)	Infective dose	% mortality	Surviving fish
0/24	<40	0	1000 b, i.m.	42	14/24
1/14	80	30	1000 b, i.m.	36	9/14
1/9	40	60	1000 b, i.m.	33	6/9
0/6	<40	90			

This lack of circulating antibodies could correlate with a lack of protection involving general defences, as it appears in Table 4 that no significant differences were found between the three successive infections involving the same fish. If this is the case, then the main consequence would be the susceptibility of trout to furunculosis throughout their life, even after previous contacts with the pathogenic agent, and indeed, recurrent attacks of the disease have been observed in fish-culture raceways! The leuco-cytolytic factor of Fuller *et al.* (1977) could properly account for such a paralysis of immune functions, inasmuch as its activity was demonstrated to occur very early, before the infection spread to the whole organism (Klontz *et al.*, 1966). Ferguson and McCarthy (1978) did not observe *in vivo* the destructive cell lesions formerly found *in vitro* and questioned whether LF was really involved in furunculosis pathogenesis. Ellis *et al.* (1981) for their part considered its action was likely, although they also did not observe cytolytic changes in experimentally infected fish. Possibly, LF could impair the cellular functions before it exerts a destructive effect on cellular structures, thus neutralizing the immune system even in the absence of detectable lesions.

The depletion of immune competence during the disease does not mean that it is impossible to immunize fish, using purified antigens or inactivated bacterins. The production of agglutinating antibodies supports this opinion. But when challenging the fish, the virulent strain of *A. salmonicida* will also produce the leucocytolytic substance. Unless protection comes into play at the very beginning of the infection, that is during the time of local proliferation of the bacteria, the consequences for the fish are serious. It may be felt, in conclusion, that the question of the protective immunity in furunculosis is not quite clear, and that if a specific protection indeed occurs, it must include a fundamental local component.

Choice of a Challenge Technique

The easiest and most reliable method of checking the efficacy of a vaccination procedure consists in reproducing the disease under controlled conditions and comparing the losses in treated and untreated animals. With regard to furunculosis, a great many techniques have been described but, due to the difficulties encountered in creating reproducible infections and to the heterogeneity of the reported results, there is no agreement among the authors to suggest the use of a particular method. Two kinds of technique have been generally developed depending on whether the parental or the bath route were preferred for infecting the fish. Both have their respective advantages and disadvantages.

Parenteral routes of infection require virulent strains of *A. salmonicida* from which the pathogenicity can be previously estimated in terms of lethal doses (LD50). It is possible to inject, both i.m. or i.p., a known dose of bacteria and to produce an expected effect in fish. If the experimental facilities allow a good control of the environmental conditions, the standardization of a model of infection can be achieved (Michel, 1980). Such a model will enable statistically valuable studies using a minimal number of fish, but some workers have pointed out that its efficacy and its severe toxic character are not suitable if a limited protection has to be demonstrated. Another and more serious criticism concerns the full significance of the model, which lies in the artificial introduction of bacteria into the fish, which allows them to avoid the crucial phase of penetration. If local specific or non-specific mechanisms are involved in protection against furunculosis, this aspect of the response will remain unaccounted for in such studies.

At the opposite extreme, the bath challenge techniques do appear milder in their effect and necessitate the penetration of the pathogen agent through a natural route of infection. They thus resemble in their pathogenesis the natural furunculosis, and in certain cases, natural furunculosis itself has been taken as a challenge test, the vaccinated fish being exposed in field conditions. Table 5 affords an example of the problems associated with statistical analysis, of the results of bath infection experiments. The recorded mortalities at the end of the experiment were in no way correlated with the concentration of bacteria added to the water. At the highest dose level, the entrance of bacteria into fish was probably effective in every case, since the losses occurred in less than 10 days as is usual with parenteral injection. In the other batches, losses were delayed, and it seems that secondary infections were mainly responsible for the mortality. So, the results can differ between similarly treated groups of fish, and unless there is a large number of experimental batches, it is hazardous to attribute to them a quantitative value.

There is then, presently, no reliable system for detection of immune protection against furunculosis in fish. A lot of precautions must be taken when experimenting with animals, and it would be very valuable if there were less cumbersome methods. It is to be hoped that the studies concerning the basic understanding of general and local immunity in fish currently under way will provide some immunological tests, easy to use, which correlate with the protection exhibited by vaccinated animals. If this happens a major problem would be solved!

Table 5. Experimental infection of 4g rainbow trout using a virulent *A. salmonicida* (TG 51/79) administered in water at different concentrations. (Water temperature 16°C)

Batches	I (inoculated control)	II	III	IV	V
Doses	2000 b i.m.	$1.5 \times 10^4\,\mathrm{ml}^{-1}$ (1 hour)	$1.5 \times 10^5\,\mathrm{ml}^{-1}$ (1 hour)	$1.5 \times 10^6\,\mathrm{ml}^{-1}$ (1 hour)	$1.5 \times 10^7\,\mathrm{ml}^{-1}$ (1 hour)
Number of fish	30	30	30	30	30
Mortalities					
10th day	30	1	4	0	30
20th day	30	4	20	1	30
Per cent	100	13	67	3	100

What Kind of Vaccine?

It has been indicated that up to now, vaccination experiments have almost invariably used inactivated bacterial suspensions. These experiments have failed to lead to the production of a commercialized bacterin, and there is some doubt as to whether any successful vaccine will be produced from a killed bacterin. Three types of vaccine are presently known in other animal diseases: killed bacterins, live modified vaccines and purified antigens. Live attenuated vaccines have been experimented with occasionally in fish, especially in viral infections, but such a vaccine does not appear suitable for preventing furunculosis. The non-virulent strains of *A. salmonicida* do not express such good immunogenic properties as virulent strains, and the stability of the non-pathogenic state is far from being ascertained, particularly *in vivo*. The diversity of the virulent factors synthesized by *A. salmonicida* increases the risk of mutation or of induction for their production, thus rendering the use of live strains very hazardous in field conditions.

Purified antigens consist of preparations containing the main antigenic fractions of the microorganism but devoid of toxic or undesirable substances. The recent interest of many researchers in the antigenic and structural analysis of *A. salmonicida* should bring the data needed to allow a sub-unit preparation which could represent the ideal route to successful furunculosis vaccination. For the present time, however, all of this work has concerned the comprehension of the virulence and immune mechanisms. The techniques for the extraction and purification of antigens are generally sophisticated, and it is not certain that they could be produced economically or applied on an industrial scale. An interesting option could be the production of toxoids, as suggested by the preliminary results of B. Austin and co-workers (unpublished results). Toxoids are known to be easily obtained using physical or chemical agents like formalin and to induce a very strong protective immunity. The protein nature of certain of the factors associated with the virulence of *A. salmonicida* certainly suggests the possibility of the production of such preparations. It should be possible to neutralize the toxic action of the substances excreted by the bacteria and to support the natural defences of the host. The neutralization of the leucocytolytic factor could be of particular interest: possibly the production of a toxoid prepared from LF and associated to an inactivated bacterin would permit the expression of the protective immunity whose existence has been so much debated.

Finally, even if a really efficacious vaccine became available, some questions would still have to be settled concerning its practical use such as the ideal administration route, addition of adjuvant substances and the possibility of association with other specific vaccines. In the present state of our knowledge, further investigations are certainly needed before there is available an efficacious and practically usable vaccine. Three directions of research seem to be of prior interest: recognition and purification of the immunogenic fractions of the bacterium, comprehensive study of the local mechanisms of specific defences in fish, and improvement or design of quantifiable and reliable challenge methods or immunological tests in order to measure the degree of protection of fish. Only the first point appears presently to have good prospects of achievement. Retrospectively, a large part of previous work seems to have proceeded on purely empirical methods. These results have played a decisive role in the choice of new trends in furunculosis research, but it is to be hoped that future research will be based on more rational understanding of the basic problems posed by this highly significant pathogen.

References

Amend, D. F. and Fender, D. (1976). Uptake of bovine serum albumin by rainbow trout from hyperosmotic solutions: a model for vaccinating fish. *Science* **192**, 793–794.

Anderson, D. P. (1972). Investigations of the lipopolysaccharide fractions from *Aeromonas salmonicida* smooth and rough forms. *In* "Symposium on the Major Communicable Fish Diseases in Europe and Their Control". FI: EIFAC, 72/SC II — *Symposium* **20**.

Anderson, D. P. and Klontz, G. W. (1970). Precipitating antibody against *Aeromonas salmonicida* in serum of inbred albino rainbow trout. *Journal of the Fisheries Research Board of Canada* **27**, 1389–1393.

Antipa, R. and Amend, D. F. (1977). Immunization of Pacific Salmon: comparison of intraperitoneal injection and hyperosmotic infiltration of *Vibrio anguillarum* and *Aeromonas salmonicida* bacterins. *Journal of the Fisheries Research Board of Canada* **34**, 203–208.

Bullock, G. L. and Stuckey, H. M. (1975). *Aeromonas salmonicida*: detection of asymptomatically infected trout. *Progressive Fish Culturist* **37** (4), 237–239.

Cipriano, R. C. (1980). An analysis of the extracellular growth products of *Aeromonas salmonicida* as virulence factors and potential immunogens. Ph.D. Thesis, Department of Biological Sciences, Fordham University, New York.

Corbel, M. J. (1975). The immune response in fish: a review. *Journal of Fish Biology* **7**, 539–563.

Dahle, H. K. (1971a). The purification and some properties of two *Aeromonas* proteinases. *Acta Pathologica et Microbiologica Scandinavica (Section B)* **79**, 726–738.

Dahle, H. K. (1971b). Regulation of the proteinase production in two strains of *Aeromonas*. *Acta Pathologica et Microbiologica Scandinavica (Section B)* **79**, 739–746.

Dorson, M., Torchy, C. and Michel, C. (1979). Rainbow trout complement fixation used for titration of antibodies against several pathogens. *Annales de Recherches Vétérinaires* **10** (4), 529–534.

Duff, D. C. B. (1937). Dissociation in *Bacillus salmonicida*, with special reference to the appearance of a G form of culture. *Journal of Bacteriology* **34**, 49–67.

Duff, D. C. B. (1942). The oral immunization of trout against *Bacterium salmonicida*. *Journal of Immunology* **44** (1), 87–94.

Ellis, A. E., Hastings, T. S. and Munro, A. L. S. (1981). The role of *Aeromonas salmonicida* extracellular products in the pathology of furunculosis. *Journal of Fish Diseases* **4**, 41–51.

Emmerich, R. and Weibel, E. (1894). Uber eine durch Bakterien erzeugte Seuche unter den Forellen. *Archive für Hygiene* **21**, 1–24.

Ferguson, H. W. and McCarthy, D. H. (1978). Histopathology of furunculosis in brown trout *Salmo trutta* L. *Journal of Fish Diseases* **1**, 165–174.

Frost, G. D. (1968). Oral immunization for possible control of furunculosis in fish. M.Sc. Thesis, Oregon State University. Corvallis, U.S.A.

Fuller, D. W., Pilcher, K. S. and Fryer, J. L. (1977). A leucocytolytic factor isolated from cultures of *Aeromonas salmonicida*. *Journal of the Fisheries Research Board of Canada* **34**, 1118–1125.

Hara, T. and Inoue, K. (1976). Vaccination trials for control of furunculosis of Salmonids in Japan. *Fish Pathology* **10** (2), 227–235.

Herman, R. L. (1968). Fish furunculosis 1952–1966. *Transactions of the American Fisheries Society* **97**, 221–230.

Kimura, T. (1970). Studies on a bacterial disease occurring in the adult "Sukuramasu" (*Oncorhynchus masou*) and pink salmon (*O. gorbuscha*) reared for maturity. *Scientific reports of the Hokkaïdo Salmon Hatchery* no. 24, 9–100.

Klontz, G. W. and Anderson, D. P. (1968). Fluorescent antibody studies of *Aeromonas salmonicida*. *Bulletin de l'Office International des Epizootics* **69**, 1149–1157.

Klontz, G. W. and Anderson, D. P. (1970). Oral immunization of Salmonids: a review. *In* "A Symposium of Diseases of Fishes and Shellfishes. Special Publication No. 5, pp.16–20. American Fisheries Society, Washington D.C.

Klontz, G. W., Yasutake, W. T. and Ross, A. J. (1966). Bacterial diseases of the Salmonidae in the western United States: Pathogenesis of Furunculosis in rainbow trout. *American Journal of Veterinary Research* **27** (120), 1455–1460.

Krantz, G. E., Reddecliff, J. M. and Heist, C. E. (1963). Development of antibodies against *Aeromonas salmonicida* in trout. *Journal of Immunology* **91** (6), 757–760.

McCarthy, D. H. (1978). A study of the taxonomic status of some bacteria currently assigned to the genus *Aeromonas*. Ph.D. Thesis, Council of National Academic Awards, Great Britain.

McCarthy, D. H. and Roberts, R. J. (1980). Furunculosis of fish. The present state of our knowledge. *In* "Advances in Aquatic Microbiology." (Eds. M. R. Droop and H. W. Jannasch), Vol. 2, pp.293–341. Academic Press, London.

McCraw, B. M. (1952). Furunculosis of fish. U.S. Fish and Wildlife Service, Special Scientific Report: Fisheries no. 84, 87pp.

McInnes, J. I., Trust, T. J. and Crosa, J. H. (1979). Deoxyribonucleic acid relationships among members of the genus *Aeromonas*. *Canadian Journal of Microbiology* **25**, 579–586.

Michel, C. (1979). Furunculosis of Salmonids: vaccination attempts in rainbow trout (*Salmo gairdneri*) by formalin-killed germs. *Annales de Recherches Vétérinaires* **10** (1), 33–40.

Michel, C. (1980). A standardized model of experimental furunculosis in rainbow trout (*Salmo gairdneri*). *Canadian Journal of Fisheries and Aquatic Sciences* **37**, 746–750.

Munro, A. L. S., Hastings, T. S., Ellis, A. E. and Liversidge, J. (1980). Studies on an ichthyotoxic material produced extracellularly by the furunculosis bacterium *Aeromonas salmonicida*. *In* "Fish Diseases." 3rd COPRAQ Session, (Ed. W. Ahne), pp.98–106. Springer Verlag, Berlin.

Palmer, R. and Smith, P. R. (1980). Studies on vaccination of Atlantic salmon against furunculosis. *In* "Fish Diseases." 3rd COPRAQ Session (Ed. W. Ahne), pp.107–112. Springer Verlag, Berlin.

Paterson, W. D. and Fryer, J. L. (1974a). Effect of temperature and antigen dose on the antibody response of juvenile coho salmon (*Oncorhynchus kisutch*) to *Aeromonas salmonicida* endotoxin. *Journal of the Fisheries Research Board of Canada* **31**, 1743–1749.

Paterson, W. D. and Fryer, J. L. (1974b). Immune response of juvenile coho salmon (*Oncorhynchus kisutch*) to *Aeromonas salmonicida* cells administered intraperitoneally in Freund's complete adjuvant. *Journal of the Fisheries Research Board of Canada* **31**, 1751–1755.

Paterson, W. D., Douey, D. and Desautels, D. (1980). Relationships between selected strains of typical and atypical *Aeromonas salmonicida*, *Aeromonas hydrophila* and *Haemophilus piscium*. *Canadian Journal of Microbiology* **26**, 588–598.

Shieh, H. S. and McLean, J. R. (1975). Purification and properties of an extracellular protease of *Aeromonas salmonicida*, the causative agent of furunculosis. *International Journal of Biochemistry* **6**, 653–656.

Smith, P. D., McCarthy, D. H. and Paterson, W. D. (1980). Further studies on furunculosis vaccination. *In* "Fish Diseases." 3rd COPRAQ Session (Ed. W. Ahne), pp.113–119. Springer Verlag, Berlin.

Snieszko, S. F. and Friddle, S. B. (1949). Prophylaxis of furunculosis in brook trout (*Salvelinus fontinalis*) by oral immunization and sulfamerazine. *Progressive Fish Culturist* **11**, 161–168.

Spence, K. D., Fryer, J. L. and Pilcher, K. S. (1965). Active and passive immunization of certain salmonid fishes against *Aeromonas salmonicida*. *Canadian Journal of Microbiology* **11**, 397–405.

Trust, T. J., Courtice, I. D. and Atkinson, H. M. (1980a). Haemagglutination properties of *Aeromonas*. *In* "Fish Diseases", 3rd COPRAQ Session, (Ed. W. Ahne), pp.218–223. Springer Verlag, Berlin.

Trust, T. J., Howard, P. S., Chamberlain, J. B., Ishiguro, E. E. and Buckley, J. T. (1980b). Additional surface protein in autoaggregating strains of atypical *Aeromonas salmonicida*. *FEMS Microbiology Letters* **9**, 35–38.

Udey, L. R. and Fryer, J. L. (1978). Immunization of fish with bacterins of *Aeromonas salmonicida*. *Marine Fisheries Review* **40** (3), 12–17.

Udey, L. R. and Guzman, R. (1980). Temperate and lytic bacteriophages specific for a virulence factor of *Aeromonas salmonicida*. Abstracts for the annual meeting of the American Society for Microbiology, B 78.

9

The Pathogenicity of
Vibrio Anguillarum (Bergman)

MICHAEL T. HORNE

*Department of Biology and Institute of Aquaculture,
University of Stirling, Stirling, Scotland, U.K.*

Introduction

Vibriosis of fish was described by Bonaveri in 1718 (see Hofer, 1904). The causative agent was first isolated by Canestrini (1893) and named *Bacillus anguillarum* from its source, the eel *Anguilla anguilla*. The present name *Vibrio anguillarum* derives from the detailed description of the pathology and bacteriology of the disease given by Bergman (1909) since which time it has become one of the most intensively studied of the bacterial diseases of fish and one of the few such diseases for which acceptably effective vaccines are available commercially (Hayashi *et al.*, 1964; Fryer *et al.*, 1978; Harrel, 1978; Amend and Eshenour, 1980; Amend and Johnson, 1981). Descriptions of its pathology and epidemiology are to be found in a number of sources (Håstein, 1975; Muroga, 1975; Roberts, 1978).

The Causative Organism

Vibrio anguillarum (Bergman) is one of the halophilic group of vibrios and has two major biotypes which have been recognized by a number of epithets by different authors. Both are capable of çausing disease (Evelyn, 1971; Harrel *et al.*, 1976; Ohnishi and Muroga, 1977; Schiewe *et al.*, 1977; Baumann *et al.*, 1978; Ezura *et al.*, 1980). It has been proposed by Schiewe (1981) that the consistent taxonomic differences between these two taxa warrant formal designation as two separate species, *Vibrio anguillarum*, Bergman (previously phenon or biotype I) and *Vibrio ordalii*, Schiewe (previously phenon or biotype II).

The many distinct serotypes determined by agglutination studies with thermostable (O) antigens, appear to cross this taxonomic boundary.

Table 1. The serotypes of *Vibrio anguillarum* (from Ezura *et al.*, 1980)

Serotype	NCMB Number	Pacha and Kiehn (1969)	Harrel (1969)	Johnsen (1977)	Strout *et al.* (1978)	Kitao (1975)	Kusuda (1975)	Ezura (1980)
1	—	Group I	—	—	—	—	—	—
2	6,829	Group II	Type II	Group I	569 Group	A	1	J-O-1
3	1,336	Group III	—	Group III	507 Group	—	—	—
4	571,813	—	Type I	Group II	775A Group	C	111	J-O-3
5	—	—	—	—	—	B	11	J-O-2

Serological studies have been made by Cisar and Fryer, 1969; Pacha and Kiehn, 1969; Fryer *et al.*, 1972; Conroy and Withnell, 1974; Harrel *et al.*, 1976; Egidius and Anderson, 1977; Johnsen, 1977; Schiewe and Hodgins, 1977; Strout *et al.*, 1978; Gould *et al.*, 1980; Ezura *et al.*, 1980; Johnson, 1980; Kitao *et al.*, 1982. Although each author uses his own terminology, the comparative study of Ezura *et al.* (1980) makes it possible to determine some of the interrelationships between these strains (Table 1). Four main serotypes are evident of which types 2 and 4 are common to both Japan and North America. Types 3 (American) and 5 (Japanese) are either differential or sufficiently rare in the corresponding areas as to be absent from the samples taken. Kitao *et al.* (1982) report three further, but rare serotypes at frequencies of 1% and 0.4%. There is no evidence to indicate the existence of ecological boundaries or specific host preferences between serotypic types; all of the major groups are found in both marine and freshwater isolates and they each also occur in many species of fish. In the japanese isolates, Ezura's types J-O-1 and J-O-2 are approximately equal in the species *Vibrio anguillarum*, but *Vibrio ordalii* contains only type J-O-1 (Table 2). The necessity of establishing which serotypes are the predominant disease strains in particular areas in order to formulate vaccines which are neither wasteful, by including unnecessary phenotypes, or ineffective, through failure to include locally important strains, has caused a number of laboratories to initiate intensive serological surveys and more comprehensive data should soon be available.

Table 2. The distribution of serotypes between the two pathogenic fish *Vibrio* species in Japanese isolates (from Ezura *et al.*, 1980)

Species	Serotypes	Percentage
Vibrio anguillarum	J-O-1	59
(Bergman)	J-O-2	6.5
	J-O-3	56
Vibrio ordalii	J-O-1	100
(Schiewe)	J-O-2	0
	J-O-3	0

Occurrence of Vibriosis

A very wide range of tropical and temperate farmed fish are affected by the disease. In Japan and in parts of North America and Europe it is the most economically damaging infectious disease of cultured marine fish (Rucker *et al.*, 1953; Mattheis, 1964; Kusuda, 1966; Muroga, 1975) and it also occurs widely in freshwater cultured species (Hacking and Budd, 1971; Muroga and Egusa, 1970; Muroga *et al.*, 1976). Although taxonomically grouped with the halophilic vibrios and generally considered to be a marine organism, experimental work is frequently carried out in rainbow trout (*Salmo gairdneri*) in fresh or brackish water (Saito *et al.*, 1964; Baudin-Laurencin and Tangtrongpiros, 1980; Agius *et al.*, 1982). No apparent differences have been found in the pathology or virulence of the disease when marine and freshwater models have been compared.

If fish are maintained under conditions of good husbandry — water quality is good, stocking densities are not excessive and the diet is properly balanced — microbially induced diseases are rare. When fish are stressed, at certain stages of maturity or when they are transported and subjected to certain management procedures, but above all when water quality or quantity is poor, then the disease frequently appears (Roberts and Shepherd, 1974). When the disease has become established, even if the conditions which favoured it are reversed, it may continue to spread, having established sufficient numbers to maintain infectivity. These statements, in general, apply to a large proportion of animal diseases but from where, in the case of vibriosis, does the infective agent come? The answers proposed to this by previous workers fall into two main groups. Firstly, that the disease arises from a change in the balance between the host and the bacteria, which normally exist commensally as part of the indigenous microflora, but are able to exploit the lowered fitness of the host. Secondly, that the disease strains are more specifically infectious agents, transmitted from one infected population to another and, although closely related to, are distinct from the commensals.

As long ago as 1911, Plehn (Plehn, 1911; Arkwright, 1912) described latent carriers as playing an important role in the epizootiology of furunculosis (*Aeromonas* spp.). Whenever the natural gut and skin microflora of healthy fish have been described, large numbers of different strains of bacteria from species known to be important in causing disease have been isolated. From freshwater fish these are mostly of the genera *Pseudomonas* and *Aeromonas* whereas in marine isolates *Vibrio* spp. are more frequent (Thjøtta and Sømme, 1943; Evelyn and McDermott, 1961; Mattheis, 1964; Horsley, 1973; Yoshimizu *et al.*, 1976; Yoshimizu and Kimura, 1976). Biochemical characterization of the vibrio component of such microfloras and especially of those from the natural "non-fish" marine environment causes the majority of them to be relegated to the ill-defined category of "non-specific" marine vibrios or marine aeromonads within which new taxa are gradually being defined (Lee *et al.*, 1981). Only a small proportion of these isolates are clear-cut unambiguous members of *Vibrio anguillarum* or *Vibrio ordalii*.

Nevertheless, this small component may be a reservoir of potential pathogens. In order to determine whether these commensals have a latent ability to cause disease in stressed fish or whether they are pathogenic when administered in high doses we took a number of young salmon (*Salmo salar*) cultured in seawater and sampled the microflora of the posterior gut without harming the fish. From the isolates, strains which were identified biochemically as *Vibrio anguillarum* were cultured and reinjected intramuscularly, at a high dose, into individuals of the salmon population from which they had been isolated. Eight bacterial strains were used in this way on different batches of ten fish each; duplicate batches of fish, previously inoculated with cortisone, were treated in the same way. In no case did disease ensue; similarly, negative results were obtained with the same strains injected into rainbow trout (*Salmo gairdneri*).

On the other hand, when bacteria are isolated from the lymphoid organs of moribund fish during an outbreak of vibriosis, pure cultures of strains which are mostly readily assignable to one or other of the two bacterial species are easily obtained. When reinjected these strains usually initiate disease in the same host species. Where more than one host species is involved, the picture is less clear. Strout *et al.* (1978) found that from a total of 81 isolates from confinement-reared salmonids, 42% were pathogenic for coho salmon (*Oncorhynchus kisutch*) compared with only 5% of the vibrios recovered from moribund feral fish. From a total of 29 isolates from moribund cultured fish, 22 proved pathogenic when reinjected into healthy fish. These results may be a consequence of host-range specificity. Egidius and Andersen (1978) showed that *Vibrio anguillarum* strains isolated from salmonids are pathogenic to salmonids but only to a very low degree to saithe (*Pollachius virens*). Conversely, strains isolated from diseased saithe were pathogenic when injected into healthy saithe, but non-pathogenic to the salmonids.

The extent of this phenomenon is not yet apparent. Many of the vibrio strains used in experimental work have been studied in hosts from which they were not originally isolated and it is to be expected that a range of host tolerances, from those with a very restricted range to those which show very little host specificity, may well be uncovered by more detailed work. Its significance for the epidemiology of vibriosis will depend on these findings. On the one hand it may act as a barrier to infection which lowers the likelihood of cultured stocks being infected from wild populations; on the other, the commensals of one fish species may be the pathogens of another. Further, there is always the possibility of laboratory artefacts. Subculturing on artificial laboratory media, even once, can impair the pathogenicity of some microorganisms particularly where adhesion is an important component of the pathogenicity (Gibbons and Houte, 1975; Smith, 1977) and a gradual loss of virulence, through repeated subculture, is common.

Despite the ambiguity and scarcity of the evidence it is still widely held that the commensal strains of *Vibrio* sp. found in healthy fish are a common origin of disease outbreaks either in their own host or another species.

The second philosophy is that vibriosis is to be considered more as an infectious disease and that the disease-causing variants are a small and genetically different portion of the population. Any contact with the marine environment, such as the maturing of freshwater bred fish in seawater, exposes populations to the ubiquitous marine vibrios including this potentially pathogenic component. Initiation of infection from the natural environment is complemented by such sources as, for example, the feeding of poorly processed, vibrio-contaminated fish offal to farmed fish (Rucker, 1959; Ross *et al.*, 1968), transmission by sea-birds of the disease from an infected farm to a neighbouring clean facility or non-observance of routine quarantine procedures. The debate is not so much the mode of transmission of the disease, as the origin of the disease strains. If they are variants of the normal marine microflora which are genetically predisposed to pathogenicity (see below) their relative rarity in environmental and gut samples may indicate a lower fitness than the more commonly isolated types. The extent to which isolates from diseased animals have a 'typical' *Vibrio anguillarum* biochemistry must be seen in the context that this definition of the species has been derived mainly from disease isolates (Kiehn and Pacha, 1969; Evelyn, 1971; Håstein and Smith, 1977; Hendrie *et al.*, 1971; McCarthy *et al.*, 1974; Kusuda *et al.*, 1979) and may simply be defining those groupings of biochemical pathways which, while they favour the strain when it is growing in a fish host, are not the fittest types in the natural environment. This would lead to an incorrect definition of the true species since it is centred on only a small part of the variation curve, not necessarily the modal characteristics. The consequences of this would be consistent with the taxonomic information currently presented for *Vibrio anguillarum*. Further taxonomic studies should show whether this is indeed so and whether the typical *Vibrio anguillarum* strains isolated from diseased animals differ sufficiently from the broader groups of marine vibrios to justify a separate taxonomic status (as at present) or whether pathogenicity and its associated biochemical syndrome is simply a part of the variation pattern of a much larger species whose modal properties are not yet fully described.

It is probable that both types of pathogenesis—the breakdown of commensalism and the infectious spread of specific pathogens—are part of the epidemiology of vibriosis. Outbreaks of disease may arise from the random conjunction of a susceptible host and a pathogenic strain in the environment or from the failure of an individual to suppress a commensal strain which may be potentially pathogenic or which may mutate to pathogenicity and whose offspring, as they multiply, are subjected to genetic selection and improvement in their ability to grow in that host species. Their increased numbers and virulence then favour infectious spread.

Route of Entry into the Host

When a few individuals in a farm facility become infected the environment rapidly becomes heavily contaminated—the water, mud and especially filters are rich sources of vibrios. Infected individuals secrete live, infective bacteria in their faeces and possibly, also, through abdominal pores (Bridge, 1879; Bles, 1898; George *et al.*, 1982). The mode of transmission from one individual to another is not clear. The ingestion of infected particulate matter, especially faeces, and the intake of bacteria through a number of sites on the body surface are the two obvious categories.

Infection by the ingestion of bacteria is difficult to demonstrate experimentally and the very high numbers which can be administered without producing disease leave doubt as to whether this route of entry is of significance in the natural spread of disease. A number of workers have included live, oral challenges in their tests of the efficacy of vaccines. Invariably these have been less effective and consistent than other forms of challenge carried out concurrently. For example Baudin-Laurencin and Tangtrongpiros (1980) found that 6.7×10^{10} viable cells administered orally in the diet daily for 5 days killed only four fish (*Salmo gairdneri*) from a total of 142. Previously 1.3×10^4 viable cells, injected intraperitoneally, had killed 34% of the fish in 15 days. We have found that the introduction directly into the stomach by catheter of a dose of pathogenic vibrio thirty times stronger than that which which gave 80% mortality in 2 days when administered intraperitoneally, produced no evidence of disease. The acidity of the stomach may be a factor in reducing the number of viable cells which pass to the gut, but Chart and Munn (1980) introduced viable cells directly into the foregut and rectum of eels (*Anguilla anguilla*) but still failed to establish infection. Cells of the same strain when given either intraperitoneally or intramuscularly resulted in rapid and high rates of mortality.

In order to remove some of the artificiality of injected challenges from their experiments without resorting to the unpredictability of purely natural challenge, many authors have successfully employed bath challenges, where fish are immersed in solutions containing viable cells in suspension (Croy and Amend, 1977; Schiewe and Hodgins, 1977; Gould *et al.*, 1979; Harbell *et al.*, 1979; Amend and Johnson, 1980). The route of entry of cells in such baths and of antigens similarly administered during vaccinations has been widely studied. R. W. Ament and Fender (1977), using the hyperosmotic infiltration method to administer bovine serum albumin concluded that the main portal of entry was the lateral line system of the fish. The other possibly important adsorptive surface, the gills, was thought not to be significant. In order to differentiate uptake by the lateral line system from uptake by the gills, Alexander *et al.* (1981) immersed only the anterior (head and gills) or the posterior (body and lateral line) in separate experiments. They concluded that the gill and not the lateral line was the main port of entry for the *Escherichia coli*, whole cells, which they used as tracers. When gill lamellae were removed from the fish and tested separately, *in vitro*, bacteria were shown to be absorbed by them and passed to the blood stream. Negative results were obtained with skin sections. The use of a hyperosmotic pretreatment (D. F. Amend and Fender, 1976; Fender and Amend, 1978) which causes small haemorrhages on the gill surface, enhanced the uptake. Evidence was also given to indicate that oral ingestion of bacteria during the head immersion was not significant to the results. Thus, although the route of entry has not been investigated with respect to disease transmission *per se*, it is probable that oral ingestion or infection through minor skin abrasions are not the major routes of infection, but that the gill surface may well be.

The Pathogenesis of Vibriosis

The pathogenesis of infections by many of the enterobacteriaceae and vibrionaceae, particularly *Escherichia* and *Vibrio* has been extensively studied in mammalian situations and, in view of the close relationships and genes held in common by these groups, it is worth considering to what extent this information is applicable to vibriosis in fish.

The environment of the host is essentially hostile to would-be invasive microbes even in the absence of specific, immune protective mechanisms. Of particular interest in the case of the pathogenicity of the enterobacteriaceae, is the ability to proliferate in the conditions of low free-iron concentration found in animal tissues (Bullen *et al.*, 1978). The greater part of the iron content of living tissues is locked up in ferritin, haemosiderin, myoglobin and haemoglobin (Lanskowsky, 1976) and is not freely available to bacteria. The amount of residual, free iron is far too low for bacterial growth and the iron-binding proteins transferrin and lactoferrin, which have a very high affinity for iron, hold even this amount in equilibrium, while themselves remaining unsaturated. This passive role of the proteins in making the host-tissue environment unsuitable for growth is complemented by positive mechanisms of protection since there is evidence that they also play an essential role in the bacteriocidal activity of polymorphonuclear lymphocytes (Bullen and Wallis, 1977); complement-mediated lysis does not function effectively in their absence. Those bacteria which are able to grow pathogenically in such environments have mechanisms which enable them to compete successfully for the free iron (Weinberg, 1978). For example, a large proportion of *Escherichia coli* strains which cause disease possess the colicin V (Col V) plasmid and these have a markedly enhanced virulence compared with plasmid free variants (Smith, 1974; Smith and Huggins, 1976). The plasmid encodes genes for an iron-sequestering system (Williams, 1979) in which a low molecular weight, extracellular, iron-chelating system competes successfully with transferrin *in vivo* (Saunders, 1981). In addition, there is a chromosomally determined, highly efficient iron-uptake system.

A very similar, possibly the same, plasmid-determined system has been shown to exist in *Vibrio anguillarum* (Crosa, 1980). Many of the highly virulent strains isolated from epizootics contain a 50 megadalton plasmid (pJM11) the removal of which markedly attenuates their virulence in experimental infections (Crosa *et al.*, 1977; 1980; Crosa and Hodges, 1981). The growth kinetics of a highly virulent strain and its plasmid-cured derivative were studied in a minimal medium which contained trace amounts of iron adequate for normal growth. Both strains grew well in the medium but, when 2.3μM transferrin was added, only the plasmid-containing, virulent strain grew. This difference was nullified by the addition of 0.2mM ferric chloride. The advantage, *in vivo*, of this ability to sequester iron in the presence of transferrin was shown by challenge experiments. When non-plasmid (avirulent) bacteria were used and iron was included in the challenge inoculum (86μg as ferric ammonium citrate) a 300-fold reduction in the viable count could be used to achieve the same LD_{50} value obtained in the absence of iron. The same experiment when carried out using a plasmid-containing (virulent) strain resulted in only a 1.3-fold increase.

In many species of bacteria, plasmid-mediated properties have been shown to be significant components of pathogenicity and the demonstration of differences in virulence between some plasmid and non-plasmid containing strains of *Vibrio anguillarum* may be relevant to the distinction between isolates obtained from commensal situations and diseased animals. A fuller description of the plasmids of *Vibrio anguillarum*, their genes and the extent to which they may be exchanged both within the genus and between *Vibrio* and other genera is very much needed.

A second factor which may be decisive in allowing infection to establish is the ability of bacteria to attach to a substrate on which to multiply (Smith, 1977). The adhesive mechanisms of the genus *Vibrio*, particularly *Vibrio cholerae*, have received considerable attention (Freter and Jones, 1976; Jones *et al.*, 1976; Nelson *et al.*, 1976) and their role in the pathogenesis of *Vibrio anguillarum* and as a tool for the study of vibriosis in fish have also been described (Horne and Baxendale, 1982). An important component of the pathogenicity of *Vibrio cholerae* is the production of a powerful exotoxin which has an adhesive subunit. The toxin has two subunits — a single 'A' subunit of molecular weight 28,000 which is responsible for the toxic activity, but which, in pure form, cannot bind to intact cells, and an aggregate of five smaller subunits each of molecular weight 11,600 which bind strongly to the G_m ganglioside receptor sites in the walls of the mucosal cells (Van Heyningen *et al.*, 1971; King and Van Heyningen, 1973). The cytotoxic activity of this exotoxin is well understood (Holmgren, 1981), although its exact role in the initiation of infection is not so clear.

No similar exotoxin has been demonstrated in the halophilic vibrios although they do contain an endotoxin membrane. *Vibrio anguillarum*, for example, possesses an endotoxin which is lethal for mice (Abe, 1972) although this produced only superficial haemorrhage when inoculated intramuscularly into chinook salmon (*Oncorhynchus tschawytscha*) and no clinical signs at all when injected intraperitoneally. Other authors too have noted the comparatively high resistance of fish to supernatant and exotoxin extracts of *Vibrio anguillarum* (Wedemeyer *et al.*, 1968; Wedemeyer, 1969; Harbell *et al.*, 1979) although there may be variation in this resistance between different fish species since goldfish (*Carassius* spp.) have been reported to be susceptible (Umbriet and Ordal, 1972; Umbriet and Fripp, 1975). In the search for exotoxins, many authors have demonstrated that halophilic vibrios produce extracellular products which are haemolytic (Yanagase *et al.*, 1970 for *Vibrio parahaemolyticus*; Munn, 1980 for *Vibrio anguillarum*). Some strains of both *Vibrio parahaemolyticus* (Miyamoto *et al.*, 1973; Miwatani *et al.*, 1969) and *Vibrio anguillarum* (Horne *et al.*, 1977) show the form of haemolysis described as the 'Kanagawa phenomenon" when grown on Wagatsuma's medium (Wagatsuma, 1968) and some authors have used this to distinguish between pathogenic and non-pathogenic strains (Kato *et al.*, 1965; Sakazaki, 1968).

However, the role of haemolysins in pathogenicity has often been questioned. Bacterial species which have pathogenic strains commonly show haemolytic activity and this may frequently be one of a group of characters which distinguish pathogenic and non-pathogenic variants (Cook and Ewins, 1975; Minishew *et al.*, 1978). However, many non-pathogenic bacteria, as part of their normal saprophytic metabolism, produce extracellular enzymes which are capable of lysing erythrocytes. The distinction of these from haemolysins, which can be said to be more specifically part of the pathogenic ability of a bacterium, is difficult (Smith and Taylor, 1964). Welch *et al.* (1981) isolated a DNA fragment encoding a haemolysin from *Escherichia coli* K12 and introduced this into a hybrid plasmid. Introduction of this hybrid plasmid to a non-haemolytic strain of *Escherichia coli* significantly enhanced its lethality for rats. Insertion of a mutant of the plasmid which contained most of the plasmid genetic background, but which was not haemolytic, did not have this effect, isolating the haemolytic ability specifically as the factor promoting virulence. While careful not to claim that the distinction between virulent and avirulent naturally occurring strains is predominantly the possession or not of the haemolysin, they conclude nevertheless that it does have a primary role in the establishment of infection in this instance. With so little data the importance of adhesins, haemolysins or, possibly, uncharacterized toxins in the pathogenesis of *Vibrio anguillarum* cannot be similarly attributed, but the evidence of Welch and co-workers suggests that the haemolysins may be more than merely a part of the bacterial, saprophytic metabolism.

The direction of research on vibriosis has, understandably, been towards accurate diagnosis and description of the disease followed, latterly, by work on antibiotic therapy and vaccines. As a consequence our knowledge of this much studied organism includes almost no information on its pathogenesis. The comprehensive descriptions of the pathology of the disease now need to be supplemented by a better knowledge of the mechanism of action of the bacterium itself—how it circumvents the protective mechanisms of its host and what affects its subsequent multiplication has on the physiology of the fish, ultimately resulting in its death. Not only will this information provide a background for the more effective combatting of the disease, but the study of model systems such as that of the rainbow trout and *Vibrio anguillarum* are capable of yielding, in a convenient experimental situation, information on host–disease relationships which has a much wider application than the field of fish disease.

References

Abe, P. M. (1972). Certain chemical and immunological properties of the endotoxin from *Vibrio anguillarum*. M.Sc. Dissertation. Oregon State University Corvallis, Oregon.

Agius, C., Horne, M. T. and Ward, P. (1982). Immunisation of rainbow trout (*Salmo gairdneri*) against vibriosis. Comparison of an extract antigen with whole cell bacterins by oral and IP routes. *Journal of Fish Diseases* (in press).

Alexander, J. B., Bowers, A. and Shamshoom, S. M. (1981). Hyperosmotic infiltration of bacteria into trout: route of entry and fate of the infiltrated bacteria. *In* "Developments in Biological Standardisation" (Eds. D. P. Anderson and W. Henessen), Vol. 49, pp.441–445. Karger, Basel.

Amend, D. F. and Eshenour, R. W. (1980). Development and use of commercial fish vaccines. *Salmonid* (March/April), 8–12.

Amend, D. F. and Johnson, K. A. (1981). Current status and future needs of *Vibrio anguillarum* bacterins. *In* "Developments in Biological Standardisation" (Eds. D. P. Anderson and W. Henessen), Vol. 49, pp.403–417. Karger, Basel.

Amend, D. F. and Fender, D. C. (1976). Uptake of bovine serum albumin by rainbow trout from hyperosmotic solutions: a model for vaccinating fish. *Science* **192**, 793–794.

Ament, R. W. and Fender, D. C. (1977). Immersion method for treating aquatic animals. U.S. Patent 4,009,259.

Arkwright, J. A. (1912). An epidemic disease affecting salmon and trout in England during the summer of 1911. *Journal of Hygiene* **XII**, 391–413.

Baudin-Laurencin, F. and Tangtrongpiros, J. (1980). Some results of vaccination against vibriosis in Brittany. *In* "Fish Diseases" (Ed. W. Ahne), pp.60–68. Springer-Verlag, Berlin.

Baumann, P., Bang, S. S. and Baumann, L. (1978). Phenotypic characterisation of *Beneckea anguillara* biotypes I and II. *Current Microbiology* **1**, 85–88.

Bergman, A. (1909). Die rote beulenkrankheit des Aals. *Bericht aus der Königlichen Bayerischen Versuchsstation* **2**, 10–54.

Bles, E. J. (1898). On the openings in the wall of the body cavity of vertebrates. *Proceedings of the Royal Society of London* **62**, 232–247.

Bridge, T. W. (1879). Pori abdominales of vertebrates. *Journal of Anatomical Physiology* **14**, 81–100.

Bullen, J. J. and Wallis, S. N. (1977). Reversal of the bacteriocidal effect of polymorphs by a ferritin-antibody complex. *FEMS Letters* **1**, 117–120.

Bullen, J. J., Rogers, H. J. and Griffiths, E. (1978). Role of iron in bacterial infection. *Current Topics in Microbiology and Immunology* **80**, 1–35.

Canestrini, G. (1893). La malattia dominante delle anguille. *Atti Ist Veneto* **7**, 809–814.

Cisar, T. O. and Fryer, J. L. (1969). An epizootic of vibriosis in chinook salmon. *Bulletin of the Wildlife Disease Association* **5**, 73–76.

Chart, H. and Munn, C. B. (1980). Experimental vibriosis in the eel (*Anguilla anguilla*). *In* "Fish Diseases" (Ed. W. Ahne), pp.39–44. Springer-Verlag, Berlin.

Conroy, D. A. and Withnell, G. C. (1974). The use of slide agglutination as an aid in the diagnosis of vibrio disease in fish. *Rivista Italiana di Piscicoltura E Ittiopatalogia* **IX**, 69–74.

Cooke, E. M. and Ewins, S. P. (1975). Properties of strains of *Escherichia coli* isolated from a variety of sources. *Journal of Medical Microbiology* **8**, 107–111.

Crosa, J. H. (1980). A plasmid associated with virulence in the marine fish pathogen *Vibrio anguillarum* specifies an iron-sequestering system. *Nature, London* **284**, 566–568.

Crosa, J. H. and Hodges, L. L. (1981). Outer membrane proteins induced under conditions of iron limitation in the marine fish pathogen *Vibrio anguillarum, 775. Infection and Immunity* **31**, 223–227.

Crosa, J. H., Schiewe, M. H. and Falkow, S. (1977). Evidence for plasmid contribution to the virulence of the fish pathogen *Vibrio anguillarum. Infection and Immunity* **18**, 509–513.

Crosa, J. H., Hodges, L. L. and Schiewe, M. H. (1980). Curing of a plasmid is correlated with an attenuation of virulence in the marine fish pathogen *Vibrio anguillarum. Infection and Immunity* **27**, 897–902.

Croy, T. R. and Amend, D. F. (1977). Immunisation of sockeye salmon (*Oncorhynchus nerka*) against vibriosis using hyperosmotic infiltration. *Aquaculture* **12**, 317–325.

Evelyn, T. P. T. (1971). First records of vibriosis in Pacific salmon cultured in Canada and taxonomic status of the responsible bacterium, *Vibrio anguillarum. Journal of the Fisheries Research Board of Canada* **28**, 517–525.

Evelyn, T. P. T. and McDermott, L. A. (1961). Bacteriological studies of freshwater fish. I. Isolation of aerobic bacteria from several species of Ontario fish. *Canadian Journal of Microbiology* **7**, 375.

Egidius, E. and Andersen, K. (1977). Norwegian reference strains of *Vibrio anguillarum. Aquaculture* **10**, 215–219.

Egidius, E. and Andersen, K. (1978). Host-specific pathogenicity of strains of *Vibrio anguillarum* isolated from rainbow trout (*Salmo gairdneri*) and saithe (*Pollachius virens*). *Journal of Fish Diseases* **1**, 45–50.

Ezura, Y., Tajima, K., Yoshimizu, M. and Kimura, T. (1980). Studies on the taxonomy and serology of causative organisms of fish vibriosis. *Fish Pathology* **14**, 167–179.

Fender, D. C. and Amend, D. F. (1978). Hyperosmotic infiltration: factors influencing uptake of bovine serum albumin by rainbow trout (*Salmo gairdneri*). *Journal of the Fisheries Research Board of Canada* **35**, 871–874.

Freter, R. and Jones, G. W. (1976). Adhesive properties of *Vibrio cholerae*: nature of the interaction with intact mucosal surfaces. *Infection and Immunity* **14**, 246–256.

Fryer, J. L., Nelson, J. S. and Garrison, R. L. (1972). Vibriosis in fish. *In* "Progress in Fishery and Food Science" (Ed. Moore, E. W.), Vol. **5**, pp.129–133. University Publication in Fisheries. New Series. Seattle, Washington.

Fryer, J. L., Nelson, J. S. and Garrison, R. L. (1978). Immunization of salmonids for control of vibriosis. *Marine Fisheries Review* **40**, 20–23.

George, C. J., Ellis, A. E. and Bruno, D. W. (1982). On remembrance of the abdominal pores in rainbow trout and some other salmonid spp. *Journal of Fish Biology* (In press).

Gibbons, R. J. and Houte, J. van (1975). Bacterial adherence in oral microbial ecology. *Annual Reviews of Microbiology* **29**, 19–44.

Gould, R. W., Antipa, R. and Amend, D. F. (1979). Immersion vaccination of sockeye salmon (*Oncorhynchus nerka*) with two pathogenic strains of *Vibrio anguillarum. Journal of the Fisheries Research Board of Canada* **36**, 222–225.

Hacking, M. A. and Budd, J. (1971). Vibrio infection in tropical fish in a freshwater aquarium. *Journal of Wildlife Diseases* **7**, 273–280.

Harbell, S. C., Hodgins, H. O. and Schiewe, M. H. (1979). Studies on the pathogenesis of vibriosis in coho salmon (*Oncorhynchus kisutch*), *Journal of Fish Diseases* **2**, 391–404.

Harrel, L. W. (1978). Vibriosis and current salmon vaccination procedures in Puget Sound, Washington. *Marine Fisheries Review* **40**, 24–25.

Harrel, L. W., Novotny, A. J., Schiewe, M. H. and Hodgins, H. O. (1976). Isolation and description of two vibrios pathogenic to Pacific salmon in Puget Sound, Washington. *Fishery Bulletin* **74**, 447–449.

Hayashi, R., Kobayashi, S., Tikamata and Ozaki, H. (1964). Studies on vibrio disease of rainbow trout (*S. gairdneri*) II. Prophylactic vaccination against vibrio disease. *Journal of the Faculty of Fisheries, Prefectural University of MU* **6**, 181–191.

Håstein, T. (1975). Vibriosis in Fish. Ph.D. Dissertation, University of Stirling, Scotland.

Håstein, T. and Smith, J. F. (1977). A study of *Vibrio anguillarum* from farmed and wild fish using principal components analysis. *Journal of Fish Biology* **11**, 69–75.

Hendrie, M. S., Hodgkiss, W. and Shewan, J. M. (1971). Proposal that the species *Vibrio anguillarum, Vibrio piscium* and *Vibrio ichthyodermis* be combined as a single species, *Vibrio anguillarum*. *International Journal of Systematic Bacteriology* **21**, 64–68.

Heyningen, W. E. van, Carpenter, C. C. J., Pierce, N. F. and Greenough, W. B. (1971). Deactivation of cholera toxin by ganglioside. *Journal of Infectious Disease* **124**, 415–418.

Hofer, B. (1904). Handbuch der Fischkrankheiten. Fischerie-Zeitung.

Holmgren, J. (1981). Actions of cholera toxin and the prevention and treatment of cholera. *Nature, London* **292**, 413–417.

Horne, M. T. and Baxendale, A. (1982). The adhesion of *Vibrio anguillarum* to host tissues and its role in pathogenesis. *Journal of Fish Diseases* (In press).

Horne, M. T., Richards, R. H., Roberts, R. J. and Smith, P. C. (1977). Peracute vibriosis in juvenile turbot (*Scophthalmus maximus*). *Journal of Fish Biology* **11**, 355–361.

Horsley, R. W. (1973). The bacterial flora of the Atlantic salmon (*Salmo salar*) in relation to its environment. *Journal of Applied Bacteriology* **36**, 377–386.

Johnsen, G. S. (1977). Immunological studies on *Vibrio anguillarum*. *Aquaculture* **10**, 221–230.

Johnson, K. A. (1980). Development of an effective vibrio vaccination program for salmonid culture. *Fish Pathology* **14**, 181.

Jones, G. W., Abrams, G. D. and Freter, R. (1976). Adhesive properties of *Vibrio cholerae*: adhesion to isolated rabbit brush border membranes and haem-agglutinating activity. *Infection and Immunity* **14**, 232–234.

Kato, T., Obara, Y., Tchinoe, H., Nagashima, K., Akiyama, S., Takizawa, K., Matsushima, A., Yami, S. and Miyamoto, Y. (1965). Grouping of *Vibrio parahaemolyticus* with haemolytic reactions. *Shokuhin Eisei Kenkyn* **15**, 83–86.

Kiehn, E. D. and Pacha, R. E. (1969). Characterization and relatedness of marine vibrios pathogenic to fish: deoxyribonucleic acid homology and base composition: *Journal of Bacteriology* **100**, 1248–1255.

King, C. A. and Heyningen, W. E. van (1973). Deactivation of cholera toxin by a sialidase-resistant, monosialosyl-ganglioside. *Journal of Infectious Disease* **127**, 639–647.

Kitao, T., Aoki, T., Fukudome, M., Kawano, K., Wada, Y. and Mizuno, Y. (1982). Serotyping of *Vibrio anguillarum* isolated from diseased freshwater fish in Japan. *Journal of Fish Diseases* (In press).

Kusuda, R. (1966). Studies on the ulcer disease of marine fishes. *Proceedings of the 1st US-Japan Joint Conference on Marine Biology, Tokyo*, pp.1–13.

Kusuda, R., Sako, H. and Kawai, K. (1979). Classification of vibrios isolated from diseased fishes — 1. On the morphological, biological and biochemical properties. *Fish Pathology* **13**, 123–137.

Lanzkowsky, P. (1976). Iron metabolism in the new-born infant. *Clinics in Endocrinology and Metabolism* **5**, 149–173.

Lee, J. V., Shread, P., Furniss, A. L. and Bryant, T. N. (1981). Taxonomy and description of *Vibrio fluvialis* sp. nov. (Synonym Group F Vibrios, Group EF6). *Journal of Applied Bacteriology* 50, 73–94.

Mattheis, T. (1964). Ökologie der bakterien in Darm von Süsswassernutzfischen. *Zeitschrift fur Fischerei* 12, 507–600.

McCarthy, D. H., Stevenson, J. P. and Roberts, M. S. (1974). Vibriosis in rainbow trout. *Journal of Wildlife Diseases* 10, 2–7.

Minishew, B. H., Jorgensen, J., Swanstrum, M., Grootes-Reuvecamp, G. A. and Falkow, S. (1978). Some characteristics of *Escherichia coli* strains isolated from extraintestinal infections of humans. *The Journal of Infectious Diseases* 137, 648–654.

Miwatani, T., Sakuri, J., Takeda, Y. and Shinoda, S. (1974). Studies on direct haemolysins of *Vibrio parahaemolyticus* "International Symposium on Vibrio parahaemolyticus". Saikon Publishing Co., Tokyo.

Miyamoto, Y., Kato, T., Obara, Y., Akiyama, S., Takizawa, K. and Yamai, S. (1969). *In vitro* haemolytic characteristic of *Vibrio parahaemolyticus*: its close correlation with human pathogenicity. *Journal of Bacteriology* 100, 1147–1149.

Munn, C. B. (1980). Production and properties of a haemolytic toxin by *Vibrio anguillarum*. *In* "Fish Diseases" (Ed. W. Ahne), pp.69–74. Springer-Verlag, Berlin.

Muroga, K. (1975). "Studies on *Vibrio anguillarum* and *Vibrio anguillarum* Infection". Faculty of Fisheries and Animal Husbandry, Hiroshima University, Japan.

Muroga, K. and Egusa, S. (1970). *Vibrio anguillarum* isolated from Ayu in fresh-water farm-ponds. *Fish Pathology* 5, 16–20.

Muroga, K., Jo, Y. and Nishibuchi, M. (1976). *Vibrio anguillarum* isolated from the European eel (*Anguilla anguilla*) cultured in Japan. *Journal of the Faculty of Fisheries and Animal Husbandry, Hiroshima University* 15, 29–34.

Nelson, E. T., Clements, J. D. and Finkelstein, R. A. (1976). *Vibrio cholerae*; adherence and colonisation in experimental, electron microscope studies. *Infection and Immunity* 14, 527–547.

Ohnishi, K. and Muroga, K. (1977). *Vibrio* sp. as a cause of disease in rainbow trout cultured in Japan. 1. Physiological characteristics and pathogenicity. *Fish Pathology* 12, 51–55.

Pacha, R. E. and Kiehn, E. D. (1969). Characterisation and relatedness of marine vibrios pathogenic to fish: physiology, serology and epidemiology. *Journal of Bacteriology* 100, 1242–1247.

Plehn, M. (1911). Die Furunkulose der Salmoniden. *Zentrablatt für Bakteriologie, Parasitenkunde, Infectionskrankheiten und Hygiene, Abt. 1.* 60, 609–624.

Roberts, R. J. (1978). "Fish Pathology" Baillière, Tindall and Cassell, London.

Roberts, R. J. and Shepherd, C. J. (1974). "Handbook of Salmon and Trout Diseases". Fishing News (Books) Ltd., London.

Ross, A. J., Martin, J. E. and Bressler, V. (1968). *Vibrio anguillarum* from an epizootic in rainbow trout (*Salmo gairdneri*) in the U.S.A. *Bulletin of the International Office of Épizootics* 69, 1139–1148.

Rucker, R. R. (1959). Vibrio infections among marine and freshwater fishes. *Progressive Fish Culturist* 21, 22–25.

Rucker, R. R., Earp, B. J. and Ordal, E. J. (1953). Infectious diseases of Pacific salmon. *Transactions of the American Fisheries Society* 83, 297–312.

Saito, Y., Otsuru, M., Furukawa, T., Kanda, K. and Sato, A. (1964). Studies on infectious diseases of rainbow trout. *Acta Medica et Biologica* 11, 267-295.

Sakazaki, R., Tamura, K., Kato, T., Obara, Y., Yamei, S. and Hobo, K. (1968). Studies on the enterpathogenic, facultatively halophilic bacteria, *Vibrio parahaemolyticus*. III. Enteropathogenicity. *Japanese Journal of Medical Science and Biology* 21, 325-331.

Saunders, J. R. (1981). Plasmids and bacterial pathogens. *Nature, London* 290, 362.

Schiewe, M. H. (1981). Taxonomic status of marine vibrios pathogenic for salmonid fish. *In* "Developments in Biological Standardisation" (Eds. Anderson, D. P. and Henessen, W.), Vol. 49, pp.149-158. Karger, Basel.

Schiewe, M. H. and Hodgins, H. O. (1977). Specificity of protection induced in coho salmon (*Oncorhynchus kisutch*) by heat-treated components of two pathogenic vibrios. *Journal of the Fisheries Research Board of Canada* 34, 1026-1028.

Schiewe, M. H., Crosa, J. H. and Ordal, E. J. (1977). Deoxyribonucleic acid relationships among marine vibrios pathogenic to fish. *Canadian Journal of Microbiology* 23, 954-958.

Smith, H. (1977). Microbial surfaces in relation to pathogenicity. *Bacteriological Reviews* 41, 475-500.

Smith, H. and Taylor, J. (1964). "Microbial Behaviour *in Vivo* and *in Vitro*". Cambridge University Press, Cambridge, U.K.

Smith, H. W. (1974). A search for transmissable pathogenic characters in invasive strains of *Escherichia coli*: the discovery of a plasmid controlled toxin and a plasmid controlled lethal character closely associated, or identical, with colicine V. *Journal of General Microbiology* 83, 95-111.

Smith, H. W. and Huggins, M. B. (1976). Further observations on the association of the colicine V plasmid of *Escherichia coli* with pathogenicity and with survival in the alimentary tract. *Journal of General Microbiology* 92, 335-350.

Strout, R. G., Sawyer, E. S. and Coultermarsh, B. A. (1978). Pathogenic vibrios in confinement-reared and feral fishes of the Maine-New Hampshire coast. *Journal of the Fisheries Research Board of Canada* 35, 403-408.

Thjøtta, T. and Sømme, O. M. (1943). The bacterial flora of normal fish. *Shrifter Norske Videnskaps-Akademi, Oslo* 4, 1-86.

Umbreit, W. W. and Ordal, E. J. (1972). Infection of goldfish with *Vibrio anguillarum*. *American Society for Microbiology News* 32, 93-96.

Umbreit, W. W. and Tripp, M. R. (1975). Characterisation of the factors responsible for the fish infected with *Vibrio anguillarum*. *Canadian Journal of Microbiology* 21, 1271-1274.

Wagatsuma, S. (1968). A medium for the test of haemolytic activity of *Vibrio parahaemolyticus*. *Media Circle* 13, 159-161.

Wedmeyer, G. (1969). Pituitary activation by bacterial endotoxins in the rainbow trout (*Salmo gairdneri*). *Journal of Bacteriology* 100, 542-543.

Wedmeyer, G., Ross, A. J. and Smith, L. C. (1968). Some metabolic effects of bacterial endotoxins in salmonid fishes. *Journal of the Fisheries Research Board of Canada* 26, 115-122.

Weinberg, E. D. (1978). Iron and Infection. *Microbial Reviews* 42, 45-66.

Welch, R. A., Dellinger, E. P., Minshew, B. and Falkow, S. (1981). Haemolysin contributes to virulence of extra-intestinal *E. coli* infections. *Nature, London* 294, 665-667.

Williams, P. H. (1979). Novel iron uptake system specified by Col V plasmids: an important component in the virulence of invasive strains of *Escherichia coli*. *Infection and Immunity* **26**, 925–932.

Yanagase, Y., Inoue, K., Ozaki, M., Ochi, T., Amano, T. and Chazono, M. (1970). Haemolysins and related enzymes of *Vibrio parahaemolyticus* 1. Identification and partial purification of enzymes. *Biken Journal* **13**, 77–92.

Yoshimizu, M. and Kimura, T. (1976). Study on the intestinal microflora of salmonids. *Fish Pathology* **10**, 243–259.

Yoshimizu, M., Kimura, T. and Sakai, M. (1976). Studies on the intestinal microflora of salmonids — 1. The intestinal microflora of fish reared in freshwater and seawater. *Bulletin of the Japanese Society of Scientific Fisheries* **42**, 91–99.

10

Fungal Disease of Aquatic Animals

D. J. ALDERMAN

Ministry of Agriculture, Fisheries and Food, Directorate of Fisheries Research, Fish Diseases Laboratory, Weymouth, Dorset, U.K.

Introduction

Diseases of fungal aetiology have long been recognized in fish, but despite this, far less is known about this type of disease than is known about those of bacterial or viral origin. Major problems often occur in identifying the fungus responsible and in determining whether it is truly pathogenic or simply a saprophyte taking advantage of an existing lesion. Even when there is good evidence that a disease is truly of fungal origin, in several cases the organism responsible is so poorly understood that its identity even as a fungus is less than certain.

The literature of fungal diseases in aquatic animals is widely spread and rather "patchy". A number of reviews have been published, but there has been an inevitable tendency either to concentrate on aquatic vertebrates (Wolke, 1975; Neish and Hughes, 1980) or to limit consideration either to marine (Johnson and Sparrow, 1961; Alderman, 1976), or freshwater hosts only. An examination of the genera and species of fungi reported from aquatic animals shows that in general the parasites themselves recognize no boundary between vertebrate and invertebrate or marine and freshwater hosts, so that reviews limited by these considerations present only a partial picture of the role of fungi as pathogens in the aquatic environment. Even if the full range of published work is considered, there is a considerable and inevitable bias towards species which are commercially important or have commercial potential.

Within these limits, the fungi reported as being responsible for or associated with diseases of aquatic animals belong to a wide range of taxa. The most frequent in all types of host and environment are the so-called water molds—the Oomycetes—but in recent years there has been an increasing recognition of the importance of various members of the higher fungi as parasites of aquatic animals. Some organisms, amongst which are two of the most important fungal pathogens, *Branchiomyces* and *Ichthyophonus*, are still of uncertain taxonomic affinity. Another, *Perkinsus* (formerly *Dermocystidium*), which was discussed extensively in earlier reviews (Wolke, 1975; Alderman, 1976; Neish and Hughes, 1980), has now been shown to be a member of the Apicomplexa (protozoa), and no longer belongs in a discussion of fungal diseases (Perkins, 1976; Levine, 1978).

The majority of reviews of this type have been arranged on a taxonomic basis, although Alderman (1976) used a host/tissue type format and Lauckner (1980) based his excellent synthesis of marine animal diseases entirely on host taxa. In this review, a taxonomically-based sequence will be followed, but the fungi of uncertain affinity will be considered after the lower fungi, to which the great majority undoubtedly have their closest affinity.

Isolation and Culture

One of the major difficulties in the investigation of aquatic animal diseases of fungal aetiology is the problem of isolating the fungus observed. In dermal infections the lesion may be infested by more than one aquatic fungus and even if unifungal there will be present a range of spores of saprophytes whose rapid growth could mask the primary species. This type of problem will be exacerbated if the tissues selected for isolation are not suitable. The more advanced an infection, the greater the possibility of involvement of secondary saprophytes. Once the animal has died then the value of isolates obtained from the carcass must be questionable.

Willoughby (1978), with infected salmonids, examined small pieces of infected tissue in sterile lake water at 7°C for up to 5 days, observing for the forms present before deciding whether to isolate from zoospores or from hyphae. No matter what the type of fungus involved, isolates should, whenever possible, be made from single spores or single hyphal tips to ensure that the isolate is truly unifungal.

Before the advent of antibiotics, there were major difficulties in securing isolates free from bacterial contamination. Numerous washings and subcultures were employed, together with glass rings to limit bacterial growth (Raper, 1937). Currently, most workers employ antibiotics in their initial isolation media. Probably the most popular combination is penicillin and streptomycin at 0.5g each per litre of agar. Some other antimicrobials which have been used are potassium tellurite and carbenicillin, but there is no conclusive evidence that these have any significant advantages. Some fungi, such as *Aphanomyces astaci* (Unestam, 1965) are too sensitive to antibiotics to permit their use in isolation. Since this fungus grows in the host's exoskeleton, it is possible to surface-sterilize infected fragments with alcohol and thereby overcome many of the problems of contamination.

Suitable isolation media are very varied, but as a general indication it is advantageous if media for this purpose are relatively low in nutrients. Media for marine organisms should be prepared with sea water. Such low nutrient media tend to inhibit the growth of the adventitious saprophytes and bacteria. Provided bacterial contamination can be kept down by means of antibiotics and provided that yeasts are not a problem, it is often advantageous for isolation agar plates to have a thin layer of fresh water (or sea water) on their surface. A general survey of the literature indicates that, except in a very few cases, there is no specific advantage to the various types of media which have been used. In the case of *Aphanomyces astaci*, growth in agar media soon ceases.

Knowledge of the physiology and nutrition of fungal parasites of aquatic animals is rather sparse. *Saprolegnia* has been intensively investigated, although not specifically those species of fish origin. *Aphanomyces astaci* has also been thoroughly investigated (Unestam, 1965, 1968), as have the marine fungi *Lagenidium callinectes* and *Haliphthoros milfordensis* (Bahnweg and Bland, 1980). In general however, little or nothing is known of the requirements of most of the other parasitic fungi which would relate to their role as parasites.

Pathogenicity

Investigations into the pathogenicity of the various fungi which have been associated with diseases of aquatic animals have, in general, shown that the majority of fungi involved are at best facultative parasites. Only *Aphanomyces astaci*, *Ichthyophonus* and *Trichomaris invadens* appear to be obligate parasites and have not been found in non-parasitic circumstances, and all three of these fungi are responsible for diseases which can be highly virulent for susceptible hosts, where very rapid infection at high levels occurs in natural populations. *Lagenidium callinectes* has been isolated from marine algal surfaces (Fuller *et al.*, 1964) and it is uncertain whether it was saprophytic there, but otherwise it is responsible for very severe mortalities in a wide range of crustacea both in natural and cultivated populations (Bland, 1975).

Willoughby (1968, 1969, 1970, 1971, 1972, 1977, 1978) has clearly shown that there is a specific type of *Saprolegnia* associated with salmonid fish lesions. Under appropriate conditions, severe fungal infections can occur in fish populations, particularly when these are densely stocked. However, as Neish (1976) amongst others has shown, obtaining infection under laboratory conditions can be very difficult. The other lower fungi seem largely to be opportunistic parasites, appearing especially under the intensive and abnormal conditions found in aquaculture or research facilities.

As regards the higher fungi, although sporadic mortalities have been directly attributed to them, attempts to induce infection under laboratory conditions have not been spectacularly successful. In many cases, injections of spores do initiate infections, but the intraperitoneal injection of fungal spores in large numbers does not equate to natural conditions of infection. The injection of large numbers of spores of *Fusarium* into crustacea for example produces mortalities, but with quite atypical pathology. It seems probable that many of the higher fungi are only opportunists capable of infecting fish under relatively unusual conditions. An example of this is *Ochroconis tshawytschae*, which although first isolated from fish, was subsequently described as a new species, *Scolecobasidium macrosporum* from soil and only subsequently reduced to synonomy. Experimental infections of salmonids with *Ochroconis humicola* incorporated in food, succeeded only when ground glass was included (Ross and Yasutake, 1973). Currently, the only known example of a higher fungus being an obligate aquatic animal parasite is that of *Trichomaris invadens* which produces the black mat disease of tanner crabs.

Myxomycota

Thraustochytriales

Members of this group are obligately marine, holocarpic, have biflagellate heterokont zoospores and possess an apparently unique ectoplasmic net/ sagenogenetosome structure in place of rhizoids (Perkins, 1972; Alderman *et al.*, 1974). The group is generally regarded as saprophytic, although the closely related Labyrinthulales are significant pathogens of marine plants (Johnson and Sparrow, 1961). Indeed, as has been pointed out (Alderman *et al.*, 1974; Olive, 1975), there is considerable doubt as to the validity of placing the Thraustochytriales and Labyrinthulales within the Eumycota as advocated by Sparrow (1973) and Dick (1973), amongst others, since this depends on the common possession of laterally biflagellate heterokont zoospores and ignores other distinctive features. Probably the best review of possible taxonomic niches for this rather orphan group is that of Olive (1975). For the moment, however, these organisms continue to be treated and examined by mycologists and are therefore included here. One genus, *Schizochytrium* Goldstein, which is characterized by regular bipartition of

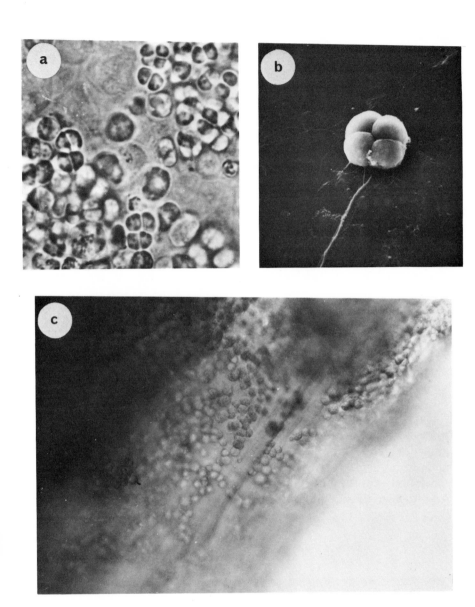

Fig. 1. Micrographs of *Schizochytrium aggregatum*: (a) vegetative growth showing characteristic tetrad form; (b) scanning electron micrograph of a single tetrad form; (c) its presence on the gill of a moribund oyster.

its vegetative thallus (Figs 1a, 1b) has been frequently found and associated with marine animals (Alderman and Gras, 1969) but without any specific evidence of pathogenicity (Fig. 1c). The organism *Thanatostrea polymorpha* described by Franc and Arvy (1970) from Portuguese oysters, *Crassostrea angulata*, suffering from gill disease, may have, in part, represented stages of *Schizochytrium*. In the United States, Quick (1972) described a number of thraustochytrid-like organisms from American oysters, *Crassostrea virginica* to which he attributed pathogenic ability. Uzmann and Haynes (1968) described a mycosis of the gills of the pandalid shrimp *Dichelopandalus leptocerus* which they attributed to a 'chytrid-like' parasite. This organism apparently possessed the *Schizochytrium*-like character of regular bipartition of the vegetative thallus which is intra-matrical in the shrimp gill. The large size of the mature thallus (up to 350μm diameter) before cleavage is, however, too great for known Thraustochytrids. A disease of the American lobster (*Homarus americanus*), known as 'leopard lobster' (Herrick, 1895, 1911; Sindermann, 1970) is also attributed to a 'chytrid-like' fungus with Schiff-positive subspherical heavy walled bodies, 30–60μm in diameter, in the diseased tissues.

Very recently thraustochytrid fungi, identified as *Schizochytrium* and *Ulkenia ammoeboidea*, have been shown to be intimately associated with necrotic epidermal lesions in the lesser octopus *Eledone cirrhosa* (Polglase, 1980, 1981) in the North Sea. *Schizochytrium* has also been observed in gill lesions in the squid *Illex illecebrosus* (Jones, 1981) in Nova Scotian waters. Polglase (1981) has also reported the isolation of a thraustochytrid, exhibiting division characteristic of *Schizochytrium*, from epidermal lesions in rainbow trout, *Salmo gairdneri* grown in marine cages. Since the Thraustochytriales and in particular *Schizochytrium* are extremely common marine fungi, it is obvious that such reports need to be examined critically, but it seems certain that, with the recognition of their involvement in cephalopod skin lesions, a new and potentially important role for the Thraustochytriales in the marine environment has been identified.

Eumycota, Mastigomycotina, Oomycetes

Saprolegniales, Saprolegniaceae

Members of this family are the most frequent and important fungal parasites in aquatic animals. *Saprolegnia* and related genera have been thoroughly reviewed by Neish and Hughes (1980) and *Saprolegnia* is dealt with extensively elsewhere in this volume and therefore, to avoid repetition, will not be considered here. The only major genus not covered by these authors is *Aphanomyces*.

Aphanomyces

Although members of the genus *Aphanomyces* have been found growing parasitically on fish, they are not generally regarded as playing a major role in fish mycoses in fresh water. However, in recent years, a series of papers originating in Japan (Miyazaki and Egusa, 1972, 1973a, b, c; Hatai *et al.*, 1977; Hatai and Egusa, 1978a, 1979) have described a fungal disease in a number of fish which the authors refer to as a mycotic granuloma and to the fungus responsible as the MG-fungus. The MG-fungus has recently been identified (Hatai, 1980) as a member of the genus *Aphanomyces*. However, the most important role of *Aphanomyces* in aquatic animal pathology is in the crustacea, where *A. astaci* is responsible for catastrophic mortalities of feral crayfish in mainland European waters.

Aphanomyces astaci. The mycelium of *Aphanomyces astaci* is from 7.5 to 10μm in diameter and is sparingly branched. Zoosporangia are formed from vegetative hyphae and there are of the same diameter and do not proliferate. Zoospores develop in a single row, emerging apically in an elongated form, then encysting around the tip of the sporangium (Fig. 2). The primary zoospore cyst germinates to give secondary zoospores.

The disease, crayfish plague (Krebspest in German), caused by *A. astaci* has been spreading through Europe for over 100 years. In the 1870s it entered Germany from France (Schaperclaus, 1954) and destroyed the majority of the crayfish populations. Early workers disputed whether the disease was of bacterial or fungal aetiology. After the fungus reached Sweden in 1929, Nybelin (1931, 1934, 1936) was able to isolate *A. astaci* into culture and satisfy Koch's postulates by producing infection under controlled conditions and then reisolating the fungus. The disease appears to occur in peaks with periods of remission. Resistance has not developed in native European species, perhaps partly because mortality is so severe. *A. astaci* does not appear to produce resistant spores so that once all the crayfish in an area have succumbed, it is possible to introduce new animals (Unestam, 1968).

Nyhlen and Unestam (1980) demonstrated that *A. astaci* zoospores would preferentially encyst in the vicinity of fresh superficial wounds of the exoskeleton of crayfish. These cysts became encapsulated by melanin. In the American crayfish *Pacifastacus leniusculus*, which is resistant to *A. astaci* except when the epicuticle is damaged, melanization is rapid, but in susceptible European species such as *Astacus astacus*, melanization is

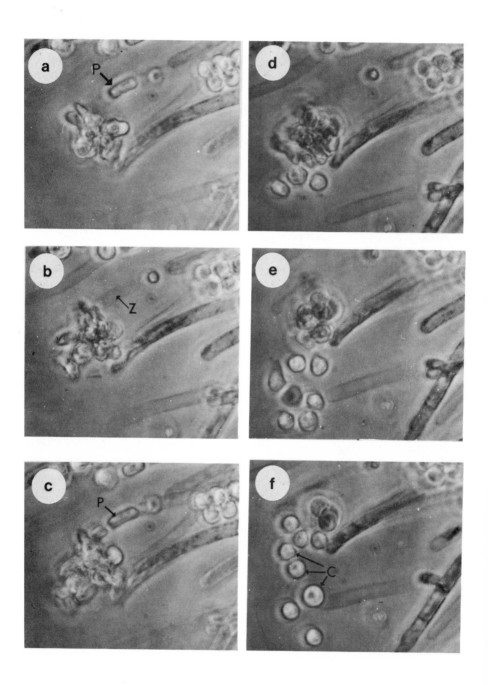

slower. In these species there is little resistance to fungal infection, which mainly involves the exoskeleton and central nervous system (Schaperclaus, 1954). Although *P. leniusculus* is resistant to *A. astaci*, it is apparently capable of spreading the fungus. Therefore the introduction of this species into any areas and waters in which there are susceptible populations of crayfish, may carry with it severe risks of a catastrophic mortality in the feral population.

Smith (1940) reported another *Aphanomyces* species—*A. laevis* DeBary —as an occasional and mild parasite of *Cambarus clarkii* Girard in an experimental population of crayfish in Massachusetts, U.S.A. Other species of *Aphanomyces* reported from freshwater crustacea are *A. pattersonii* reported as causing a dramatic decline of *Daphnia* populations (Scott, 1956), *A. daphnii*, again on *Daphnia* (Prowse, 1953) and *A. ovidestruens* on *Diaptomus* (Gicklehorn, 1923).

Hatai (1980) reported that an outbreak of mycotic granulomatosis in pond-cultured ayu (*Plecoglossus altivelis*) in Shiga Prefecture Japan, was due to an *Aphanomyces* which had previously been referred to as MG-fungus. No sexual stages were found, but Hatai indicates that he believes it to be a new species. Isolated into pure culture, inoculation experiments using ayu and goldfish showed that the fungus was the causative agent of the mycotic granulomatosis. Infection was achieved by injection of hyphae intramuscularly producing granulomata from which the fungus was re-isolated.

Aphanomyces spp. have also been identified sporadically from a range of fish species (Shanor and Saslow, 1944; Scott and O'Bier, 1962; Scott, 1964; Vishniac and Nigrelli, 1957; Willoughby, 1970), but without any clear evidence that significant aggressive pathogenicity is involved. Vishniac and Nigrelli demonstrated that *Aphanomyces* would infect wounded platyfish.

Saprolegniales, Leptolegniaceae and Leptolegniellaceae

Dick (1971) separated the Leptolegniellaceae from the Leptolegniaceae primarily on the basis of oospore protoplasmid structure and oospore wall morphology.

Leptolegniella marina. L. marina is a mycelial fungus reported by Atkins

---

Fig. 2. Zoospore release in *Aphanomyces astaci* shown in sequence from (a) to (f). Primary zoospores (P) escape through the tip of zoosporangium (Z) in succession and accumulate in a slowly moving aggregate at its tip, where they slowly round up and encyst (C).

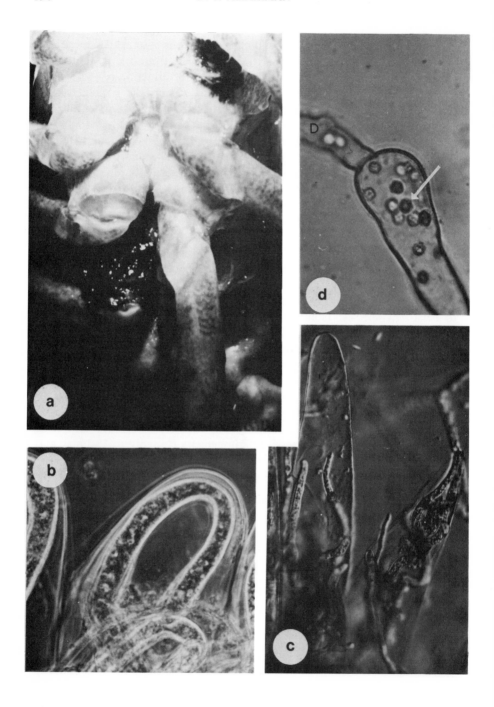

(1954a) as *Leptolegnia marina* from the eggs and gills of *Pinnotheres pisum* and in *Barnea candida* and *Cardium echinatum*. Johnson and Pinschmidt (1963) subsequently identified it on eggs of the blue crab *Calinectes sapidus*. Hyphae are both intra- and extra-matrical, 6–14μm in diameter and freely branched. Sporangia, which themselves may be branched, are delimited from both intra- and extra-matrical hyphae, but do not differ morphologically from vegetative hyphae. The zoospores are dimorphic and diplanetic, the primary zoospores being pyriform 8–11 × 3–4μm in diameter, encysting then re-emerging as reniform secondary zoospores, 8–14 × 3–6μm. Oogonia are developed intramatrically and are 16–40 μm in diameter, mainly spherical to globose. Oogonial walls are generally smooth and antheridia are predominantly hypogynous. Each oogonium has a single oospore (15–39μm in diameter) which largely fills it.

Johnson and Sparrow (1961) suggested that this organism might not belong in *Leptolegnia* and that *Leptolegniella* might be more appropriate. Dick (1971) in a paper in which he erected the new family *Leptolegniellaceae* transferred Atkins genus to *Leptolegniella* as *L. marina*.

Leptolegnia baltica. *L. baltica* which was described by Hohnk and Vallin (1953), was reported as being associated with a massive mortality of the copepod *Eurytemora hirundoides* Nordquist in the Northern Baltic (Vallin, 1951). Hyphae were both intra- and extra-matrical (5–20μm wide), freely branching, with zoosporangia which are filamentous and proliferous. Zoospores were biflagellate, dimorphic and measured 11 × 17μm. Oogonia were 27–35μm in diameter on short lateral branches with single oospheres and diclinous antheridia.

Saprolegniales, Haliphthoraceae

The family Haliphthoraceae was erected by Vishniac (1958) to contain a new marine biflagellate fungus isolated from the egg cases of the oyster drill *Urosalpinx cinerea*. Vishniac also included *Atkinsiella*, a new genus which she erected to contain the fungus which Atkins (1954b) had previously described as *Plectospira dubia*. The present state of uncertainty with regard to the systematic position of *Atkinsiella* is described under that organism.

Haliphthoros milfordensis. This rather romantic generic name (the name

---

Fig. 3. Photographs of *Haliphthoros milfordensis* showing a gross lesion caused by this organism in a larval lobster (a), vegetative mycelia in the gill of a larval lobster (b and c) and zoospores (arrowed) in (d) an holocarpic sporangium (D = discharge tube).

means the destroyer on the sea, pirate) describes an obligately marine, filamentous, holocarpic biflagellate fungus. The hyphae are 10–13 (–25) μm wide with cytoplasm which is at first granular, later vacuolate (Figs 3b, c). The mycelium is aseptate, but after 5 to 7 days culture at 25°C, gemmae with non-vacuolate protoplasm and thickened cell walls may be formed. Zoosporulation can be induced by placing actively growing mycelium in sterile sea water. Vishniac observed some stages of zoosporulation and noted that at the time of zoospore discharge the entire contents of the thallus had been cleaved into a close packed mass of zoospores. Since no septa were formed this was holocarpy. Zoospores were free swimming, laterally biflagellate and reniform (8–9μm in diameter). Exit tubes were irregularly wavy to partly coiled structures usually originating on one end of the thallus (Fig. 3d).

The fungus was isolated in pure culture and Vishniac (1958) and Ganaros (1957) stated that they were able to demonstrate infection of both ova and early developing stages of *Urosalpinx cinerea* and eggs of *Pinnotheres*. Subsequently Fisher *et al.* (1975) reported the involvement of *Halipthoros milfordensis* in a mycosis of American lobsters *Homarus americanus* in an experimental facility in California. The fungus was isolated and infection experiments were carried out. One thousand juvenile *H. americanus* placed in a fungus-contaminated semiclosed system showed 46% mortality after 22 days, with 95% of the dead showing symptoms of *H. milfordensis* infection. In a controlled infection experiment with nine juvenile lobsters in a system arranged such that only *H. milfordensis* zoospores could reach the lobsters, all nine experimental animals died within 11 days. The fungus was reisolated. The European lobster *H. gammarus* was also found to be susceptible. Mortality for both American and European lobsters as a result of infection was restricted to small juvenile lobsters between 5 and 27mm carapace length. Histopathologically, the heaviest involvement occurred at the point where the fungus first entered the tissue, with mycelium spreading in all directions throughout muscle and gill tissues. Heavy melanization characterized the lesion, with the mycelium being encapsulated (Fig. 3a).

Further evidence of the pathogenicity of *H. milfordensis* for crustacea was presented by Tharp and Bland (1977) who reported the fungus as causing mortalities in aquarium populations of *Penaeus setiferus*. These workers were also able to infect the eggs and larvae of *Artemia* and ova of *Callinectes sapidus*. Tharp and Bland provided new information on the developmental morphology and life cycle of *H. milfordensis*. Their isolate differed from Vishniac's original description in that the zoospores were capable of repeated emergence and were not of consistent shape. Although flagellar attachment was subapical, they pointed out that these zoospores had a lateral groove which was characteristic of the secondary zoospore type. The zoospore cysts possess spines basically similar to those described for *Saprolegnia parasitica* (Meier and Webster, 1954) amongst other saprolegnids. The zoospore discharge of the Tharp and Bland isolate was basically akin to that of *Atkinsiella*, and *Leptolegniella*, but vegetative thallus structure was characteristically lagenidiaceous. On this basis, the authors agree with Sparrow's (1976) suggestion that *H. milfordensis* should be placed in the Lagenidiales and probably in the family Sirolpidiacae.

Haliphthoros philippinensis. *H. philippinensis* was described by Hatai *et al.* (1980) from the mysis stage larvae of the jumbo tiger prawn *Penaeus monodon* in laboratory culture in the Philippines. The authors separate this species from *H. milfordensis* on a number of bases. Firstly that zoosporulation was initiated only 2.5 hours after transfer of hyphae into sea water (*H. milfordensis* 7 days, 8 hours, or 22–48 hours according to Vishniac, 1958, Fuller *et al.*, 1964 and Tharp and Bland, 1977, respectively). The second major feature identified by Hatai *et al.* (1980) is that their species has polyplanetic and polymorphic zoospores. It is of note that Tharp and Bland (1977) comment that their *H. milfordensis* has zoospores of this type, pointing out that "obviously there is great variation in zoospore shape amongst the various strains of *H. milfordensis* investigated to date". On this basis it would seem that *H. philippinensis* could fall within *H. milfordensis* as recognized by Tharp and Bland (1977).

Saprolegniales, Haliphthoraceae

Atkinsiella

As with *Lagenidium* species there has been an increasing recognition of the role and potential of *Atkinsiella* sp. as aquatic animal parasites. There are now three species in the genus. The first, *Atkinsiella dubia* was originally described by Atkins (1954b) as *Plectospira dubia* and was renamed by Vishniac (1958) and placed by her in her newly created family Haliphthoraceae. The taxonomic position of *Atkinsiella* still remains to be agreed. Sparrow (1976) created the Atkinsiellaceae in a new order Eurychasmales in the saprolegnian "galaxy". In contrast, Martin (1977) again allied *Atkinsiella* with *Eurychasmium* but in a Eurychasmacae to be placed in the Lagenidiales. A major difficulty lies in the lack of detailed information on the lesser known taxa, and until these organisms are adequately understood a general agreement on the various interrelationships is unlikely to be obtained.

Atkinsiella dubia. Atkins discovered this fungus parasitizing the eggs of

Pinnotheres pisum and *Gonoplax rhomboides*. In the eggs the hyaline aseptate mycelium is from 27–50μm in diameter. Growth soon becomes irregular and the hyphae "inflate" up to a width of 100μm and the whole forms a sporangium which is largely intramatrical. Discharge tubes can be short or elongate (up to 400μm) and are flared at the orifice. Zoospores are diplanetic and dimorphic, the first motile stage being pyriform and the second elongate, both are laterally biflagellate and heterokont. The primary zoospores swim within the sporangium and encyst there, subsequently germinating to give secondary zoospores which are ultimately discharged through the exit tubes. Atkins (1954b) was able to infect the eggs of other marine crustacea (*Trypton spongicola*, *Crangon vulgaris*, *Leander serratus*, *Portunus depurator* and *Macropodia* sp.). Fuller et al. (1964) were able to isolate *Atkinsiella* from algal surfaces and investigated zoosporangial development. No sexual stages were observed.

Atkinsiella entomophaga. This species was found to be parasitic on the eggs of eight species of midges (Chironomid and Tanytodid) in fresh water in Virginia, U.S.A. (Martin, 1977). The thallus is spherical to ovate, 20–319 × 18–118μm, holocarpic with one to four discharge tubes which may be more than 3.5mm in length. Primary zoospores are formed endogenously and swarm within the sporangium before release, encysting immediately outside the sporangium. These zoospores are pyriform, 11 × 7μm and heterokont, the anterior flagellum being tinsel. The secondary zoospores are reniform, 7 × 9μm and laterally biflagellate. No sexual stages were observed.

Atkinsiella hamanaensis. Parasitic on larvae and ova of the mangrove crab in Japan (Bian and Egusa, 1980). The hyphae are stout, abundant and sparingly septate. *A. hamanaensis* is holocarpic with tapering discharge tubes 12–20μm in diameter, and up to a millimetre in length. Primary zoospores are pyriform measuring 6 × 4μm and are laterally biflagellate, usually encysting within the zoosporangium. The secondary zoospores are also pyriform, 6 × 5μm with no detected morphological differences from the primary zoospores. The fungus was isolated and readily infected crab eggs under laboratory conditions. Experiments with brine shrimps showed that *A. hamanaensis* was a more effective pathogen than *Lagenidium scyllae*. Physiological investigation showed the fungus to be euryhaline with an optimum temperature for growth between 29 and 32°C.

Lagenidiales

The order Lagenidiales contains a primarily parasitic group of endobiotic fungi occurring both in fresh and marine waters. There are three families.

The Lagenidiaceae, the Olpidiopsidaceae and the Sirolpidiaceae. The majority of members of the Lagenidiaeles are parasites of aquatic plants, but species of *Lagenidium* and *Sirolpidium* are significant parasites of aquatic animals.

Lagenidiaceae

These fungi have endobiotic, holocarpic thalli. Zoospores are of the secondary type developing either entirely within the sporangium or exogenously, with or without surrounding vesicles. A number of species have been described as parasites of nematodes and rotifers, but a more important role is played by the two marine species, *Lagenidium callinectes* and *Lagenidium chthamalophilum*.

Lagenidium callinectes. First recognized by Newcombe (Sandoz *et al.*, 1944) as an internal parasite of the eggs of the blue crab, *Callinectes sapidus*, this fungus was formally described by Couch (1942) and has been the subject of considerable investigation in recent years. Johnson and Bonner (1960) found it on the ova of the barnacle *Cheloniba patula*, and it was successfully isolated into pure culture from algal surfaces (Fuller *et al.*, 1964) and from blue crab eggs (Bland and Amerson, 1973). C. E. Bland (personal communication) found the fungus to be common in North Carolina waters—in late spring 1972, he found 95% of ovigerous crabs to be infected. The fungus consists of intramatrical branched, sparingly septate irregular hyphae, 5–12μm in diameter which will eventually fill the egg or body of the young crab (Figs 4a, b). Zoosporangia are formed on short extramatrical hyphae which penetrate through the host wall and act as discharge tubes. At the tip of the discharge tubes, a gelatinous vesicle up to 100μm in diameter is formed. Cytoplasm moves into this vesicle and zoospores are differentiated within. Successive protoplasmic units move into the extramatrical hyphae until nearly all the vegetative mycelium has been converted (Figs 4c, d, e). Bland and Amerson (1973) described this process in detail. Zoospores are pyriform, $9 \times 12\mu m$ with two laterally attached flagella, the anterior being tinsel, the posterior whiplash.

Lagenidium chthamalophilum. Johnson (1958, 1960) identified this fungus developing in the ova of *Chthamalus fragilis* at Beaufort Inlet, North Carolina. The stout (10–18μm) irregularly branched hyphae fill the infected ova and emerge from them. Sporangia are normally produced on intramatrical hyphae with one stout emergent discharge tube which expands apically into a spherical vesicle. Zoospores are reniform, laterally biflagellate, approximately $9 \times 7\mu m$, cleaved within the vesicle and

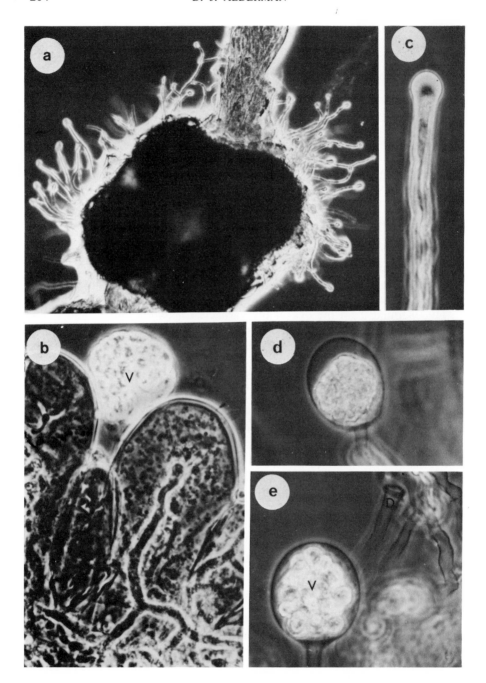

discharged at its rapid deliquescence. Oogonia, which were rarely observed, were 19–47μm in diameter, developing on intramatrical hyphae containing one or occasionally two oospores (18–25μm). No antheridia were observed.

Lagenidium scyllae. This fungus was found (Bian *et al.*, 1977) to be responsible for a lethal disease of ova and larvae of the mangrove crab *Scylla serrata* in experimental facilities in the Phillipines. The hyphae were stout, sparingly septate, branched with a diameter of 7.5 to 17μm. The fungus is holocarpic with vesicles formed at the end of discharge tubes which may measure up to 500μm in length. Zoospores are monoplanetic, biflagellate, pyriform in shape and 12.5 × 10μm in size. Release is by deliquescence of the vesicle or singly through an opening in the vesicle.

Lagenidium spp. In addition to the identified species of *Lagenidium* there have been numerous recent reports concerning the infection of larval marine crustacea, under artificial culture conditions, including shrimp in Texas (Lightner and Fontaine, 1973), Florida, Mexico, Tahiti and Honduras and in Dungeness crab from Oregon and American lobster larvae from California (Bland, 1975).

The outbreak reported by Lightner and Fontaine (1973) was in *Penaeus setiferus* in a shrimp hatchery in Texas, where larval mortality reached 12.4%. Those larvae that succeeded in reaching the first mysis stage survived and mortality ceased although fungal spores were still present in water samples. The mycosis was invasive, resulting in massive tissue destruction. Hyphae were contorted, irregular, branched, sparingly septate, thin-walled and 8–10μm in diameter. The only tissue reaction to invasion was the presence of a few melanized areas found associated with the hyphae. Discharge tubes with vesicles were formed and the fungus seemed to be very close to *Lagenidium callinectes*, although the authors report that there are some biochemical and morphological differences.

A similar mycosis of larval lobster (*Homarus americanus*) was reported by Neilson *et al.* (1976) in an experimental rearing system where 34 out of 42 hatches gave very low post-larval yields with more than 90% of animals in an affected system dying within 72 hours. Initial invasion was through the epidermal layer of the carapace with subsequent formation of mycelial mat

---

Fig. 4. *Lagenidium callinectes* is a parasitic endobiotic fungus found in crabs. (a) Eggs of blue crab infected by *L. callinectes* (dark field), (b) *L. callinectes* mycelium in gill of blue crab larva (V = vesicle), (c) shows an early vesicle of *L. callinectes*, (d) a vesicle with cleaving cytoplasm and (e) a mature vesicle with zoospores (V = vesicle; D = tip of discharge vesicle).

beneath. Larvae usually died by the second and third stages. The organism was a typical *Lagenidium*, but no specific identification has yet been published. Armstrong *et al.* (1976) described a similar mortality of the Dungeness crab.

All of the above outbreaks have been described from marine crustacea, largely in artificial or experimental rearing systems and they indicate that fungi of the genus *Lagenidium* have the potential to be severe parasites of artificially cultured crustacea in larval stages and that, in the blue crab at least, *Lagenidium callinectes* is a severe pathogen of the eggs and larvae of feral crabs.

Although the species of *Lagenidium* so far described are parasites of marine crustacea, Redfield and Vincent (1979) reported a *Lagenidium*-like fungus as a virulent parasite of the eggs of a calanoid copepod (*Diaptomus novamexicanus*) in an alpine lake in California. The authors estimated that in one year (1976), due to the onset of a severe epizootic in the early summer growing season, the fungus was responsible for an almost 50% decrease in potential copepod recruitment. Zoospore release is from a discharge tube which emerges through the egg sac membranes. No vesicle is formed, although thick-walled resting spores (20μm in diameter) were observed in up to 10% of the infected eggs but no antheridia were observed and the authors were uncertain whether or not these might have been sexual stages.

Lagenidiales, Sirolpidiaceae

Sirolpidium zoophthorum. This species was described (Vishniac, 1955) as the cause of sporadic mycoses of clam and oyster (*Mercenaria mercenaria* and *Crassostrea virginica*) larvae in laboratories at Milford, Connecticut, U.S.A. (Davis *et al.*, 1954). The fungus has a branched, septate thallus and hyphae 10–15μm wide when young, up to 80μm when mature. It is holocarpic, with sporangia being formed from enlarged terminal cells. Zoospores are monoplanetic, pyriform 5 × 2μm, endogenously cleaved. Thick-walled, gold-coloured resting spores up to 80 × 90μm, occur in older cultures. Grown on "dry" agar surfaces, "olpidioid" thallae were formed, separating the genus from *Pontisma*. Only one other species, *Sirolpidium bryopsidis* from marine algae has been described (Petersen, 1905).

Leptomitales

Willoughby (1970) and Pickering and Willoughby (1977) found that *Leptomitus lacteus* was an early and important member of the fungal flora, invading epidermal lesions of perch from Lake Windermere, Cumbria, England. The aetiology of the lesions was uncertain, but fungal involvement was not suspected although *L. lacteus* was the predominant fungus, whilst *Achyla*, *Aphanomyces* and *Saprolegnia* developed later. *Leptomitus lacteus* was also observed by Scott and O'Bier (1962) on eggs of *Salmo gairdneri* and *Esox lucius*. The authors commented that the fungus flourished on the fish eggs but rapidly deteriorated when that source of nourishment was depleted. They were unable to isolate it.

Peronosporales, Pythiaceae

The Peronosporales are coenocytic mycelial fungi, many of which are important plant parasites, whereas others are soil or water inhabiting saprophytes. Only one genus has been reported as being parasitic on aquatic animals — *Pythium*.

Atkins (1955), as part of a study of the pea crab *Pinnotheres pisum*, found a fungus inhabiting the egg masses of a few crabs which she described as *Pythium thalassium*. Its mycelium is largely intramatrical, 5–20μm in diameter and heavily branched (Fig. 5c). Extramatrical hyphae may reach 1mm in length. The zoosporangia are filamentous, single or branched, with extramatrical evanescent vesicles, 70–90μm in diameter. After zoospore release the vesicle membrane disintegrates and further sporangia may proliferate within the walls of the dehisced sporangium. Zoospores normally swim away actively but have also been observed to encyst within the sporangium and at the rupture of the vesicle. Zoospores are numerous, grooved, laterally biflagellate, 15μm long; when encysted they are 10.5–12μm in diameter and round to oval in shape. Spherical asexual resting bodies, 25–50μm in diameter occur occasionally. Atkins achieved experimental infection of viable eggs of *Crangon vulgaris*, *Leander serratus*, *Portunus depurator* and *Macropodia* spp. No sexual stages were observed and Atkins described *Pythium thalassium* as a new species on the basis of its marine habitat and proliferating filamentous sporangia.

In addition to Atkins' work, Delves-Broughton and Poupard (1976) described an epidemic systemic fungal disease of *Palaemon serratus*, a marine caridean prawn. The fungus isolated from the lesion did not produce sexual stages but on the basis of thallus morphology and asexual reproductive stages the authors suggested it to be *Pythium afertile* (Figs 5a, b). The gross signs in affected animals were the presence of an opaque zone with reddening spreading internally from the pre-existing wound. The disease could be transmitted by injection of hyphal fragments or by feeding the fungus incorporated into normal diet. Infection occurred in 50% of the experimental animals within 17 days, whether by injection at 18°C or by feeding at 7°C. Re-isolation after experimental infection was achieved.

Pythium daphnidarum was described as a destructive parasite of

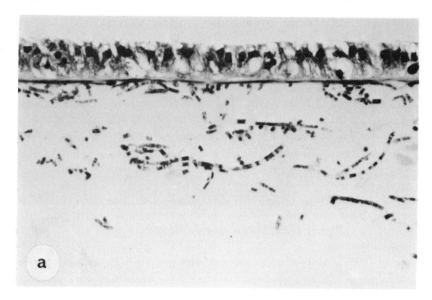

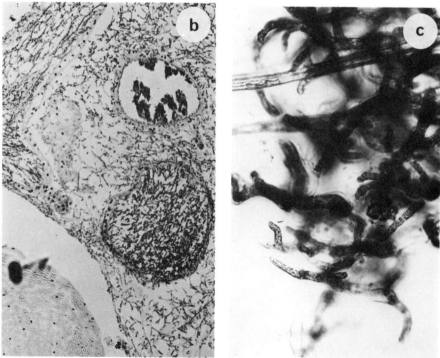

Fig. 5. In the Peronosporales, only *Pythium* spp. have been found as parasites on aquatic animals. (a) Shows *Pythium afertile* mycerlia in sub-exoskeletal tissues of shrimp and (b) shows mycelia ramifying through viscera of shrimp. (c) Shows *Pythium marinum* in an egg of the pea crab.

cladoceran crustaceans from Danish freshwater lakes by Petersen (1910). Khulbe and Sati (1979) isolated *Pythium undulatum* from adult *Carassius auratus* and reported successful attempts to infect artificially wounded fish under laboratory conditions. Shah *et al.* (1977) reported 10% of trout eggs and 5% of fry, on a survey of infections of Indian fresh water commercial species, to be infected with *Pythium*. Scott and O'Bier (1962), in their survey of fungi growing on fish eggs, isolated six strains of *Pythium* of which only *Pythium ultimum* was identified. The authors regarded their isolates as being saprophytes on dead eggs.

Eumycota, Zygomycotina, Zygomycetes

Entomophthorales

Basidiobolus. Neish and Hughes (1980) pointed out that the inclusion of the genus *Basidiobolus* in lists of fungal species parasitic on fish dates back to Leger's (1927) suggestion that *Ichthyophonus* should be transferred to the genus *Basidiobolus*. This suggestion appears to have been based on a

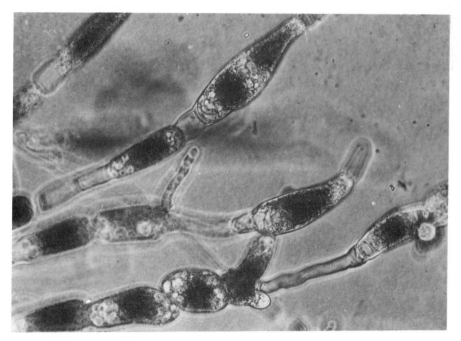

Fig. 6. Vegetative hyphae of *Basidiobolus ranarum*.

misunderstanding of the nature of *Ichthyophonus* on Leger's behalf. Neish and Hughes (1980) conclude that "at our present level of understanding there is little reason to suspect that *Basidiobolus* and *Ichthyophonus* will ever be shown to be congeneric." Nickerson and Hutchinson (1971) reported *B. ranarum* (Fig. 6) from fish, whilst Yang (1962) reported that *B. meristosporus* infected young carp (*Cyprinus carpio*). Tills (1977) in a survey for *B. ranarum* in the Southern Appalachian region of the U.S.A. found the species only in amphibia and not in fish or reptiles. It seems unlikely that *Basidiobolus* species are ever significant fish pathogens.

Zygomycotina, Trichomycetes

The Trichomycetes are a class of obligate symbionts of arthropods which grow attached to the chitinous linings of the gut or exoskeleton of the host. The relationship is generally regarded as purely symbiotic, but recently a new species of *Smittium*, *S. morbosum* Sweeney (1981) has been described which grows in the larval hind gut and penetrates the cells of the mid gut epithelium of the mosquito *Anopheles hilli*. It is regarded as causing the death of some larvae.

Fungi Incertae Sedis

Ichthyophonus

The genus *Ichthyophonus* Plehn and Mulsow (1911) has a very complex taxonomic history, resulting largely from a tendency to use the genus as a convenient "waste basket" for partially observed organisms, often with only superficial resemblances to each other, much as has occurred with *Perkinsus* (*Dermocystidium*). *Ichthyophonus* is considered in detail particularly in relation to life cycle and to recent outbreaks in Scottish waters elsewhere in this volume (McVicar, p.243) and therefore only limited discussion of a taxonomic and historical aspect of this important organism will be included here.

Plehn and Mulsow (1911) described the species *Ichthyophonus hoferi* parasitic in the rainbow trout (*Salmo gairdneri*), regarding it as a fungus with chytridiaceous affinities. This was probably the same organism observed by Hofer in cases of Taumelkrankheit ("Whirling Disease" or loss of balance) in trout, whilst Robertson (1909) had clearly observed *Ichthyophonus* in sea trout (*Salmo trutta*), flounder (*Platichthys flesus*) and haddock (*Gadus aeglefinus*). Previously Caullery and Mesnil (1905) had described two species in a new genus *Ichthyosporidium*. One of these species was *Ichthyosporidium phymogenes* and the other *Ichthyosporidium gastrophilum*. Robertson considered that the organism which she had observed was *Ichthyosporidium gastrophilum*. Pettit (1913) tried to overcome the confusion by transferring *Ichthyophonus hoferi* to become *Ichthyosporidium hoferi*. Over the years various authors have accepted, rejected, misunderstood or ignored this transfer.

Sprague (1965) has ably collated these confusions and proposed a logical solution. Neither of Caullery and Mesnil's (1905) two species of *Ichthyosporidium* were designated as type species by these authors. *Ichthyosporidium phymogenes* was corrected by Swarczewsky (1914) to *Ichthyosporidium giganteum* (Thelohan). *Ichthyosporidium giganteum* is generally accepted to be a protozoan (Sprague, 1965), whilst *Ichthyosporidium gastrophilum* and *Ichthyophonus hoferi* have fungus-like characters. Sprague therefore proposed accepting *Ichthyosporidium giganteum* as the type species of a genus *Ichthyosporidium*. As a result, *Ichthyosporidium gastrophilum* cannot remain in that genus since it is not in any way related to the type species of the genus. The first validly published name of this type of fungus is therefore *Ichthyophonus* Plehn and Mulsow (1911) and Plehn and Mulsow's description of *Ichthyophonus hoferi* will be the description of the type species. Undoubtedly Sprague's (1965) logical way out of the confusion into which science has been thrown should be accepted.

During this period of taxonomic confusion two other species of *Ichthyophonus* have been described — *Ichthyophonus intestinalis* Leger and Hesse (1923) and *Ichthyophonus lotae* Leger (1924). Neish and Hughes (1980) point out that there was no evidence that either of these fungi were associated with any pathological condition and that Leger (1927) subsequently transferred them to the genus *Basidiobolus*. Unless new cases of these fungi are found, no adequate comment on their validity can be made.

Although *Ichthyophonus* has been known since Hofer (1893), has been grown in culture (Sindermann and Scattergood, 1954), and various authors have proposed elaborate life cycles (Sindermann, 1956, Dorier and Degrange, 1961), the organism (Fig. 7) has never really become part of the mainstream mycological literature. Probably the main reason for this is that it has always been studied by zoologists or pathologists and is not an organism which easily fits into any well known mycological taxon. The only proposal for an affinity for *Ichthyophonus* is with *Basidiobolus* and the Entomophthorales which probably originates with Leger's (1927) transfer of his *Ichthyosporidium intestinalis* to *Basidiobolus intestinalis*. Certainly there are aspects of *Ichthyophonus* which are reminiscent of the Entomophthorales, but there is really no good evidence at present to make any

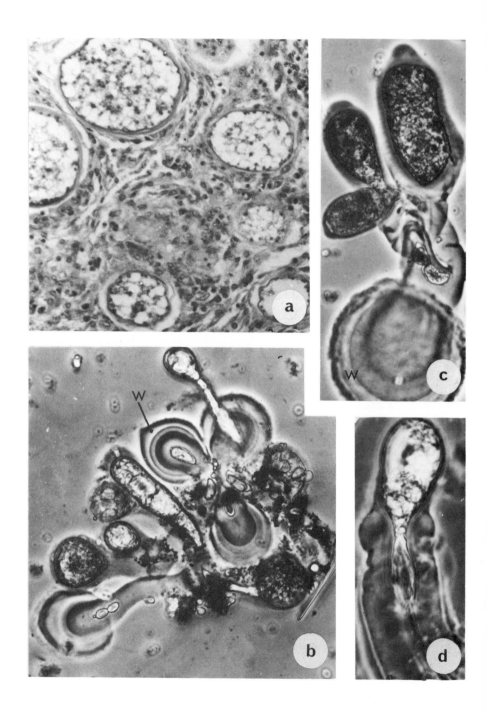

coherent suggestion for any relationship for *Ichthyophonus*. Indeed, as Neish and Hughes (1980) pointed out, the evidence favouring fungal affinities for *Ichthyophonus* is far from overwhelming. Equally, however, no adequate alternative affinity (excepting the original *Ichthyosporidium* confusion) has so far been proposed.

In recent years, investigations of fungal ultrastructure have led to the clarification of the affinities of a number of organisms (for example the *Thraustochytriales* and *Perkinsus* (*Dermocystidium*)). So far no extensive investigation of the ultrastructure of *Ichthyophonus* has been made. Preliminary investigations show some interesting points. The multiple cyst walls of *Ichthyophonus* under the light microscope are strongly reminiscent of the walls of the Thraustochytrids which consist of multiple layers of scales. However, *Ichthyophonus* cyst walls appear to be fibrous in nature (Fig. 8a). With the light microscope it is apparent that the *Ichthyophonus* cyst is multi-nucleate. The electron microscope shows that each of the multiple nuclei is accompanied by its own group of organelles — golgi, mitochondria and endoplasmic reticulum (Fig. 8b). These preliminary observations need further confirmation and unfortunately have not so far provided any new taxonomic pointers. A much greater understanding of the life cycle and structure of *Ichthyophonus* will be required.

Apart from the problem of the external taxonomic affinities of *Ichthyophonus*, there is the secondary problem of speciation within the genus. If Leger's species are ignored, two species, *I. hoferi* and *I. gasterophilum* have been described. Neither has been described in sufficient detail to permit modern workers to be really certain whether the organisms that they themselves are investigating belong to either of these species. The original descriptions were from freshwater fish but the most detailed investigations in recent years (Sinderman and Scattergood, 1954; McVicar, this volume) have been into epizootics of marine fish. In the main, the marine *Ichthyophonus* seem to be fairly consistent, bearing in mind the wide range of hosts involved. Recent descriptions from freshwater fish have been much more variable. For example, the organism described by Chauvier (1979) does not seem to fit *Ichthyophonus* as currently understood. Dorier and Degrange (1961) were clearly investigating an organism which fits into *Ichthyophonus*, but is significantly different from the forms in marine fish. It is clear that major epizootics occur in feral marine fish (Sindermann and Scattergood, 1954) whereas epizootics in freshwater fish are largely from

---

Fig. 7. Photographs of *Ichthyophonus* sp. showing (a) cysts in muscle of herring, (b) and (c) germinating cysts in culture (note the multiple layers in the old cyst walls (W)) and (d) the growing tip of a 'mycelium', showing trailing strands of cytoplasm leading back to the cyst.

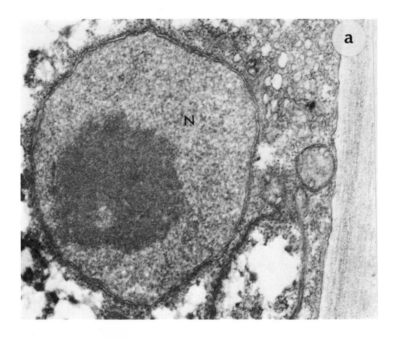

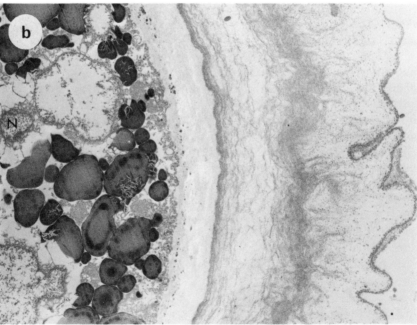

Fig. 8. Electron micrographs of *Ichthyophonus* showing (a) nucleus and associated organelles and (b) the thick multi-layered fibrous cyst wall (N = nucleus).

farmed fish (Rucker and Gustafson, 1953; Dorier and Degrange, 1961), where contaminated marine trash fish in the diet is a potential source of infection. Whether natural unaided infections of *Ichthyophonus* occur in the freshwater environment is uncertain.

Chatton (1920) and Jepps (1937) have described what may well be *Ichthyophonus* from marine copepods and Sindermann and Scattergood (1954) proposed that infected copepods might be a natural means of transmitting infection in the sea.

So confused are the descriptions of *Ichthyophonus* from different workers that only a systematic investigation based on cultures derived from a wide range of hosts will be adequate to determine speciation in *Ichthyophonus* and indeed to determine whether or not the wide range of organisms which are described as *Ichthyophonus* actually belong in the same taxon. From this point of view it is essential that cultures of *Ichthyophonus*, if obtained, should be made available to future workers by deposition in one or more of the major fungal culture collections.

Branchiomycosis

Despite the fact that *Branchiomyces* is considered a major problem in Eastern European commercial fish production (Meyer, 1973), the organism responsible continues to be a mycologist's enigma. Although two species have been described—*Branchiomyces sanguinis* and *Branchiomyces demigrans*—and although various authors have indicated that *Branchiomyces* may easily be cultured (Neish and Hughes, 1980), descriptions of its asexual (and sexual, if any exist) reproductive structures have been inadequate for mycotaxonomic comment. The genus is ignored by Ainsworth *et al.* (1973), and Ainsworth (1963) lists it as questionable.

Branchiomyces is known only as a parasite of gill tissues, *B. sanguinis* from carp, tench and stickleback and *B. demigrans* from pike and tench. Hyphae are coenocytic and *B. demigrans* is described as the possessor of thicker hyphal walls, somewhat larger spores and a tendency to spread beyond the vascular system of the gills. Bespalyi (1950) believed that he had observed both forms in a single culture and Lucky (1970) indicated that he felt that the described differences between the two species related more to host and environment than to any difference in species *per se*. The most recent extensive investigation of *Branchiomyces* has been in fish from alpine lakes (Grimaldi *et al.*, 1973) in which species identification was not possible.

Branchiomyces appears to produce terminal sporangia with spores which are 5–9μm in diameter. No adequate evidence as to the nature of these spores and as to whether they really are aplanospores has been produced. Many aspects of the spores as described appear very similar to spores of

Saprolegnia encysted within zoosporangia. Without adequate evidence as to the type and nature of the mycelium, the type and nature of the spores and the presence or absence of sexual reproductive stages, no adequate comment may be made as to the significance or taxonomic position of this fungus. Currently no evidence exists which could differentiate between inadequate descriptions of *Saprolegnia* spp. and *Branchiomyces*. For example, specimens observed at the Fish Diseases Laboratory, Weymouth, of *Saprolegnia* invasion of fish gills could mimic quite adequately existing descriptions of *Branchiomyces*. Peduzzi (1973) showed that the antigenic structure of his isolate of *Branchiomyces* was very similar to that of four different *Saprolegnia* isolates, leading him to suggest that the genus belonged in the *Saprolegniaceae*. If this is so, then *Branchiomyces* should have motile heterokont zoospores — features which are totally absent from the published descriptions of *Branchiomyces* to date.

The majority of descriptions of branchiomycosis is from fish farms in Eastern Europe (Plehn, 1924; Reichenback-Klinke and Elkan, 1965; van Duijn, 1956). A *Branchiomyces* in cultured eel in Taiwan was reported by Chien *et al.* (1978) who regarded the fungus responsible as being similar to *B. sanguinis*. The fungal hyphae grew in filamental arteries and the lamellar capillaries in the gills. Spore formation within hyphae was observed. There is no indication that isolation was attempted. Currently therefore, despite quite extensive investigation of *Branchiomyces* by zoologists and fish pathologists, and despite evidence that the fungus may be isolated into culture, there is inadequate evidence from the mycological aspect to allow adequate identification of *Branchiomyces*. Clearly this is an area which would repay further investigation.

Ostracoblabe implexa

This organism is a coenocytic mycelial fungus which has been shown (Alderman and Jones, 1971) to be responsible for shell disease in oysters. Although the fungus is capable of invading the shells of most molluscs, the severe irritation and subsequent reaction which produces shell disease apparently occurs only in the European flat oyster *Ostrea edulis* L.

O. implexa is endemic in Western European coastal waters and its discovery in *O. edulis* in New Brunswick, Canada, associated with shell diseases adds Eastern Canadian waters to the distribution given by Alderman (1976). Despite some taxonomic confusion (Bornet and Flahault, 1889; Bornet, 1891; Santesson, 1939; Feldmann, 1937) which led to the acceptance of *O. implexa* as a synonym for the lichen *Arthropyrenia* Leight, no reproductive stages have adequately been linked to the *O. implexa* mycelium. *O. implexa* is a shell-inhabiting organism utilizing the organic

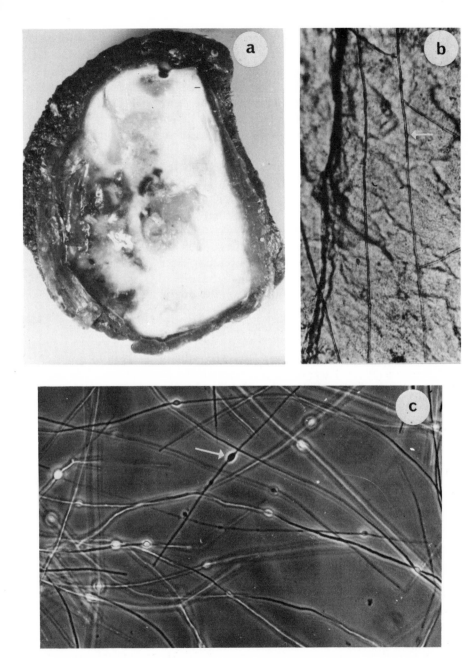

Fig. 9. Shell disease in the European flat oyster (*Oestrea edulis*) (a) is caused by *Ostracolabe implexa*. (b) Thin section of oyster shell showing mycelium of *O. implexa*. (c) Vegetative mycelium of *O. implexa* in culture. Arrows in (b) and (c) indicates 'prochlamydospore'.

matrix of the shell as nutrient. In *O. edulis* the penetration of the fungal mycelium between the shell and the oyster mantle causes irritation to which the living mantle tissues respond by laying down shell of high organic content. *Crassostrea* species may also be attacked by *O. implexa* but do not react to the irritation of the fungus by laying down highly proteinacious shell. The high levels of protein laid down by *O. edulis* result in increased growth by the fungus and the inevitable increased reaction from the oyster (Fig. 9a).

Both in the oyster and in culture *O. implexa* has a thin, straight mycelium 2μm in diameter. At regular (40–100μm) intervals the mycelium bears enlargements (termed by Alderman and Jones, 1971, proclamydospores) each of which contains a nucleus and other organelles. The mycelium is coenocytic, with septa being formed only in senescent regions (Figs 9b, c).

Significant levels of severe shell disease only occur on shallow water oyster beds over which water temperatures may exceed 18°C for significant periods of time. This agrees well with the behaviour of *O. implexa* in culture where there is very little growth at 15°C and an optimum of 30°C.

Nephromyces Giard

This was included as an imperfectly known or doubtful taxon by Johnson and Sparrow (1961). There are four species which have been described using the name *Nephromyces*. *Nephromyces* spp. Giard were from the kidney or renal organ of marine ascidians. Lacaze-Duthiers (1874) recorded the presence of "filaments confervoides" associated with concretions of uric acid and urates which are stored in the lumen of this organ in these animals. Alderman (1976) suggested that *Nephromyces* Giard must be regarded as extremely doubtful unless adequate new evidence becomes available.

Nephromyces piscinus Plehn (1916) was described by Plehn (1916) from the kidney of a freshwater carp; later Plehn (1924) used the form of the name *Nephromyces piscium*. It would seem clear from the various descriptions that Plehn did not intend to refer her organism to *Nephromyces* Giard, since she considered that the fungus that she isolated was similar to *Aspergillus*.

Reichenbach-Klinke (1956) reported a fungus which he believed to be *Nephromyces piscium* Plehn, which was in fact a *Penicillium*. Neish and Hughes (1980) consider that *Nephromyces* Plehn (1916) was "some sort of Hyphomycete" but with "only the most superficial resemblance to either *Aspergillus* or *Penicillium*". It would seem clear that neither *Nephromyces* Giard nor *Nephromyces* Plehn can be adequately identified on the basis of their original authors descriptions.

Spongiophaga

Carter (1878) described under this name some filaments which he observed in sponges, which he regarded as "Saprolegnious mycelium". Other reports by Lieberkuhn (1859) Schmidt (1862) and Polejaeff (1884) have also been made. Galtsoff (1942) reported on a mass mortality of adult commercial sponges (*Spongia* and *Hippospongia*) in which 60–90% of the sponge population on the coast of the West Indies died. He reported the presence of masses of fine aseptate hyphae growing in dead and dying sponges. No isolations were made, but Galtsoff suggested that the organism might be *Spongiophaga*.

Eumycota Deuteromycotina

The Deuteromycetes are the imperfect fungi. None are obligate parasites of fish, but there seems to be clear evidence that, in appropriate circumstances, some members are capable of acting as primary invaders of healthy fish. The Deuteromycetes consist of three groups—the Coelomycetes whose spores are produced in or on special fruiting structures, Hyphomycetes which are sterile mycelia or bear conidia and the Blastomycetes which are the Ascomycetous and Basidiomycetous yeasts for which sexual stages have yet to be demonstrated.

A number of different terms have been used in the description of diseases of deuteromycete aetiology and there has clearly been some confusion. The term phaeohyphomycosis has been used by Ajello (1975) to describe an infection caused by a dematiacious (= dark mycelium) hyphomycete. Ajello *et al.* (1977), however, also use this term to describe infections by *Phoma herbarum* which has hyaline hyphae and is a Coelomycete and not a Hyphomycete. Therefore neither phaeohyphomycosis nor chromomycosis applies. The term deuteromycosis might be used to apply to mycoses caused by imperfect fungi, or, should there really be a requirement for a specific term to cover *Phoma*-type mycoses, the term hyalocoelomycosis would appear appropriate.

Blastomycetes

These are the yeasts for which sexual stages have yet to be recognized, and therefore include both ascomycetous and basidiomycetous forms. A wide range of different Blastomycete species can be isolated from fish skin, mucus, gut etc. as has been demonstrated by workers such as Ross and Morris (1965) and Bruce and Morris (1973). *Cryptococcus* spp. were found

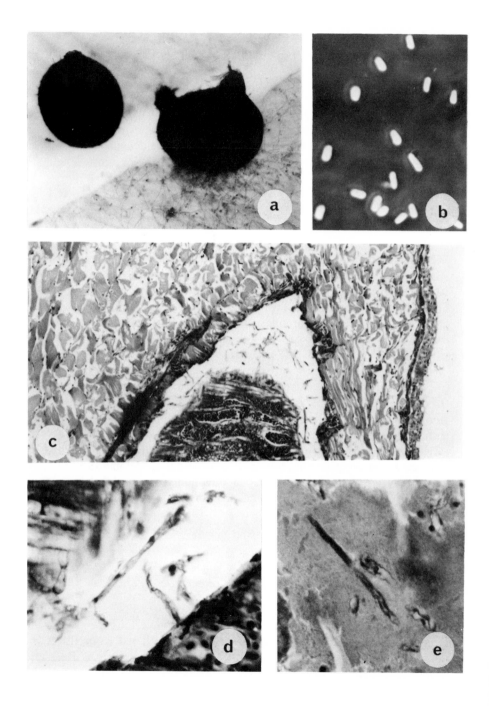

associated with exophthalmos of tench (Pierotti, 1971) and Hatai and Egusa (1975) described a condition which they term gastro-tympanites, in amago (*Oncorhynchus rhodurus*); they identified the yeast species as *Candida sake*. The disease is characterized by the presence of an extremely distended stomach, full of a viscid, turbid fluid and gas bubbles. The authors state that the stomach fluids contained large numbers of yeast cells which were readily isolated and identified. No indication of the diet of the fish was given.

Coelomycetes

Only one genus of Coelomycetes has been reported as responsible for disease in aquatic animals. The genus concerned is *Phoma*, species of which have been suggested to be responsible for two widely different diseases. *Phoma herbarum* (Figs 10a, b), fungal plant saprophyte has several times been reported from salmonid fry and fingerlings (Wood, 1974; Ross *et al.*, 1975). In contrast, Van Hyning and Scarborough (1973) described *Phoma fimeti* Brun, as the cause of the black mat syndrome of the tanner crab *Chionoecetes bairdi*. More recently, Hibbits *et al.* (1981) have suggested that an ascomycete, *Trichomaris invadens* is responsible. This disease is therefore discussed under that name.

Phoma herbarum

P. herbarum has been found infecting salmonid fry and fingerlings in the Pacific North West of the United States of America and in South West England. In one American site, losses of 2.6% over 6 years were attributed to this infection. External signs consisted of swollen and haemorrhagic vent and compression of the abdominal area. Caudal fin haemorrhaging was sometimes extensive with petechiae occurring occasionally on the lateral and ventral body surfaces. Severely affected animals rest on their sides on the bottom but are capable of righting themselves when startled. Histopathological investigation has indicated that the earliest detectable mycelium appears to occur in the pneumatic duct area of the swim bladder, with the infection becoming systemic thereafter. The swim bladder is usually free of fluid whilst the stomach may contain a watery fluid. Penetration of the swim bladder walls results in extensive inflammatory

Fig. 10. *Phoma herbarum* has been reported from salmonid fry and fingerlings. (a) Shows *P. herbarum* pycnidia and (b) *P. herbarum* conidia, (c), (d) and (e) are micrographs showing mycelium of *P. herbarum* infecting tissues of rainbow trout fry.

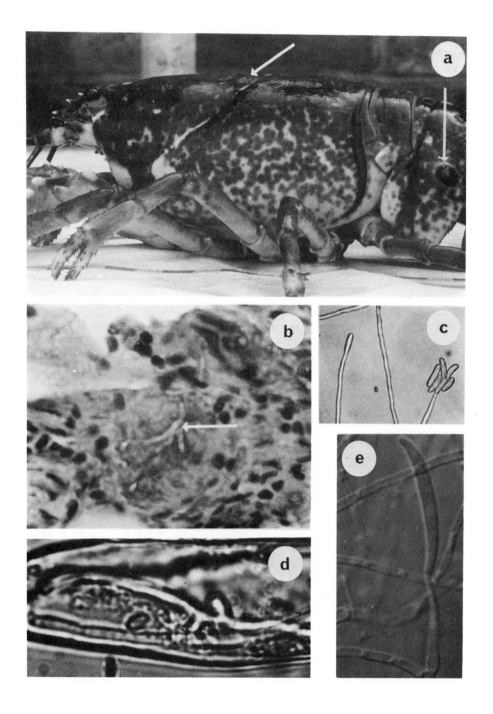

reaction in the surrounding tissues as the fungus invades the visceral organs (Figs 10c, d, e). Ross *et al.* (1975) succeeded in producing laboratory infections in chinook salmon fry both by feeding *Phoma* spores mixed with fish food (one infection in 24 animals) and by spraying an aerosol of *P. herbarum* conidia over the surface of a container in which anaesthetized salmon fry were recovering from MS222 anaesthesia (4 in 100 became infected).

Hyphomycetes

The hyphomycetes are those deuteromycetes in which the mycelium is either sterile or bears its asexual spores on hyphae which are not formed into a distinct and characteristic fruiting body.

Fusarium

The form genus *Fusarium* is very large in numbers of species. It consists of those Hyphomycetes with fusoid macroconidia with a foot cell which bears some kind of "heel". Microconidia and terminal or intercalary chlamydosopores may or may not be present. The authoritative taxonomic work on this genus is Booth (1971).

One species, *F. culmorium* has been reported as being responsible for mortality of 200 carp in a new earthen pond (Horter, 1960), the infection possibly being derived from a large inoculum of spores present because of layers of beech leaves on the pond bottom.

Within the last 10 years, a much more important role has been recognized for *Fusarium* in the marine environment. In the crustacea, *F. solani* in particular is increasingly accepted as a significant parasite, especially under conditions of intensive aquaculture. The condition known as burn spot disease or *Brandenfleckenkrankheiten* of crustacean exoskeletons is a single condition which may be of either fungal or bacterial aetiology and in the past 10 years there have been an increasing number of reports which associate *Fusarium* with this type of lesion.

In lobsters (Fisher *et al.*, 1978; Alderman, 1980), *Fusarium* infection takes the form of a chronic localized erosion of the exoskeleton, often accompanied by penetration of encapsulated fungal mycelium deep into the

---

Fig. 11. *Fusarium* infection in lobsters often takes the form of localized erosions: (a) 'burn spot disease' lesions (arrowed) on lobster; (b) encapsulated hyphae (arrowed) of *Fusarium solani* in deap burn spot lesion; (c) conidia of *F. solani*; (d) *Fusarium* hyphae in lobster larva gills; (e) conidia of *F. solani* isolated from lobster larvae.

underlying tissues (Fig. 11). Alderman (1980) reported the involvement of the fore gut in some infections. Death may be due to a combination of factors such as fungal toxins, secondary bacterial invasions, or a prevention of moulting as a result of large adhesions caused by the penetrating fungal hyphae. It was also possible to show that the introduction of mycelium of *F. solani* into artificial wounds in crabs would produce typical burn spot lesions whilst injections of *F. solani* at 40,000 spores per animal and higher produced a rapid mortality. Investigation of animals which died in this acute way showed that death resulted from thrombosis and infarction of branchial blood vessels due to encapsulated *F. solani* spores rather than to any active fungal growth.

In Japan, Egusa and Ueda (1972) reported the isolation of a *Fusarium* species from the Kuruma prawn, *Pennaeus japonicus*. The prawns were infected with what has become known as black gill disease which is characterized by the presence of many black spots in the gills, accompanied in severe cases by necrosis or collapse of the gills. In culture, the fungus produced four-celled canoe-shaped macroconidia and one-celled ovoid or oblong microconidia. The authors felt that the isolate probably represented a new species of *Fusarium* but temporarily designated it BG-*Fusarium*, standing for Black Gill *Fusarium*. Subsequently, Hatai *et al.* (1978) and Hatai and Egusa (1978b) carried out further work on BG-*Fusarium* and identified it as *Fusarium solani*. Lightner (1975) and Solangi and Lightner (1976) investigated large-scale mortalities of raceway reared Californian brown shrimps *Pennaeus californiensis* and carried out an investigation of artificial infections produced by the *Fusarium* species from *P. californiensis* in *P. aztecus* and *P. setiferus*. When *Fusarium* conidia were injected into the haemocoeles of the shrimps, very high numbers of conidia (in excess of 10^6 conidia per animal) were required to produce an infection. At lower levels, melanized and encapsulated conidia accumulated in the gills. The gross lesions in natural infections were much like those described for the black gill disease of Kuruma prawn. The failure of Solangi and Lightner to obtain infection except at very high levels by injection is perhaps explicable in that it would seem most likely for natural *Fusarium* infection to become established on the outer surfaces of the exoskeleton, perhaps at wounds, and then to penetrate deeply therefrom. Once established externally, invasion by vegetative mycelium would be quite different from the condition produced by injected conidia which might well be encapsulated before they germinated.

Burns *et al.* (1979) described an isolate of *Fusarium* from cuticular lesions on the Malaysian freshwater prawn *Macrobrachium rosenbergii*. Infections were observed in the abdominal pleura, carapace, swimmeretts, uropods and walking and feeding appendages. No 'black gill' condition was present but extensive tissue reaction, particularly melanin deposition around invading fungal hyphae was observed. Although the fungus was not identified to specific level the authors comment on its similarity to Egusa and Ueda's (1972) and Lightner and Fontaine's (1973) isolates.

Other Fungi Associated with Burn Spot Disease

Mann and Pieplow (1938) described three new hyphomycetes associated with burn spot lesions on crustaceans. *Didmaryia cambari* from *Cambarus affinis* had hyaline 4–6μm wide mycelium, unbranched conidiophores bearing uniseptate conidia 10–12 × 5–6μm which tend to form a cluster at the end of the conidiophore. The second species was *Ramularia astaci* from *Astacus astacus* which had 3–3.5μm diameter hyphae, and short conidiophores with four-celled conidia 3.5–4.5 × 20–40μm which were ellipsoidal in shape. Finally *Septocylindricum eriocheir* was isolated from *Eriocheir sinensis*, forming pale pink colonies with two- to four-celled conidia, 4.5–5.5 × 20–24μm and ellipsoidal in shape.

In 1958, Sordi described *Ramularia branchialis* from burn spot lesions on aquarium lobsters *Homarus gammarus* and *Didymaria palinuri* from crawfish *Palinuris vulgaris*.

Aureobasidium

A single case involving a species of *Pullularia* was described by Otte (1964) from a stingray, *Trygon pstonacea*, in a marine aquarium. The fungus involved can probably be more accurately reassigned to the genus *Aureobasidium*. The infection was typical of hyphomycete infection with soft, whitish-grey focal masses involving the liver. Tissue response was granulomatous. Otte reported isolation of the fungus, and experimental infection of carp and subsequent re-isolation of fungus.

Dematiaceous Hyphomycetes

The dematiaceous hyphomycetes have pigmented hyphae and systemic mycoses produced by dematiaceous species have been termed phaeohyphomycoses or chromomycoses. There are two main dematiaceous genera reported with some consistency from fish — *Exophiala* and *Ochroconis*.

Ochroconis

As a result of the work of Kirilenko and All-Achmed (1977) the genus *Ochroconis* de Hoog & von Arx (1973) now contains two species found to be pathogenic to fish and whose rather complex taxonomic history is outlined by Neish and Hughes (1980).

Ochroconis tshawytschae. This was isolated by Doty and Slater (1946) from young chinook salmon (*Oncorhynchus tshawytschae*). It was found in the posterior half of a kidney in less than 1% of the fish from one fisheries station in California. Doty and Slater were unable to induce experimental infection in salmon with their isolates. The species has subsequently been isolated from soil (Barron and Bush, 1962; Roy *et al.*, 1962) as well as from the surface of tomato roots (Kirilenko and All-Achmed, 1977). Conidia are 3.5 × 14μm, three septate, ovoid, cylindric and minutely echinulate.

Ochroconis humicola. In 1973, Elkan and Philpot reported *O. humicola* to be a pathogen of frogs. Shortly afterwards, Ross and Yasutake (1973) reported the same species as causing weakly contagious disease of laboratory held juvenile coho salmon (*Oncorhynchus kisutch*). External lesions were not consistently present, and in their absence the only indication of disease was an enlarged abdomen. The body cavity usually contained watery fluid and adhesions frequently occurred between the various visceral organs, some of which exhibited grey coloured lesions. Histopathologically, the condition was found to be systemic with the fungal mycelium responsible for the development of numerous large lesions throughout the tissues (Fig. 12). The kidney was apparently particularly susceptible. The authors attempted experimental infection, but were successful only when ground mycelial matt was mixed in a commercially prepared dry meal diet with ground glass. Only three of ten experimental fish were infected in this way.

Subsequently Ajello *et al.* (1977) reported a series of epizootics in rainbow trout (*Salmo gairdneri*) in a Tennessee fish hatchery from 1969 to 1973. Disease outbreaks began shortly after egg hatch (September), reaching a peak in October and November with infections rarely being observed during June, July and August. External signs consisted of vesicular areas on the flank, together with small to medium size ulcers, oedema and exophthalmus. Haemorrhages were found throughout the entire body cavity and internal organs were studded with mycelial aggregates. Histopathological investigation showed abundant dematiaceous septate hyphae in all infected tissues. In particular, the kidneys contained massive chronic granulomata which progressively displaced normal tissue. Conidia were 2.5–4 × 6–11.5μm, pale to olive-brown in colour, two-celled and finely echinulate, developing sympodially from the unbranched conidiospores. The outbreaks caused by this fungus occurred seasonally over a 4-year period but ceased when a new source of hatchery water was

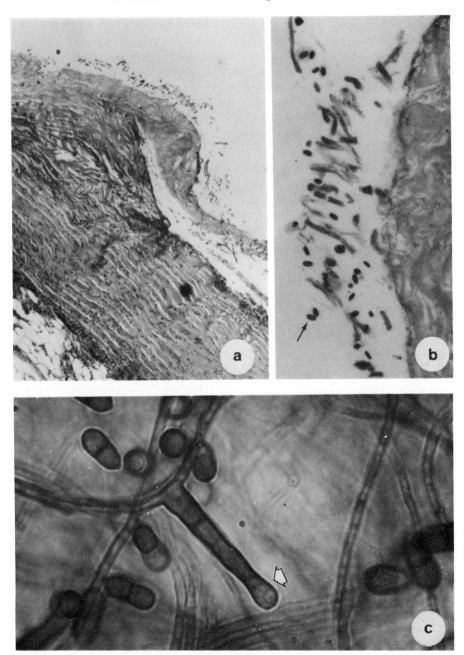

Fig. 12. *Ochroconis humicola* can infect the dermis of rainbow trout (a and b; arrow indicates conidium). (c) Shows a conidiophore (arrow) and conidia of *O. humicola*.

obtained, the old being contaminated with septic tank seepage. Attempts to produce infections by placing yearling rainbow trout in strong suspensions of *O. humicola* mycelium and spores failed, but intra-peritoneal injections succeeded within 3 days, death generally occurring within 7–10 days after inoculation with similar clinical and histopathological features to those of natural infections.

Exophiala

There are four separate reports of members of this genus being found as parasites of fish.

E. salmonis (Fig. 13) was reported (Carmichael, 1966) from three widely separated mass mortalities at one hatchery in Alberta, Canada. The years concerned were 1948, 1956 and 1960 and all outbreaks were in winter. Gross signs were exophthalmos and cranial ulcers, with infection levels up to 40%.

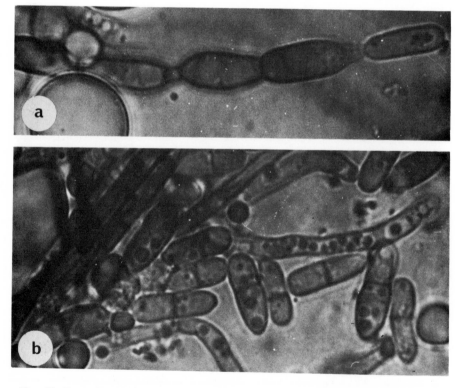

Fig. 13. Some *Exophiala* spp. are parasitic on fish. (a) Shows a conidiophore and (b) a mature 2-celled conidia of *Exophiala salmonis*.

Histopathological investigation showed necrotic and granulomatous response with the presence of giant cells in the brain. No other organs were involved. Both Wolke (1975) and Ajello (1975) point out that the description of this pathology as a mycetoma by Carmichael is inaccurate.

Richards *et al.* (1978) reported a further mortality due to *E. salmonis*, this time in *Salmo salar* L. second year smolts in sea cages on the Scottish West Coast. The outbreak was limited to one cage, in which approximately 10% of fish died during a 4-month period. Affected fish had grossly swollen posterior abdomens due to enlargement of the posterior kidney, which itself showed large (circa 3.5cm) greyish white nodules with, in two cases, necrotic lesions extending into the dorsal musculature. Histopathological investigations showed proliferating mycelium invading the kidney, with a variable degree of involvement of heart, liver, spleen, pancreas and muscle. The tissue reaction was granulomatous and giant cells were present. The authors gave extensive and detailed description of the histopathology of this mycosis. Isolates were made and identified as *E. salmonis*. Since only one cage of fish was infected, the authors suggested that infection might have been as a result of a focal fungal contamination of the artificial diet. De Hoog (1977) indicated that *E. salmonis* had also been isolated from *Aurucaria* wood and that *E. brunnea* Papendorf isolated from soil is synonymous with *E. salmonis*.

Conidia are 3 × 5–8 or 3 × 11–14μm, typically uniseptate, cylindrical clavate in shape with stipitate proximal end, constricted at the (refractile) septum and formed on annellides.

The third *Exophiala* outbreak was described by Fijan (1969) amongst channel catfish (*Ictalurus punctatus*) in Alabama. Tissue response was either non-proliferative or proliferative and granulomatous. Isolations were made and the pathology was reproduced in healthy fish by means of intraperitoneal injection. The organism was subsequently described as *E. pisciphila* McGinnis & Ajello (1974). Conidia are 2–3 × 3–5μm, aseptate, subglobose or ovoid with rounded distal end, stipitate and truncate at the proximal end.

The most recent *Exophiala* outbreak was described by Blazer and Wolke (1979) from a marine aquarium in New England. Five natural infections were found in *Steneotomus versicolor*, *Gadus morhua*, *Hippocampus hudsonius*, *Xanthichthys ringens* and *Amphiprion sebae*. The authors give detailed descriptions of both the natural infection and experimentally induced ones. Externally, two fish (*X. ringens* and *H. hudsonius*) showed external dermal masses which the authors attributed to fungus. Internally, two animals (*S. versicolor* and *G. morhua*) had internal lesions—raised (1 to 5mm) round yellow to white areas in the liver, kidney, myocardium, swim bladder and spleen. All natural cases except for *G. morhua* were regarded as acute and were non-proliferative.

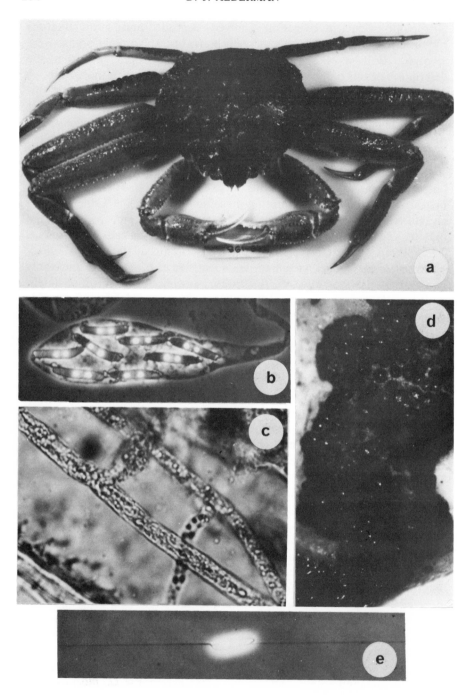

Eumycota Ascomycotina

The only known case of an Ascomycete in its perfect form parasitizing an aquatic animal is that of the newly described *Trichomaris invadens* Hibbits *et al.* (1981). Hyphomycetes such as *Exophiala*, *Ochroconis* and the coelomycete, *Phoma*, are probably the imperfect or anomorph stages of Ascomycetes, whose perfect stages are not known.

Trichomaris invadens

The snow or tanner crab, *Chinocetes bairdi*, is the subject of an industry which in 1977 was worth in excess of $50,000,000 (Sparks and Hibbits, 1979). The black mat syndrome as originally defined by van Hyning and Scarborough (1973) was described as a purely external encrustation of the exoskeleton occurring mainly on the posterior part of the carapace, but also affecting the posterior walking legs and occasionally extending over the entire carapace to cover the eyes and mouth parts (Fig. 14a). The covering, as indicated by its name, is a dense mat black colour and is nodular in appearance. As described by van Hyning and Scarborough (1973), the disease was regarded purely in terms of a non-pathogenic incrustation of the exoskeleton, which caused problems in processing. It appeared to be area and species specific, occurring with particular frequency in the Kodiak-Cordova area of Alaska, where up to 75% infection was detected in certain localities.

Sparks and Hibbits (1979), who carried out more extensive histopathological investigations of *C. bairdi* showing black mat syndrome, were able to show, by use of Grocott's fungal stain, that the black mat external signs were accompanied by a fungal invasion of tissues beneath the exoskeleton. Hyphae invading internal tissues were non-pigmented (Fig. 14c) and therefore difficult to detect except by means of Grocott's method. Virtually all of the epidermal tissues were invaded and lesions extended to the eyestalk, eyestalk muscles and the connective tissue sheaths of the oesophagus, stomach, heart, thoracic ganglion, haematopoietic tissue, ovary, hepatopancreas and antennal gland. Although Sparks and Hibbits (1979) did not isolate the fungus concerned, they expressed some doubt as to its identity. van Hyning and Scarborough (1973), in their original work

---

Fig. 14. *Trichomaris invadens* infects Tanner crabs causing 'black mat' disease which encrusts the carapace (a). Unitunicate ascus with ascospores is shown in (b) and 'black mat' subiculum and perithecia in (c). (d) Hyaline hyphae of *T. invadens* within crab tissue and (e) a single ascospore showing fine hairs at either end.

with this syndrome, isolated a coelomycete which they identified as *Phoma fimeti*. Hibbits *et al.* (1981) have now elaborated their doubt (Sparks and Hibbits, 1979) as to this original identification and consider that the *P. fimeti* isolated by van Hyning and Scarborough (1973) was a chance contaminant and that the fruiting bodies observed on the surface of infected crab exoskeletons were not those of a Coelomycete but of an Ascomycete which they describe as *Trichomaris invadens*, a new genus and species of marine ascomycete.

The external hyphae are 5μm in diameter, black, branched and sparingly septate, forming the black matt subiculum over the host carapace. In contrast, the hyphae within the living tissues are non-pigmented and only 2–2.5μm in diameter. The perithecea are embedded in the subiculum (Fig. 14d) and are thick walled 250–400μm in diameter, containing unitunicate thin walled clavate asci 85–155 × 12–17μm in size (Fig. 14b). The asci contain hyaline oblong-to-elipsoidal ascospores 15–11 × 4.6–5μm in size, largely uniseptate and bearing an unusually long hair-like appendage at either end which may be up to 360μm in length (Fig. 14e). Despite extensive attempts Hibbits *et al.* (1981) have been unable to isolate the fungus into culture. Since there is a very high level of infection of a feral population, they comment that there seems to be no doubt that *T. invadens* is a far more virulent pathogen than any of the other fungi previously implicated in the Burn Spot Disease Syndrome in crustacea.

Other Ascomycetes

It is of note that Kohlmeyer (1972) has identified the Ascomycete *Abyssomyces hydrozoicus* growing on the tubes of hydrozoans from a number of sites. There is no evidence that this organism is other than a saprophyte, but nevertheless, in view of the recent work of Hibbits *et al.* (1981) discussed above, the possibility that Ascomycetes may play more of a role in aquatic pathobiology than has hitherto been realised must be borne in mind.

Control

Control of fungal diseases can obviously be practised adequately only under fish farm or experimental conditions. Therefore, even if control measures were available for fungal diseases of feral marine fish and shellfish, it would not be practicable to attempt to control disease organisms such as *Ichthyophonus* in natural populations. In the somewhat more controllable freshwater environment and with sedentary marine species such as molluscs, one form of control, namely avoidance of the introduction of new diseases, is a very practical proposition. This can take the form of either a prohibition on all introductions or the enforcement of an adequate quarantine regime.

In the farm or laboratory environment it is possible, to varying degrees, to take disease control to the level of chemoprophylaxis and/or chemotherapy. For the most part, the fungi responsible for aquatic diseases differ markedly from species responsible for agricultural diseases and for this reason and for reasons of host sensitivity, conventional agrochemicals are not used.

The two culture systems in which fungi cause regular and severe clinical disease are in saprolegnid infections in freshwater fish culture where saprolegnid infections are a major problem and in crustacean culture. For this reason, these are the only areas into which any significant and systematic research into chemical control has been carried out.

Control of saprolegnid infections on fish and fish eggs has been successfully practised for nearly 50 years using the diarylmethane dye, malachite green. As a result of possible difficulties with continued use of malachite green, a number of workers have made extensive investigations into the possibility of developing new fisheries fungicides (Olah and Farkas, 1978; Alderman, 1982; Hatai, 1980). Only Hatai has reported the discovery of a compound which could remotely equal malachite green in terms of low toxicity to host combined with very high efficacy.

In the area of crustacean culture, there have been investigations into the control of *Aphanomyces astaci* (Häll and Unestam, 1980) and of *Lagenidium callinectes* (Armstrong *et al.*, 1976; Bland *et al.*, 1976) and again malachite green seems to be the chemical of choice both in terms of high efficacy and low host toxicity.

Other agents such as formalin, copper sulphate, potassium permanganate and furanace have been used to control or to attempt to control fungal infections of aquatic animals; however, none of these appear to be entirely satisfactory. Clearly, chemotherapy of the important fungal diseases is an area which may repay further investigation.

Acknowledgements

I would like to thank Dr A. K. Sparks and colleagues for permission to quote from their unpublished manuscript on *Trichomaris invadens* and for the use of their photographs of that organism. I am also indebted to Dr C. Bland for illustrations of *Fusarium*, *Lagenidium* and *Haliphthoros*, to Drs Bland and Richardson for the photograph of the *Haliphthoros*-infected crab and to Dr Delves Broughton for the photomicrographs of *Pythium afertile.* Fig. 4(c) is reproduced by kind permission of Mycologia and Figs. 3(a)-3(c) by kind permission of the Director, Japan Sea Regional Fisheries Laboratory.

References

Ainsworth, G. C. (1963). "Ainsworth and Bisby's Dictionary of the Fungi." Commonwealth Mycological Institute, Kew, Surrey.

Ainsworth, G. C., Sparrow, F. K. and Sussman, A. S. (1973). "The Fungi—an Advanced Treatise. Volume IVB—A Taxonomic Review with keys: Basidiomycetes and Lower Fungi." Academic Press, New York.

Ajello, L. (1975). Phaeohyphomycosis: definition and etiology. Proceedings 3rd International Conference on the Mycoses, São Paulo, Brazil, 1974. *Pan American Health Organization Scientific Publication* **304**, 126-130.

Ajello, L., McGinnis, M. R. and Camper, J. (1977). An outbreak of phaeohypnomycosis in rainbow trout caused by *Scolecobasidium humicola. Mycopathologia* **62**, 15-22.

Alderman, D. J. (1976). Fungal diseases of marine animals. *In* "Recent Advances in Aquatic Mycology" (Ed. E. B. G. Jones), pp.223-260. Paul Elek, London.

Alderman, D. J. (1980). *Fusarium solani* causing an exoskeletal pathology in cultured lobsters, *Homarus vulgaris. Transactions of the British Mycological Society* **76**(1), 25-27.

Alderman, D. J. (1982). *In vitro* testing of fisheries chemotherapeutants. *Journal of Fish Diseases* **5**, 112-123.

Alderman, D. J. and Gras, P. (1969). Gill disease of Portuguese oysters. *Nature, London* **224**, 616-617.

Alderman, D. J. and Jones, E. B. G. (1971). Shell disease of oysters. *Fishery Investigations, London, Ser.II* **26**(8), 1-19.

Alderman, D. J., Harrison, J. L., Bremer, G. B. and Jones, E. B. G. (1974). Taxonomic revisions in the marine biflagellate fungi: the ultrastructural evidence. *Marine Biology* **25**, 345-347.

Armstrong, D. A., Buchanan, D. V. and Caldwell, R. S. (1976). A mycosis caused by *Lagenidium* spp. in laboratory reared larva of the Dungeness crab, *Cancer magister*, and possible chemical treatments. *Journal of Invertebrate Pathology* **28**(3), 329-336.

Atkins, D. (1954a). Further notes on a marine member of the Saprolegniaceae, *Leptolegnia marina* n. sp. infecting certain invertebrates. *Journal of the Marine Biological Association of the United Kingdom* **33**, 613-625.

Atkins, D. (1954b). A marine fungus *Plectospira dubia* n. sp. (Saprolegniaceae) infecting crustacean eggs and small crustacea. *Journal of the Marine Biological Association of the United Kingdom* **33**, 721-732.

Atkins, D. (1955). *Pythium thalassum* sp. nov. infecting the egg mass of the pea crab, *Pinnotheres pisum. Transactions of the British Mycological Society* **38**, 31-46.

Bahnweg, G. and Bland, C. E. (1980). Comparative physiology and nutrition of *Lagenidium callinectes* and *Haliphthoros milfordensis*, fungal parasites of marine crustaceans. *Botanica Marina* **23**, 689-698.

Barron, G. L. and Bush, L. F. (1962). Studies on the soil hyphomycete *Scoleco-basidium*. *Canadian Journal of Botany* **40**, 77–84.

Bespalyi, I. I. (1950). "Zhabernaya gnil 'karpa i mery ber'by s nei." Akademii Nauk, Ukraine, SSR, Kiev. (not seen, cited by Neish and Hughes, 1980: *vide infra*).

Bian, B. Z. and Egusa, S. (1980). *Atkinsiella hamanaensis* sp. nov. isolated from cultivated ova of the mangrove crab, *Scylla serrata* (Forsskal). *Journal of Fish Diseases* **3**(5), 373–386.

Bian, B. Z., Hatai, K. P. G. L. and Egusa, S. (1977). Studies on the fungal diseases in Crustaceans. I. *Lagenidium scyllae* sp. nov. isolated from cultivated ova and larvae of the mangrove crab (*Scylla serrata*). *Transactions of the Mycological Society of Japan* **20**, 115–124.

Bland, C. E. (1975). Fungal diseases of marine crustacea. *Proceedings of the Third US–Japan Meeting on Aquaculture at Tokyo, October 1974*, 41–48.

Bland, C. E. and Amerson, H. V. (1973). Observations on *Lagenidium callinectes*: isolation and sporangial development. *Mycologia* **65**(2), 310–320.

Bland, C. E., Ruch, D. G., Salser, B. R. and Lightner, D. V. (1976). Chemical control of *Lagenidium*, a fungal pathogen of marine crustacea. *University of North Carolina Sea Grant Publication, UNC-SG-76-02*, 38pp.

Blazer, V. S. and Wolke, R. E. (1979). An *Exophiala*-like fungus as the cause of a systemic mycosis of marine fish. *Journal of Fish Diseases* **2**, 145–152.

Booth, C. (1971). The genus *Fusarium*. Commonwealth Mycological Institute, Kew, Surrey, England.

Bornet, E. (1891). Note sur l'*Ostracoblabe implexa* Born et Flah. *Journal de Botanique* **5**, 397–400.

Bornet, E. and Flahault, C. (1889). Sur quelque plantes vivant dans le test calcaire des Mollusques. *Bulletin de la Societe Botanique de France* **36**, CXLVII-CLXXVI.

Bruce, J. and Morris, E. O. (1973). Psychrophilic yeasts isolated from marine fish. *Antonie van Leeuwenhoek* **39**, 331–339.

Burns, C. D., Berrigan, M. E. and Henderson, G. E. (1979). *Fusarium* sp. infections in the freshwater prawn *Macrobrachium hendersonii*. *Aquaculture* **16**(3), 193–198.

Carmichael, J. W. (1966). Cerebral mycetoma of trout due to a *Phialophora*-like fungus. *Sabouraudia* **5**, 120–123.

Carter, H. J. (1878). Parasites of the Spongida. *Annals and Magazine of Natural History (Series 5)* **2**, 157–172.

Caullery, M. and Mesnil, F. (1905). Sur les haplosporidies parasites des poissons marins. *Comptes rendu des Seances de la Societé Biologie* **58**, 640–643.

Chatton, E. (1920). Les Peridiniens parasites. Morphologie, reproduction, ethologie. *Archives de Zoologie experimentale et generale* **59**, 1–475.

Chauvier, G. (1979). Mycose viscerale de poissons dulcaquicoles tropicaux. *Annales de Parasitologie* **54**(1), 105–111.

Chien, C.-H., Miyazaki, T. and Kubuta, S. S. (1978). *Branchiomyces* of the reared Japanese Eel in Taiwan. *Fish Pathology* **13**(4), 179–182.

Couch, J. N. (1942). A new fungus on crab eggs. *Journal of the Elisha Mitchell Scientific Society* **58**, 158–162.

Davis, H. C., Loosanoff, V. L., Weston, W. H. and Martin, C. (1954). A fungus disease in clam and oyster larvae. *Science, New York* **120**, 30–38.

De Hoog, G. S. (1977). The black yeasts and allied hyphomycetes. *Studies in Mycology*, Centraalbureau voor Schimmelcultures, Baarn, **15**, 1–140.

De Hoog, G. S. and von Arx, J. A. (1973). Revision of *Scolecobasidium* and *Pleurophragmium*. *Kavaka* **1**, 55–60.

Delves-Broughton, J. and Poupard, C. W. (1976). Disease problems of prawns in recirculation systems in the U.K. *Aquaculture* **7**, 201–217.

Dick, M. W. (1971). Leptolegniellaceae, fam. nov. *Transactions of the British mycological Society* **57**, 417–425.

Dick, M. W. (1973). Saprolegniales. *In* "The Fungi. An Advanced Treatise (Eds. G. C. Ainsworth, F. K. Sparrow and A. S. Sussman), Vol. IVB Ch. 7. Academic Press, New York.

Dorier, A. and Degrange, C. (1961). L'evolution de l'*Ichthyosporidium (Ichthyophonus) hoferi* (Plehn and Mulsow) chez les salmonides d'elevage (truite arc en ciel et saumon de fontaine). *Travaux de la Laboratoire de Hydrobiologie et Pisciculture, Université de Grenoble 1960/1961*, 7–44.

Doty, M. S. and Slater, D. W. (1946). A new species of *Heterosporium* pathogenic on young chinook salmon. *American Midland Naturalist* **36**, 663–665.

Egusa, S. and Ueda, T. (1972). A *Fusarium* sp. associated with Black Gill Disease of the Kuruma prawn, *Penaeus japonicus* Bate. *Bulletin of the Japanese Society of Scientific Fisheries* **38**(11), 1253–1260.

Elkan, E. and Philpot, C. M. (1973). Mycotic infections in frogs due to a *Phialophora* like fungus. *Sabouraudia* **11**, 99–105.

Feldmann, J. (1937). Sur les gaudies de quelques *Arthropyrenia* marins. *Revue Bryologique et Lichenologique (N.S.)* **10**, 64–73.

Fijan, N. (1969). Systemic mycosis in channel catfish. *Bulletin of the Wildlife Diseases Association* **5**, 109–110.

Fisher, W. S., Nilsen, E. H. and Shleser, R. A. (1975). Effect of the fungus *Haliphthoros milfordensis* on the juvenile stages of the American lobster *Homarus americanus*. *Journal of Invertebrate Pathology* **26**, 41–45.

Fisher, W. S., Nilson, E. H., Steenbergen, J. F. and Lightner, D. V. (1978). Microbial diseases of cultured lobsters—a review. *Aquaculture* **14**, 115–140.

Franc, A. and Arvy, L. (1970). Donnees sur l'evolution de la "maladie des branchies" chez les hutres et sur son agent causal: *Thanatostrea polymorpha* Franc et Arvy 1969. *Bulletin biologique de la France et de la Belgique* **104**, 3–19.

Fuller, M. S., Fowles, B. E. and McLaughlin, D. J. (1964). Isolation and pure culture study of marine phycomycetes. *Mycologia* **56**, 745–756.

Galtsoff, P. S. (1942). Wasting disease causing mortality of sponges in the West Indies and Gulf of Mexico. *Proceedings of the 8th American Science Congress, 1940* **3**, 411–421.

Ganaros, A. E. (1957). Marine fungus affecting eggs and embryo of *Urosalpinx cinerea*. *Science, New York* **125**, 1194.

Gicklehorn, J. (1923). *Aphanomyces ovidestruens* nov. spec.—ein parasit un den Eiern von *Diaptomus*. *Lotos* **71**, 143–155.

Grimaldi, E., Peduzzi, G., Caviccholi, G. and Spreafico, E. (1973). Diffuson infezione branchiale da funghi attribuiti al genere *Branchiomyces* Plehn (Phycomyces, Saprolegniales) a carico dell'ittiofauna di laghi situati a nord e a sud dell Alpi. I. Epidemiologia dell'infezione da *Branchiomyces* in ambiente lacustre. *Memorie Instituto italiano di Idrobiologia Marco de Marchi* **30**, 61–80.

Häll, L. and Unestam, T. (1980). The effect of fungicides on the survival of the crayfish plague fungus, *Aphanomyces astaci*, Oomycetes, growing on fish scales. *Mycopathologia* **72**, 131–134.

Hatai, K. (1980). Studies on the pathogenic agents of Saprolegniasis in fresh water fishes. *Special Report of Nagasaki Prefectural Institute of Fisheries. No. 8*, 95pp.

Hatai, K. and Egusa, S. (1975). *Candida* sake from gastro-tympanites of amago *Oncorhynchus rhodurus*. *Bulletin of the Japanese Society for Scientific Fisheries* **49**, 993.

Hatai, K. and Egusa, S. (1978a). Studies on the pathogenic fungus of mycotic granulomatosis — II. Some of the note on the MG-fungus. *Fish Pathology* **13**(2), 85–89.

Hatai, K. and Egusa, S. (1978b). Studies on the pathogenic fungus associated with Black gill disease of Kuruma Prawn, *Penaeus japonicus* — II. Some of the note on the BG-fungus. *Fish Pathology* **12**(4), 225–231.

Hatai, K. and Egusa, S. (1979). Studies on the pathogenic fungus of mycotic granulomatosis — III. Development of the medium for the MG-fungus. *Fish Pathology* **13**(3), 147–152.

Hatai, K., Egusa, S., Takahashi, S. and Ooe, K. (1977). Study on the pathogenic fungus of mycotic granulomatosis I. Isolation and pathogenicity of the fungus from cultured ayu infected with the disease. *Fish Pathology* **12**, 129–133.

Hatai, K., Furuya, K. and Egusa, S. (1978). Studies on the pathogenic fungus associated with Black gill disease of Kuruma Prawn, *Penaeus japonicus* — I. Isolation and identification of the BG-*Fusarium*. *Fish Pathology* **12**(4), 219–224.

Hatai, K. Bian, B. Z., Baticados, C. A. and Egusa, S. (1980). Studies on the fungal diseases in Crustaceans. II. *Haliphthoros philippensis* sp. nov. isolated from cultivated larvae of the jumbo tiger prawn (*Penaeus monodon*). *Transactions of the Mycological Society of Japan* **21**, 47–55.

Herrick, F. H. (1895). The American lobster, a study of its habits and development. *Bulletin of the US Fisheries Commission* **15**, 1–252.

Herrick, F. H. (1911). Natural history of the American lobster. *US Bureau of Fisheries, Bulletin* **29**, 149–408.

Hibbits, J., Hughes, G. C. and Sparks, A. K. (1981). *Trichomaris invadens* gen. et sp. nov. An Ascomycete parasite of the Tanner Crab (*Chionoecetes bairdi*) Rathbun (Crustacea, Brachyura). *Canadian Journal of Botany* (In press).

Hofer, B. von. (1893). Eine Salmoniden — Erkrankung. *Allgemeine Fischerei — Zeitung* **18**, 168–171. (Vol. 8 in N.S.)

Hohnk, W. and Vallin, S. (1953). Epidemisches Absterben von *Eurytemora* in Bothnischen Meerbusen, verursacht durch *Leptolegnia baltica* nov. spec. *Veroffentlichungen des Instituts fur Meeresforschung in Bremerhaven* **2**, 215–223.

Horter, H. (1960). *Fusarium* als Erreger einer Hautmykose bei Karpfen. *Zeitschrift fur Parasitenkunde* **20**, 355–358.

Jepps, M. W. (1937). On the protozoan parasites of *Calanus finmarchicus* in the Clyde Sea area. *Quarterly Journal of Microscopical Science (N.S.)* **79**, 589–658.

Johnson, T. W., Jr. (1958). A fungus parasite in the ova of the barnacle *Chthalamus fragilis denticulata*. *Biological Bulletin* **114**, 205–214.

Johnson, T. W., Jr. (1960). Infection potential and growth of *Lagenidium chthamalophilum*. *American Journal of Botany* **47**, 383–385.

Johnson, T. W. and Bonner, R. R., Jr. (1960). *Lagenidium callinectes* Couch in barnacle ova. *Journal of the Elisha Mitchell Scientific Society* **76**, 147–149.

Johnson, T. W., Jr. and Pinschmidt, W. C., Jr. (1963). *Leptolegnia marina* Atkins in blue crab ova. *Nova Hedwigia* **5**, 413–418.

Johnson, T. W. and Sparrow, F. K. (1961). "Fungi in Oceans and Estuaries". J. Cramer, Weinheim.

Jones, G. (1981). Thraustochytrid pathogens. Aquatic Mycology, Meeting of the British Mycological Society, Portsmouth, April 1981. *Bulletin of the British Mycological Society*. (Abstract only, in press)

Khulbe, R. D. and Sati, S. C. (1979). *Pythium undulatum* Peterson, a new pathogen of *Carassius auratus* L. *Geobios* **6**, 178.

Kirilenko, T. S. and All-Achmed, M. A. (1977). *Ochroconis tshawytschae* (Doty and Slater) comb. nov. *Mikrobiologichnii Zhurnal* **39**, 303–306.

Kohlmeyer, J. (1972). Marine fungi and deteriorating chitin of hydrozoa and keratin like annelid tubes. *Marine Biology* **12**, 277–284.

Lacaze-Duthiers, H. de (1874). Les Ascidies simple des cotes de France. *Archives de Zoologie experimentale et generale* **3**, 119–174, 257–330, 531–656.

Laukner, G. (1980). *In* "Diseases of Marine Animals. Volume I, General Aspects, Protoza to Gastropoda" (Ed. O. Kinne), Chs 3–12. John Wiley, Chichester.

Leger, L. (1924). Sur un organisme du type Ichthyophone parasite du tube digestif de la Lote d'eau douce. *Comptes rendu hebdomadaires des Seances de L'Academie des Sciences, Paris* **177**, 785–787.

Leger, L. (1927). Sur la nature et l'evolution des "spherules" decrites chez les Ichthyophones, Phycomycetes parasites de la truite. *Comptes rendus hebdomadaires des Seances de l'Academie des Sciences, Paris* **184**, 1268–1271.

Leger, L. and Hesse, E. (1923). Sur un champignon du type *Ichthyophonus* parasite de l'intestin de la Truite, *Comptes rendu hebdomadaires des Seances de l'Academie des Sciences, Paris* **176**, 420–422.

Levine, N. D. (1978). *Perkinsus* gen.n. and other new taxa in the Protozoan Phylum Apicomplexa. *Journal of Parasitology* **64**(3), 549.

Lieberkuhn, N. (1859). Neue beitrage zur anatomie der Spongen. *Archiv fur Anatomie, Physiologie und Wissenschaftlich Medizin (Muller)* pp.353–382 and 515–529.

Lightner, D. V. (1975). Some potentially serious disease problems in the culture of penaeid shrimp in North American. *Proceedings 3rd US–Japan Meeting on Aquaculture at Tokyo, Japan, October 1974*, 75–97.

Lightner, D. V. and Fontaine, C. T. (1973). A new fungus disease of the white shrimp *Penaeus setiferus*. *Journal of Invertebrate Pathology* **22**, 94–99.

Lucky, Z. (1970). The occurrence of branchiomycosis in the *Silurus glanis*. *Acta veterinaria Brno* **39**, 187–192.

McGinnis, M. R. and Ajello, L. (1974). A new species of *Exophiala* isolated from channel catfish. *Mycologia* **66**, 518–520.

Mann, H. and Pieplow, U. (1938). Die Brandenfleckenkrankheit bei Krebsen und ihre Erreger. *Zeitschrift fur Fischerei* **36**, 225–240.

Martin, W. W. (1977). The development and possible relationships of a new *Atkinsiella* parasitic in insect eggs. *American Journal of Botany* **64**(6), 760–769.

Meier, H. and Webster, J. (1954). An electron microscope study of cysts in the Saprolegniaceae. *Journal of Experimental Botany* **5**, 401–409.

Meyer, F. P. (1973). Branchiomycosis: a new fungal disease of North American fishes. *Progressive Fish-Culturist* **35**(2), 74–77.

Miyazaki, T. and Egusa, S. (1972). Studies on mycotic granulomatosis in freshwater fishes — I. The goldfish. *Fish Pathology* **7**, 15–25.

Miyazaki, T. and Egusa, S. (1973a). Studies on mycotic granulomatosis in freshwater fishes — II. Ayu, *Plecoglossus altivelis*. *Fish Pathology* **7**, 125–133.

Miyazaki, T. and Egusa, S. (1973b). Studies on mycotic granulomatosis in freshwater fishes — III. Blue gill. *Fish Pathology* **8**, 41–43.

Miyazaki, T. and Egusa, S. (1973c). Studies on mycotic granulomatosis in freshwater fishes — IV. Wild fishes. *Fish Pathology* **8**, 44–47.

Neish, G. A. (1976). Observations on the pathology of saprolegniasis of Pacific salmon and on the identity of the fungi associated with this disease. Ph.D. Thesis, University of British Colombia, Vancouver.

Neish, G. A. and Hughes, G. C. (1980). *In* "Diseases of Fishes, Book 6: Fungal Diseases of Fishes" (Eds. S. F. Snieszko and H. R. Axelrod), pp.1–159. TFH Publications, Neptune, New Jersey.

Nickerson, M. A. and Hutchinson, J. A. (1971). The distribution of the fungus *Basidiobolus ranarum* Eidam in fish, amphibians and reptiles. *American Midland Naturalist* **86**, 500–502.

Neilson, E. S., Fisher, W. H. and Schleser, R. A. (1976). A new mycosis of larval lobster (*Homarus americanus*). *Journal of Invertebrate Pathology* **27**, 177–183.

Nybelin, O. (1931). Undersökningar över kräftpestens orsak. *Ny Svensk Fiskeritidskrift*, **No. 15**, 144–149.

Nybelin, O. (1934). Nya undersökningar över kräftpestens orsak. *Ny Svensk Fiskeritidskrift*, **No. 10**, 110–114.

Nybelin, O. (1936). Untersuchungen über die Ursache der in Schweden gegenwärtig vorkommenden Krebspest. *Meddelanden fran Statens undersökningsoch försögsanstalt för sotvattensfisket, Stockholm*, **No. 9**, 29pp.

Nyhlen, L. and Unestem, T. (1980). Wound reactions and *Aphanomyces astaci* growth in crayfish cuticle. *Journal of Invertebrate Pathology* **36**, 187–197.

Olah, J. and Farkas, J. (1978). Effect of temperature, pH, antibiotics, formalin and malachite green on the growth and survival of *Saprolegnia* and *Achlya* parasitic on fish. *Aquaculture* **13**, 273–288.

Olive, L. S. (1975). "The Mycetozoans." Academic Press, New York.

Otte, E. (1964). Eine mykose bei einem Stachelrochen (*Trigon pastinaceae*). *Wiener tierarztliche Monaksschrift* **51**, 171–175.

Peduzzi, R. (1973). Diffusa infezione branchiale da funghi attribuiti al genere *Branchiomyces* Plehn (Phycomycetes, Saprolegniales) a carico dell' ittiofauna di laghi situati a nord e a sud delle Alpi II. Esigense colturali, transmissione sperimentale ed affinita tassonomiche del micete. *Memorie Instituto italiano di Idrobiologia Marco de Marchi* **30**, 81–96.

Perkins, F. O. (1972). The ultrastructure of holdfasts, "rhizoids" and "slime tracks" in Thraustochytriaceous fungi and *Labyrinthula* spp. *Archives fur Mikrobiologie* **84**, 95–118.

Perkins, F. O. (1976). Fine structure of apicomplexan organelles in the oyster pathogen *Dermocystidium marinum*. *Journal of Protozoology* **23**(2), 10A.

Petersen, H. E. (1905). Contributions a la connaissance des Phycomycetes marins (Chytridinae Fischer). *Oversigt-Kongelige Danske Videnskabernes Selskabs Forhandlinger* **1905**, 439–488.

Petersen, H. E. (1910). An account of Danish freshwater — Phycomycetes with biological and systematical remarks. *Annales Mycologiques* **8**, 494–560.

Pettit, A. (1913). Observations sur l'Ichthyosporidium et sur la maladie qu'il provoque chez la truite. *Annales de l'Institut Pasteur, Paris* **27**, 986–1008.

Pickering, A. D. and Willoughby, L. G. (1977). Epidermal lesions and fungal infections on the perch, *Perca fluviatalis* L. in Windermere. *Journal of Fish Biology* **11**, 349–354.

Pierotti, P. (1971). Su di un particolare episodio di micosi in *Tinca tinca*. *Atti Societa italiana della Scienze Veterinare* **25**, 361–363.

Plehn, M. (1916). Pathogene Schimmalpilze in der Fishniere. *Zeitschrift fur Fischerei*. **18**, 51–54.

Plehn, M. (1924). "Praktikum der Fischkrankheiten." E. Schweizerbart'sche Verlage Stuttgart.

Plehn, M. and Mulsow, K. (1911). Der Erreger der "Taumelkrankheit" der Salmoniden. *Zentblatt fur Bakteriologie Parasitenkunde (Abteilung I)* **58**, 63–68.

Polejaeff, N. (1884). Report on the Keratosa collected by HMS Challenger during the years 1873–76. *Challenger Reports, Zoology* **11**, 1–88.

Polglase, J. L. (1980). A preliminary report on the Thraustochytrid(s) and Labyrinthulid(s) associated with a pathological condition in the lesser octopus *Eledone cirrhosa*. *Botanica Marina* **23**, 699–706.

Polglase, J. L. (1981). Thraustochytrids as potential pathogens of marine animals. *Aquatic Mycology, British mycological Society, Portsmouth, April 1981*.

Prowse, G. A. (1953). *Aphanomyces daphniae* sp. nov. parasitic on *Daphnia hyalina*. *Transactions of the British Mycological Society* **37**, 22–28.

Quick, J. A. (1972). A new Thraustochytridiaceous fungus endoparasitic on the American oyster *Crassostrea virginica* Gmelin in Florida. *Society for Invertebrate Pathology Newsletter* **IV**(3), 13 (Abstract).

Raper, J. R. (1937). A method of freeing fungi from bacterial contamination. *Science, New York* **85**, 342.

Redfield, G. W. and Vincent, W. F. (1979). Stages of infection and ecological effects of a fungal epidemic on the eggs of a limnetic copepod. *Freshwater Biology* **9**, 503–510.

Reichenbach-Klinke, H.-H. (1956). Eine Aspergillacee (Fungi, Ascomycetales, Plectascales) als Endoparasit bei Susswasserfischen. *Veroffentlichungen des Instituts fur Meeresforschung in Bremerhaven* **4**, 111–116.

Reichenbach-Klinke, H.-H. and Elkan, E. (1965). "The Principal Diseases of Lower Vertebrates." Academic Press, New York.

Rennerfelt, E. (1936). Untersuchungen uber die Entioicklung und Biologie des Krebspest pilzes *Aphanomyces astaci* Shikara. *Mitterlungen der Anstalt fur Binnenfischerei bei Drottingholm, Stockholm No. 10*, 1–21.

Richards, R. H., Holliman, A. and Helgasson, S. (1978). Naturally occurring *Exophiala salmonis* infection in Atlantic salmon (*Salmo salar* L.). *Journal of Fish Diseases* **1**, 357–359.

Robertson, M. (1909). Notes on an Ichthyosporidian causing a fatal disease in sea-trout. *Proceedings of the Zoological Society of London 1909*, 399–402.

Ross, S. S. and Morris, E. O. (1965). An investigation of the yeast flora of marine fish from Scottish coastal waters and a fishing ground off Iceland. *Journal of Applied Bacteriology* **28**(2), 224–234.

Ross, A. J. and Yasutake, W. T. (1973). *Scolecobasidium humicola*, a fungal pathogen of fish. *Journal of the Fisheries Research Board of Canada* **30**, 994–995.

Ross, A. J., Yasutake, W. T. and Leek, S. (1975). *Phoma herbarum*, a fungal plant saprophyte as a fish pathogen. *Journal of the Fisheries Research Board of Canada* **32**, 1648–1652.

Roy, R. Y., Dwivadi, R. S. and Mishra, R. R. (1962). Two new species of *Scolecobasidium* from soil. *Lloydia* **25**, 164–166.

Rucker, R. R. and Gustafson, P. V. (1953). An epizootic among rainbow trout. *Progressive Fish-Culturist* **25**, 203–207.

Sandoz, M. D., Rogers, R. and Newcombe, C. L. (1944). Fungus infection of eggs of the blue crab *Callinectes sapidus* Rathbun. *Science, New York* **99**, 124–125.

Santesson, R. (1939). Amphibious Pyrenolichens I. *Arkiv fur Botanik* **29A**, 1–67.

Schaperclaus, W. (1954). "Fischkrankheiten." Akademie-Verlag, Berlin. 708pp.

Schmidt, E. O. (1862). "Die Spongien des adriatischen Meeres." *Leipzig*, 88pp (not seen, cited by Johnson and Sparrow, 1961).

Scott, W. W. (1956). A new species of *Aphanomyces* and its significance in the taxonomy of watermoulds. *Virginia Journal of Science* 7 (NS), 170–175.

Scott, W. W. (1964). Fungi associated with fish diseases. *Developments in Industrial Microbiology* 5, 109–123.

Scott, W. W. and O'Bier, A. H., Jr. (1962). Aquatic fungi associated with diseased fish and fish eggs. *Progressive Fish-Culturist* 24, 3–15.

Shah, K. L., Jha, B. C. and Jhingran, A. G. (1977). Observations on some aquatic phycomycetes pathogenic on eggs and fry of freshwater fish and prawn. *Aquaculture* 12(2), 141–148.

Shanor, L. and Saslow, H. B. (1944). *Aphanomyces* as a fish parasite. *Mycologia* 36, 413–415.

Sindermann, C. J. (1956). Diseases of fishes of the Western North Atlantic IV. Fungus disease and resultant mortalities of herring in the Gulf of St. Lawrence in 1955. *Research Bulletin of the Department of Sea Shore Fisheries of Maine* 25, 1–23.

Sindermann, C. J. (1970). "Principal Diseases of Marine Fish and Shellfish." Academic Press, New York.

Sindermann, C. J. and Scattergood, L. W. (1954). Diseases of fishes of the western North Atlantic II. *Ichthyosporidium* disease of the sea herring (*Clupea harengus*). *Research Bulletin of the Department of Sea Shore Fisheries of Maine* 19, 1–40.

Smith, R. I. (1940). Studies on two strains of *Aphanomyces laevis* found occurring as wound parasites on crayfish. *Mycologia* 32, 205–213.

Solangi, M. A. and Lightner, D. V. (196). Cellular inflammatory response of *Penaeus aztecus* and *P. setiferus* to the pathogenic fungus, *Fusarium* sp. isolated from the California brown shrimp, *P. californiensis*. *Journal of Invertebrate Pathology* 27(1), 77–86.

Sordi, M. (1958). Micosi dei crostacei decapodi marini. *Rivista di parassitologia* 19(2), 132–137.

Sparks, F. K. and Hibbits, J. (1979). Black mat syndrome: an invasive mycotic disease of the tanner crab, *Chionecetes bairdi*. *Journal of Invertebrate Pathology* 34, 184–191.

Sparrow, F. K. (1973). Mastigomycotina. *In* "The Fungi, an Advanced Treatise" (Eds. G. C. Ainsworth, F. K. Sparrow and A. S. Sussman), Vol. IVB, pp.61–73. Academic Press, New York.

Sparrow, F. K. (1976). The present status of classification of the biflagellate fungi. *In* "Recent Advances in Aquatic Mycology" (Ed. E. B. G. Jones), pp.213–222. Elek (Science) Ltd., London.

Sprague, V. (1965). *Ichthyosporidium* Caullery and Mesnil, 1905, the name of a genus of fungi or a genus of sporozoans? *Systematic Zoology* 14, 110–114.

Swarczewsky, B. (1914). Uber den Lebencyclus einiger Haplosporidien. *Archiv fur Protistenkunde* 33, 49–108.

Sweeny, A. W. (1981). An undescribed species of *Smittium* (Trichomycétes) pathogenic to mosquito larvae in Australia. *Transactions of the British Mycological Society*, 77(1), 55–60.

Tharp, T. P. and Bland, C. E. (1977). Biology and host range of *Haliphthoros milfordensis*. *Canadian Journal of Botany* 55, 2936–2944.

Tills, D. W. (1977). The distribution of the fungus *Basidiobolus ranarum* Eidem, in fish, amphibians and reptiles of the southern Appalachian region. *Transactions of the Kansas Academy of Science* 80, 75–77.

Unestam, T. (1965). Studies on the crayfish plague fungus, *Aphanomyces astaci*. *Physiologia Plantarum* **18**, 483–505.

Unestam, T. (1968). Studies on the European Crayfish Plague *Bulletin de l'Office internationale des Epizootics* **69**(7–8), 1237–1238.

Uzmann, J. R. and Haynes, E. B. (1968). A mycosis of the gills of the pandalid shrimp *Dichelopandalus leptocerus*. *Journal of Invertebrate Pathology* **12**(3), 275–277.

Vallin, S. (1951). Plankton mortality in the northern Baltic caused by a parasitic water mould. *Report of the Institute for Freshwater Research, Drottningholm* **32**, 139–148.

Van Duijn, C., Jr. (1956). Diseases of Fishes. Illife Books, London. 371pp.

Van Hyning, J. M. and Scarborough, A. M. (1973). Identification of fungal incrustations on the shell of the snow crab (*Chionoxcetes bairdi*). *Journal of the Fisheries Research Board of Canada* **30**, 1738–1739.

Vishniac, H. S. (1955). The morphology and nutrition of a new species of *Sirolpidium*. *Mycologia* **47**, 633–645.

Vishniac, H. S. (1958). A new marine phycomycete. *Mycologia* **50**, 66–79.

Vishniac, H. S. and Nigrelli, R. F. (1957). The ability of the Saprolegniaceae to parasitise platyfish. *Zoologica* **42**, 131–134.

Willoughby, L. G. (1968). Atlantic salmon disease fungus. *Nature, London* **217**, 872–873.

Willoughby, L. G. (1969). Salmon disease in Windermere and the River Leven; the fungal aspect. *Salmon and Trout Magazine* **186**, 124–130.

Willoughby, L. G. (1970). Mycological aspects of a disease of young perch in Windermere. *Journal of Fish Biology* **2**, 113–116.

Willoughby, L. G. (1971). Observations on fungal parasites of Lake District salmonids. *Salmon and Trout Magazine* **192**, 152–158.

Willoughby, L. G. (1972). UDN of Lake District trout and char: outward signs of infection and defense barriers examined further. *Salmon and Trout Magazine* **195**, 149–158.

Willoughby, L. G. (1977). An abbreviated life cycle in the salmonid fish *Saprolegnia*. *Transactions of the British Mycological Society* **68**, 91–95.

Willoughby, L. G. (1978). Saprolegniasis of salmonid fish in Windermere: a critical analysis. *Journal of Fish Diseases* **1**, 51–67.

Wolke, R. E. (1975). Pathology of bacterial and fungal diseases affecting fish. *In* "The Pathology of Fishes" (Eds. W. E. Ribelin and G. Migaki), pp.33–316. University of Wisconsin Press, Madison.

Wood, J. W. (1974). "Diseases of Pacific salmon—their prevention and treatment." 2nd Edition. Department of Fisheries, Hatcheries Division, State of Washington.

Yang, B. Y. (1962). *Basidiobolus meristosporus* of Taiwan. *Taiwania* **8**, 17–27.

11

Ichthyophonus Infections of Fish

A. H. McVICAR

Marine Laboratory, Aberdeen,
Scotland, U.K.

Introduction

Ichthyophonus is one of the few recorded fungus diseases of marine fish and in contrast to most of the fungi from freshwater fish which are discussed by Alderman in Chapter 10, it is both an internal and obligate parasite. The condition was first observed by Hofer (1893) and named *Ichthyosporidium gasterophilum* by Caullery and Mesnil (1905). The genus and species *Ichthyophonus hoferi* was described by Plehn and Mulsow (1911). Although the generic name *Ichthyosporidium* has since been frequently used for the fungus, Sprague (1965) recommended that this name be reserved for a protozoan and under the rules of nomenclature the fungus should be termed *Ichthyophonus*. There are several comprehensive reviews of the literature on the fungus (Sproston, 1944; Reichenbach-Klinke, 1954–55; Dorier and Degrange, 1960; Amlacher, 1970; Sindermann, 1970) so that it is not intended that this paper should fully cover the early information on *Ichthyophonus* and instead, emphasis will be placed on areas of discrepancy and on the more recent data, particularly that concerned with the identification, distribution, life cycle, effects on the host and economic significance of the disease.

Identification and Taxonomy

It is clear that much of the confusion which has appeared in the literature on *Ichthyophonus* was directly due to problems associated with wrongly identifying pathologically similar cyst-forming disease conditions and with the question of whether one or several species of *Ichthyophonus* existed. Alderman (1976) thought it probable that a complex of related forms was involved and Schäperclaus (1953) discussed a form of *Ichthyophonus* peculiar to aquarium fish which was sufficiently different from that in trout and marine fish to possibly constitute a different species. However, Amlacher (1965, cited by Amlacher, 1970) introduced a cautionary note when it was shown that some reports of *Ichthyophonus* in aquarium fish were mis-identification of mycobacterial infections. Similarly, Dorier and Degrange (1960) noted that the commensal fungus *Basidiobolus intestinalis* may have been confused with *Ichthyophonus* in some descriptions from salmonids.

External signs attributable to *Ichthyophonus* infection in fish have only been reported in a small number of cases. Behavioural changes in salmonids ('swinging disease'), curvature of the spine in herring and salmonids and darkening of areas of the skin all may be associated with the fungus invading the host's nervous system. Pathological changes leading to a roughening of the skin in herring (*Clupea harengus*) and rainbow trout (*Salmo gairdneri*) were noted by Sindermann and Scattergood (1954) and Reichenbach-Klinke (1973); the condition in herring leading to ulcers in later infections. Secondary effects such as severe emaciation have also been used to preliminarily identify *Ichthyophonus*-infected plaice (*Pleuronectes platessa*) by McVicar (in press). It should be stressed, however, that the above clinical signs are not specifically diagnostic of the disease and consequently any identification based solely on them or on the occurrence of multiple cysts must be considered doubtful. McVicar (in press) suggested that the characteristic germination of spores after host death could be used to provide definite field identification in the absence of cultural, histological or bacteriological studies.

Using culture studies, Reichenbach-Klinke (1973) showed that fungus isolated from discus fish (*Symphysodon* sp.) did not differ from *Ichthyophonus* described from salmonids and herring although germination may be slightly different in tropical fish. Observations of the disease in Scottish marine fish has shown morphological variations due to differing host reaction in different fish species (McVicar, in press) but experimental cross transmissions between fish species and the common antigenicity of the fungus from different hosts indicated that at least in that area only one parasite species was involved. Similarly, personal observations on *Ichthyophonus* from rainbow trout in Norway (by courtesy of S. O. Raold) and Australia (by courtesy of B. L. Munday) showed that they were morphologically identical to material from Scottish waters. The extensive studies on *Ichthyophonus* from the western North Atlantic, summarized by Sindermann (1970) and those by Myazaki and Kubota (1977b) and Chien *et al.* (1979d) from Japan, have shown similar forms in these areas, so that it is possible that only one species exists; that is *Ichthyophonus hoferi* Plehn & Mulsow, 1911. However, until specifically diagnostic intermediate stages in the life cycle are studied or further transmission experiments with

Ichthyophonus from different hosts and localities are carried out, some doubt must still remain as to whether one or several species exist. The taxonomic position of *Ichthyophonus* in relation to other fungi of fish has already been discussed by Alderman in Chapter 10.

Distribution and Epidemiology

Reichenbach-Klinke (1954–55) assembled a large list of host species for *Ichthyophonus* including fish from marine and fresh water in temperate and tropical zones and since then many new host and geographical records have been made. This wide range of hosts and the ease of transmission of the fungus between fish in fresh water (Gustafson and Rucker, 1956) between marine fish and freshwater fish (Dorier and Degrange, 1960; McVicar, 1977) and between marine fish (Sindermann and Scattergood, 1954; McVicar and MacKenzie, 1972) suggested that *Ichthyophonus* showed low host specificity. Consequently, the listing of new host records, particularly in localities where the disease is common, may only indicate that a particular fish species has been sufficiently examined to detect infection. However, there were indications of differences in susceptibility and response of different fish species to the disease. Gustafson and Rucker (1956) found that goldfish (*Carassius auratus*), guppy (*Lebistes reticulatus*), squawfish (*Ptychocheilus oregonensis*) and catfish (*Ameiurus nebulosus*) were refractory to experimental challenge with *Ichthyophonus* whereas control rainbow trout produced positive infections. Lack of susceptibility of cod (*Gadus morhua*) from the Gulf of St Lawrence was also indicated by Sindermann (1966) when, during an epidemic of the disease causing high mortalities in herring, alewives (*Alosa pseudoharengus*) and mackerel (*Scomber scombrus*), the cod showed increased growth rate which could possibly be related to the abundance of diseased and dying fish as a rich food source. Although cod could be infected in Scottish waters (McVicar, 1977), no serious effects or extensive tissue invasion were apparent. On the same fishing grounds, haddock (*Melanogrammus aeglefinus*) appeared to tolerate high prevalence levels of infection with little pathogenicity, while plaice with a lower prevalence of infection had a high mortality attributable to the disease (McVicar, 1981). Reichenbach-Klinke (1973) noted records of *Ichthyophonus*-like organisms in amphibia and copepods, but the specific identification of these need to be checked and their relationship with the disease in fish and the life cycle considered.

Most authorities accept that *Ichthyophonus* is primarily a disease of marine origin. The majority of records are from fish from both sides of the

North Atlantic (Sproston, 1944; Sindermann, 1970; McVicar, 1977) but this may only reflect the greater intensity of sampling in these regions. Munday (1976, 1979 personal communication) recorded the disease in Australian waters while Miyazaki and Kubota (1977a) and Chien *et al.* (1979a) reported its occurrence from Japan and Taiwan. It thus appears that *Ichthyophonus* has a world-wide distribution. Outbreaks of *Ichthyophonus* have occurred in freshwater fish farms in the U.S.A. (Rucker and Gustafson, 1953; Gustafson and Rucker, 1956; Ross and Parisot, 1958), Europe (Dorier and Degrange, 1960; Fijan and Maran, 1976; personal observations), Japan (Miyazaki and Kubota, 1977a) and Australia (Munday, 1976), but in most cases a direct link with the sea was established by the farm using marine fish as feed. There is no evidence that the disease has become established in freshwater environments, in spite of the fact that, as Gustafson and Rucker (1956) demonstrated, transmission between fish in fresh water is possible through the water. In addition, although *Ichthyophonus* is widespread in Scottish coastal waters and has been reported from sea trout in northern Scotland by Robertson (1909) and a migrating salmon in a Scottish east coast river by McVicar (1977) the disease has not become endemic in Scottish rivers.

Sindermann (1958, 1963, 1970) believed that *Ichthyophonus* was endemic in western North Atlantic herring stocks and that the disease was characterized by periodic outbreaks in the Gulf of Maine and Gulf of St Lawrence. Six major epidemics had occurred since the end of the nineteenth century each lasting 1 to 3 years. Prevalence of infection was about 25% of all herring sampled during epidemics and was well under 1% during intervening periods (Sindermann, 1970). The sporadic nature of outbreaks suggested to Sindermann (1965) that there were variations in the resistance of herring populations to the disease, while Sindermann and Scattergood (1954) also suggested that physical factors in the environment, as well as biological factors, could exert an influence on the disease. Host population density was selected for particular consideration although no large-scale long-term investigations were available. The higher prevalence of infection found by Sindermann and Scattergood (1954) in inshore waters, particularly during late winter and spring, could have been partly due to seasonal migrations of herring in that region. Sandholzer *et al.* (1945, cited by Johnson and Sparrow, 1961) found that the greatest number of ocean pout (*Zaorces anguillaris*) infected with *Ichthyophonus* during an epidemic were then from deep cooler water off Massachusetts.

There is evidence that the disease has also been endemic in northern European waters for a considerable time. An excellent, and subsequently largely ignored, illustrated description of the disease under the name *Dokus adus* was presented by Williamson (1913) working on material from haddock at the Marine Laboratory, Aberdeen, and it was stated that the disease was then often observed in haddock caught off the West coast of Scotland. Similarly, Johnstone (1905) described plaice infected with *Ichthyophonus* from the Isle of Man, drawing attention to its fungal nature without naming the organism. An epidemic of *Ichthyophonus* in mackerel with a high prevalence of infection being maintained for over 3 years was recorded by Sproston (1944). Details of the position of capture of the mackerel were not given but two small samples in which all fish were infected were received from Hull on the North Sea coast. No subsequent epidemics of the disease have been recorded in mackerel, although infection has been noted in this species by McVicar (1977) from the west of Scotland. Prevalence levels are currently low, for during detailed microscopic examination of the viscera of over 500 mackerel from the western English Channel and North Sea, K. MacKenzie (personal communication) has not recorded any *Ichthyophonus* infection.

A high prevalence of *Ichthyophonus* has recently been found in haddock caught off the north coast of Scotland with up to 85% of fish in individual catches being infected (McVicar, in press). This heavily infected stock showed a sharp line of demarcation in the Orkney-Shetland Channel with more lightly infected haddock stocks (2–12% prevalence) throughout the northern North Sea and a less clear distinguishing boundary with uninfected haddock off western Scotland (Fig. 1). These boundaries were maintained during 5 years of sampling between 1977 and 1981 and indicated a distinct group of haddock off the North of Scotland. Prevalence of infection was lower in plaice (maximum 25%) but not surprisingly, due to the ease of cross transmission of the disease between the species (McVicar and MacKenzie, 1972), it showed the same geographical pattern of distribution as in haddock. Unpublished records in the Marine Laboratory, Aberdeen, show *Ichthyophonus* to have been not uncommon in the Shetland–West Orkney area since 1956 and the failure to detect any major changes in prevalence levels since more detailed studies began in 1971 suggest that the disease may have been present in epidemic proportions in the area for a considerable time possibly since early this century (see Williamson, 1913). The disease was not recorded in haddock south of 56°N and only rarely in plaice in the southern North Sea (McVicar, in press). At present no reason can be suggested for the persistence of the high prevalence level of *Ichthyophonus* in haddock and plaice off the north coast of Scotland, especially as no physical barriers exist between that and other stocks of the species.

The cyclical nature of epidemics of *Ichthyophonus* in herring in the western North Atlantic illustrated that the occurrence of a low prevalence level of the disease does not necessarily mean the fungus will not cause

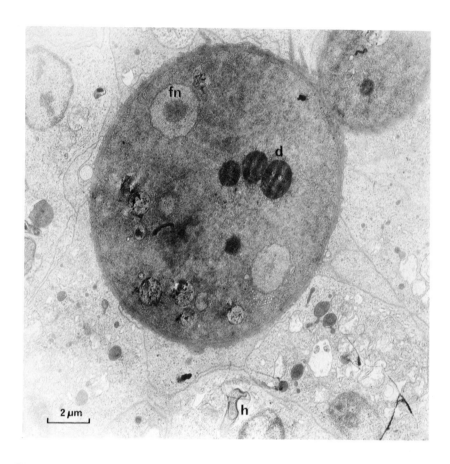

Fig. 5. Low-power electron micrograph of *Ichthyophonus* spores in plaice kidney.
d = dense bodies, h = hyphae penetrating into surrounding host cells, f.n. = fungal
nucleus.

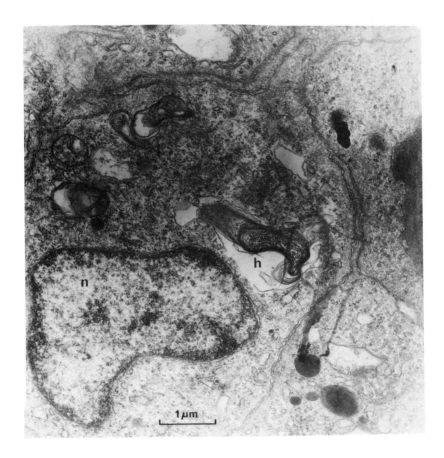

Fig. 6. Electron micrograph of hyphae (h) penetrating through the cytoplasm of a host cell. The fungus cytoplasm within the hyphae contains numerous free ribosomes. n = host cell nucleus.

infection sites, although in heavy infections the entire body can be invaded by the fungus. Squash preparations or histological sections of organs from infected fish reveal the most commonly observed developmental stage of *Ichthyophonus*, the thick-walled "resting spores", which are variable in size up to more than 200μm in diameter, and contain numerous nuclei scattered in the cytoplasm (Figs. 2, 3). These appear identical in all fish species studied. Immediately after death of the host the 'resting spores' germinate to produce branching hyphae (Fig. 4), this 'post mortem' germination being a characteristic feature noted by numerous authors. The rate of germination in plaice and haddock is clearly related to temperature and at 20°C commences within 15–30 minutes of host death. It is probable from the illustrations in many reports that there was often sufficient delay by the authors to allow germination to start before tissues were fixed, as in rapidly fixed material for light microscopy there was little evidence of extensive hyphal growth. Ultrastructurally, some hyphae can be observed penetrating into host cells surrounding *Ichthyophonus* spores (Fig. 5) and lytic activity of living tissue is often apparent in the vicinity of the hyphal tips (Fig. 6). The 'resting spore' wall consists of tightly packed fibrillar layers which in the developing hyphae are more loosely packed. Large numbers of free ribosomes, various vacuoles and prominent dense bodies are contained within the cytoplasm, while the nuclei are large with a prominent central endosome. There is as yet little information on the ultrastructure of *Ichthyophonus* during the different phases of its life cycle.

Although there have been various attempts to elucidate the life cycle of *Ichthyophonus*, notably those by Sproston (1944), Sindermann and Scattergood (1954), Dorier and Degrange (1960), Miyazaki and Kubota (1977b) and Chien *et al.* (1979d) various discrepancies and gaps in the developmental sequences proposed are still apparent. The cycle suggested by Sproston (1944) is notable in that it alone included sexual reproduction but, apart from minor details, the other studies conform to the general pattern described in detail by Dorier and Degrange (1960). With the development of new culture techniques giving good *in vitro* growth and the observation of previously poorly defined stages in the life cycle, the author has recently been able to make original observations on *Ichthyophonus* from plaice and haddock which are discussed below.

Ichthyophonus from plaice, directly or after passage through rainbow trout, was successfully cultured in two media: 1. Liquid medium—Minimum Eagles Medium (MEM) + 10% foetal calf serum + 3.5% NaCl + 100 units of penicillin and streptomycin; 2. Solid medium—Hagem's fungus medium modified to the following in 1 litre of de-ionized water: 0.5g potassium dihydrogen orthophosphate, 0.5g ammonium chloride, 0.5g magnesium sulphate, 5mg ferric chloride, 50μg thiamine hydrochloride,

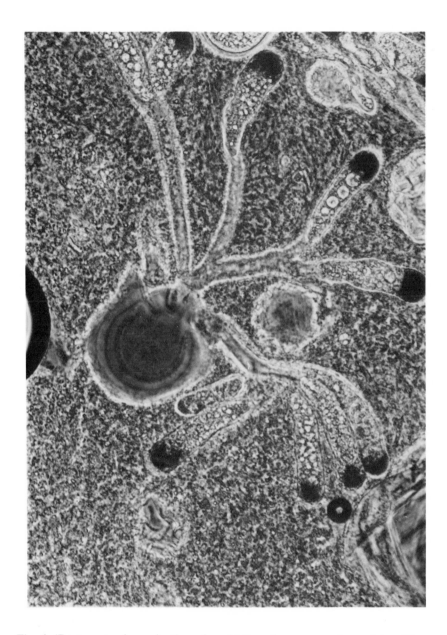

Fig. 4. 'Post mortem' germination of an *Ichthyophonus* spore from plaice. Phase-contrast illumination.

epidemics in a fish species under particular circumstances and, conversely, as was shown in haddock, high prevalence levels of the disease do not necessarily mean serious effects on the fish population.

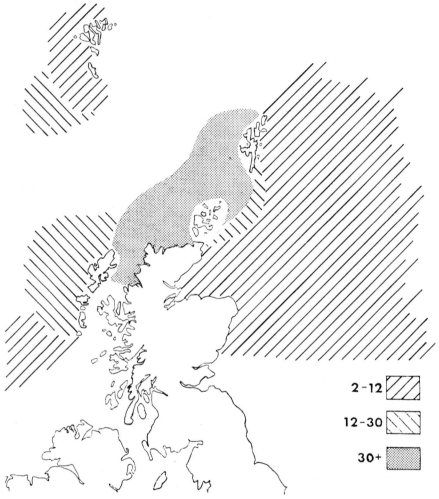

Fig. 1. Prevalence of infection of *Ichthyophonus* in haddock in Scottish waters.

Morphology and Life Cycle

The systemic nature of *Ichthyophonus* results in those organs richly supplied with blood (kidney, heart, spleen and liver) being the principal

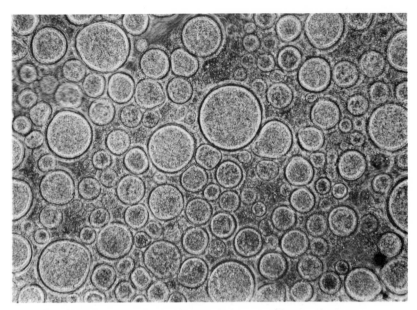

Fig. 2. Kidney squash of an infected plaice showing 'resting' spores.

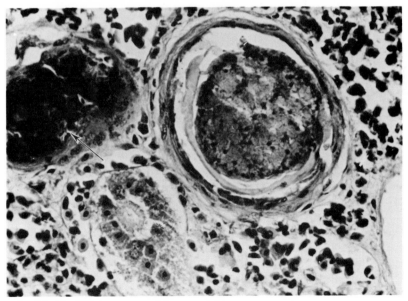

Fig. 3. Histological section of infected haddock kidney. Degeneration of a spore is apparent (arrowed).

5g malt extract, 10g dextrose, 18g nutrient agar (Oxoid CM3). Most prolific growth was obtained in MEM, but culture of *Ichthyophonus* on solid medium had the advantage that the fate of individual spores and their products could be followed over a prolonged period.

The rapid germination of spores within fish tissues after host death commences at least with *Ichthyophonus* from plaice, as a protrusion of the contents through a rupture in the spore wall, leading occasionally to the development of a single plasmodial mass, but usually to the formation of branched hyphae of varying length and number (Fig. 7). Hyphae grow both

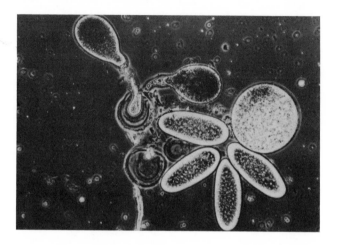

Fig. 7. Germination of hyphae and formation of hyphal bodies in MEM culture. Phase-contrast illumination.

on the surface and into the substrate of solid medium (Fig. 8). The thick connective tissue capsules which largely contained the fungus in such species as haddock and rainbow trout while the host was still alive (see under Host Reaction and Defence, p.260) appeared to be easily penetrated by the hyphae soon after host death. It is not known if this was due to a change in the capsule structure and/or a stimulation of the 'resting spore' to germinate after host death. The cytoplasmic contents of the spore were evacuated into the hyphae as they grew and accumulated in the hyphae tips (Fig. 7) which subsequently rounded up and separated off as large spherical bodies 4 to 10 days after growth had started. The further development of these large multinucleate bodies, 20 or more of which could be formed from one original 'resting spore' has been the subject of much discussion. They often developed thick walls and were then distinguishable from 'resting spores'. Clearly, they could aid dispersal by increasing the number of free fungal units available to potential hosts and possibly by the hyphae penetrating on to the surface of tissues. In most attempts to culture *Ichthyophonus*, germination did not exceed this point (Dorier and Degrange, 1960) and consequently had not improved on that which normally occurred in dead host tissue. However, Sindermann and Scattergood (1954) and Chien *et al.* (1979b) found that while some hyphal

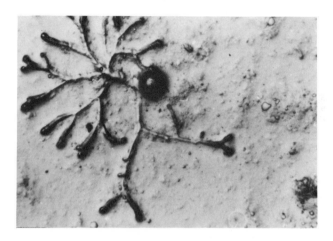

Fig. 8. Growth of *Ichthyophonus* from plaice on solid Hagem's medium.

tips formed these new thick-walled 'resting spores', others showed progressive division of the cytoplasm giving rise to as many as several hundred small hyphal bodies or "endospores". Fragmentation of the multinucleate bodies at hyphal tips to form small 'endospores', 10μm or less in diameter, was regularly achieved in MEM culture from plaice (Fig. 9) and occasionally in dead host tissues. Small bodies produced by similar division were observed in the intestine of rainbow trout infected with *Ichthyophonus* from the same species by Dorier and Degrange (1960) and from plaice (Fig. 10), and have often been noted during secondary invasion and proliferation of the disease within living host tissue (Miyazaki and Kubota, 1977b). Nuclear number was low, frequently 1 or 2 (Fig. 11). The development of similar 'endospore' bodies, in host tissues before and after host death, in the intestinal lumen of potential hosts and in culture suggested that the distinction of different developmental cycles in each situation, which has been made by various authors, may have been artificial. It is probable that any differences found, such as the extent and type of hyphal growth and the size and structure of hyphal terminal bodies largely reflect the nutrients available and the conditions surrounding the developing fungus.

No fusion of hyphae which Sproston (1944) considered to be a usual form of development preceeding spore formation has been observed in any other study on *Ichthyophonus*. Dorier and Degrange (1960) put forward the possibility that the uninucleate amoeboid forms could fuse to form a zygote but in spite of many observations made by them, and of the material cultured from plaice, this has never been observed. Thus no sexual cycle is known for *Ichthyphonus* and at present a simple life cycle can be proposed involving subdivision of multinucleate spores into small endospore bodies, with or without the prior formation of hyphae and terminal hyphal bodies, the dissemination of these motile bodies into new hosts or within the body of an already infected host, and their growth into large multinucleate spores. The formation of thick-walled 'resting' spores may depend on adverse conditions around the multinucleate body such as host reaction or lack of nutrients.

Host Reaction and Defence

Within 2 days of an initial infection in rainbow trout Dorier and Degrange (1960) reported an increase in the number of phagocytes, particularly in the perivascular connective tissue surrounding the intestinal vein and in the gills. Granules enclosed within the phagocytes resembled the amoeboid forms of *Ichthyophonus* and these authors believed that a number of units of the infective stage could be destroyed at the time of crossing the intestinal barrier. Miyazaki and Kubota (1977a) similarly illustrated the smallest stages of *Ichthyophonus* phagocytozed by the reticuloendothelial cells lining a sinusoid. Host defence at the phagocytic level may occur either during initial infection or during the continuous fragmentation and dissemination phases of the fungus within the host tissues, but would be less effective against the larger and thicker walled stages of the parasite. Sindermann and Scattergood (1954) observed that the initial reaction of herring to *Ichthyophonus* took the form of round cell infiltration concentrically around the site of localization of the parasite, and similarly in plaice aggregation of numerous macrophages occurred around small stages of the parasite (Figs 14, 15). Ultrastructurally these could be seen to contain both single small units of the fungus (? 'endospores') and larger spheres containing several fungal bodies which were probably the products of an *in situ* fragmentation of a large spore body (Fig. 16). Degeneration of fungal tissue was apparent within certain phagolysosomes so that it could be concluded that macrophages were effective in destroying some *Ichthyophonus* bodies.

It is clear, however, that the macrophage phagocytic response was not effective in preventing the rapid proliferation and spread of the fungus in the tissues of many species of fish. The inflammatory cellular response which occurred around larger developing fungal bodies in rainbow trout was illustrated in detail by Miyazaki and Kubota (1977a): mononuclear cells, probably macrophages, formed a layer to completely enclose the fungal body. This developed into a syncytium which could have associated free giant cells and finally there was proliferation of fibroblasts and fibrocytes to form a surrounding fibrous capsule and ultimately a granuloma. Similar reactions were observed in eel (*Anguilla japonica*), yellowtail (*Seriola quinqueradiata*) and black sea bream (*Acanthpogrus schlegelii*) by Chien *et al.* (1979a), in herring by Sindermann and Scatter-good (1954), in haddock by McVicar (in press) and in numerous other species by various authors. Dorier and Degrange (1960) considered that fungal cysts in rainbow trout were first surrounded by leucocytes before thickening of the reaction wall by deposition of connective tissue layers. Although it is probable that the cellular reaction is common to all fish species infected, there is evidence of variability in the degree of reaction, and this may be linked with the range of pathogenicity of the disease found in different fish. Species such as cod which characteristically produce a thick capsule around spores apparently tolerate infection without extensive invasion, species such as haddock with a moderately thick enclosing capsule (up to 47μm) were only rarely seriously affected, whereas in plaice where the capsule was always thin, the disease was highly pathogenic (McVicar, in press). In plaice, there was no evidence that spores were destroyed within the capsules, but in haddock numerous large fibrotic areas containing tissue in various stages of necrosis (Fig. 3) but occasionally recognizable as *Ichthyophonus* were commonly found. Many resting spores retained their viability after encapsulation and germinated hyphae after host death, but in living hosts such as cod and haddock the fibrotic capsules were apparently effective in restricting development of spores or the spread of the disease within the host body by limiting dissemination of the products of spore division. In some species of fish, several generations of *Ichthyophonus* were enclosed within one large granuloma (Chien *et al.*, 1979a).

Elimination of *Ichthyophonus* cysts at the level of the gills and intestinal mucosa was reported by Dorier and Degrange (1960) 22 days after an infected meal while Sindermann and Scattergood (1954) noted release of the fungus through necrotic areas of the skin. The appearance of fungal hyphae within kidney tubules of plaice (Fig. 17) indicates another route by which *Ichthyophonus* could pass to the exterior of fish, but such phenomena should probably be considered as a potential means of transmission of the fungus to new hosts, rather than as a protective benefit to the fish. Pathological changes associated with *Ichthyophonus* which have been 'endospore'-like bodies formed in the intestine of rainbow trout after an infected meal by Dorier and Degrange (1960) and in the present study (Fig. 10) were found to show activity such that the contents of the hyphal body ('amoeboblast') performed intermittent rotating movements. Dorier and Degrange (1960) observed the release of these amoeboid forms and found that under favourable conditions they showed activity for several days. They considered these to be the infective stage which somehow managed to cross the intestinal mucosa and be carried away by lymph or blood. The failure to detect the uninuclear stages crossing the intestinal wall, or in blood smears, was attributed to the probable short duration of their passage through these areas. Chien *et al.* (1979c) observed hyphae of

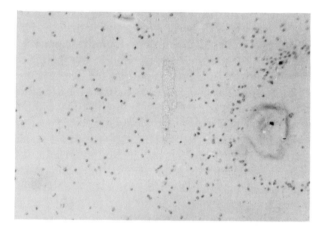

Fig. 12. Migration of motile 'endospores' through solid culture medium to form a ring after their release from a hyphal terminal body.

Ichthyophonus penetrating the stomach epithelium of *Glossogobius giuris* 3 days after feeding with viscera of diseased rainbow trout and considered that infection of new hosts occurred by this route. Further studies on the motile bodies could be rewarding, particularly with respect to the taxonomic position of *Ichthyophonus*.

Rapid growth of the invasive stage was reported by Dorier and Degrange (1960), in the tissues of rainbow trout heart, some fungal bodies attaining a diameter of more than 200μm within 20 days. In MEM culture of *Ichthyophonus* from plaice, growth of the endospore-like bodies also occurred, but rather more slowly (Table 1). Ultimately, these bodies became identical with 'resting' spores and given a suitable supply of nutrients, were capable of dividing again and repeating the complete development cycle.

Some of the motile endospores observed in Hagem's medium also showed growth to form 'resting' spores, but the smallness of the proportion which developed (approximately five per 'ring') may have been the result of limitations in the growth medium.

Massive secondary invasion of host tissues was a characteristic feature of most *Ichthyophonus* infections studied. Dorier and Degrange (1960) presented evidence which suggested the formation of new infective elements within about 8 days of a primary infection. The formation of new fungal bodies occurred either within the original cyst or in short hyphae, was also noted by Sindermann and Scattergood (1954), to form endospores 12 to 17 μm in diameter. This led to the multiplication of the parasite in the organ attacked, forming the nodules of the gross lesions, or the spread of the disease around the body in the circulatory system.

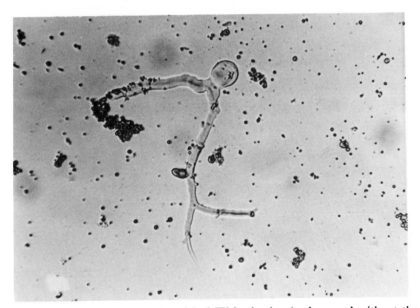

Fig. 13. Hyphae of a spore cultured in MEM releasing 'endospores' without the formation of hyphal terminal bodies.

Table 1. Percentage of fungal bodies within different size categories in MEM culture

Size (μm)	Day:	0	2	5	8	21	27
6–20		70	71	35	16	10	10
21–53		7	17	42	64	60	43
>53		23	12	23	20	30	47
Total measured		216	194	273	179	79	93

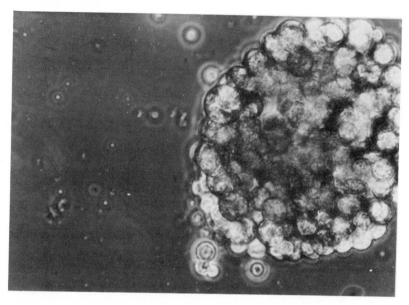

Fig. 9. Development of 'endospores' by division of hyphal terminal body in MEM culture. Phase-contrast illumination.

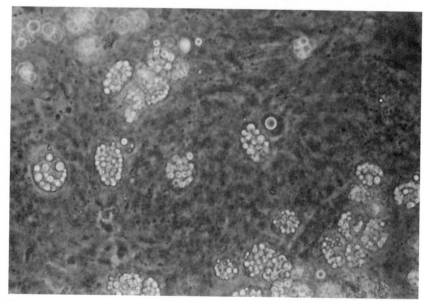

Fig. 10. Development of motile 'endospores' in the intestine of rainbow trout experimentally fed with *Ichthyophonus* from plaice. Phase-contrast illumination.

Evidence for motility of the 'endospore' has been presented by Sproston (1944) who observed that in dead host tissue some hyphal tips became rounded off and formed 'sporangia' which discharged minute 'amoeboid' bodies. Similarly, in Hagem's culture medium with *Ichthyophonus* from plaice, hyphal terminal bodies were observed, on numerous occasions, to rupture and release small bodies approximately 10μm diameter which were capable of considerable movement through the medium from their point of origin to form a concentric ring (Fig. 12). Most of these bodies travelled 1 to 2mm (maximum 4.8mm) from the hyphal tip within 2 to 3 days but then showed no further movement. It was not possible to determine if the large numbers of uninucleate bodies produced by fragmentation of the hyphal terminal bodies in MEM (Fig. 9) or these formed within living host tissues (Fig. 11) were capable of independent movement but their similarity in structure and formation suggest that they represent the same developmental stage. Infrequently, hyphae growing in MEM were observed to release small bodies without the formation of spherical hyphal bodies (Fig. 13). These may correspond to the 'unusual' type of reproduction noted by Sproston (1944) where hyphal contents sometimes broke up directly into 'endospores' which immediately showed amoeboid movement on being liberated. The

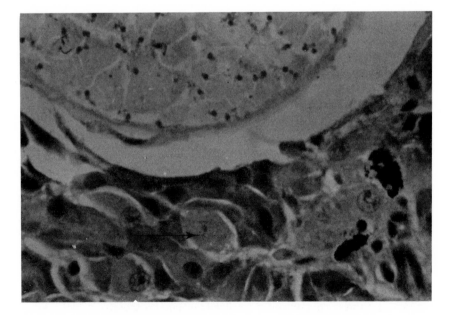

Fig. 11. Uninuclear fungal body (arrowed) close to a multinuclear spore in the liver of an experimentally infected rainbow trout. Haematoxylin Eosin stain.

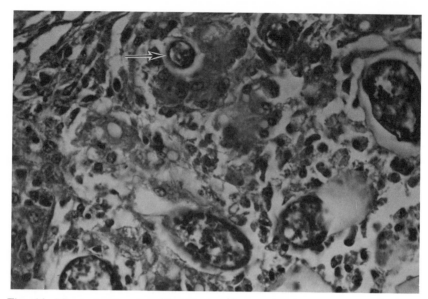

Fig. 14. Macrophage aggregation surrounding a small stage of *Ichthyophonus* (arrowed) in rainbow trout kidney.

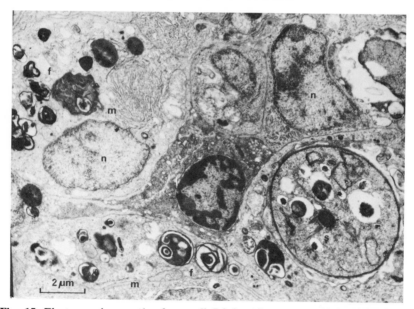

Fig. 15. Electron micrograph of a small *Ichthyophonus* spore(s) in plaice kidney surrounded by macrophages (m) containing small fungal bodies (? endospore) (f) in vacuoles. n = macrophage nucleus.

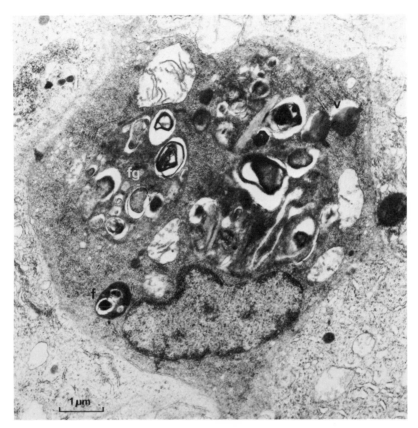

Fig. 16. Electron micrograph of a macrophage containing groups of fungal bodies (f.g.) a single small fungal body (? endospore) (f) and vesicles with structureless densely staining contents(v).

observed within various organs depend greatly on the species of fish being studied and may to a large extent reflect secondary changes associated with physical disruption and organ malfunction.

Antibody production specifically against *Ichthyophonus* has been detected by the Ouchterloney gel diffusion–precipitation technique using live spores, or an acellular extract of spores, against the serum of naturally infected plaice, but was shown to be absent from almost 500 uninfected plaice tested (McVicar in press, 1981). Single precipitin lines developed in 1 to 2 days at 4°C but varying strengths of reaction were apparent in different fish and no reaction was detected in 58% of infected plaice tested (Fig. 18). This variation was attributed to differences in the duration of infection in

Chien, C., Miyazaki, T. and Kubota, S. S. (1979c). Studies on *Ichthyophonus* disease of fishes — VI. Artificial infection. *Bulletin of the Faculty of Fisheries, Mie University* **6**, 153–159.

Chien, ·C., Miyazaki, T. and Kubota, S. S. (1979d). Studies on *Ichthyophonus* disease of fish — VII. Morphology and life cycle. *Bulletin of the Faculty of Fisheries, Mie University* **6**, 161–172.

Dorier, A. and Degrange, Ch. (1960). L'evolution de l'*Ichthyosporidium (Ichthyophonus) hoferi* (Plehn & Mulsow) chez les salmonides d'elevage (truite arc-en-ciel et saumon de fontaine). *Travaux du Laboratoire d'hydrobiologie et de Pisciculture de l'Université de Grenoble* **52**, 7–94.

Duijn, C. van, Jr. (1956). "Diseases of Fishes." Iliffe, Books Ltd, London.

Fijan, N. and Maran, B. (1976). A case of Ichthyosporidiosis in rainbow trout. *Veterinarski arhiv* **46**, 65–67.

Gustafson, P. V. and Rucker, R. R. (1956). Studies on an *Ichthyosporidium* infection in fish: transmission and host specificity. *U.S. Department of the Interior, Fish and Wildlife, Service, Special Scientific Report — Fisheries No. 166*, 1–8.

Hofer, B. von (1893). Eine Salmonidenerkrankung. *Allgemeine Fischereizeitung* **18**, 168–171.

Johnson, T. W., Jr. and Sparrow, F. K. Jr. (1961). "Fungi in Oceans and Estuaries." J. Cramer, Weinheim.

Johnstone, J. (1905). Internal parasites and diseased conditions of fishes. *Report of the Lancashire Sea-fisheries Laboratory* **14**, 151–185.

McVicar, A. H. (1977). *Ichthyophonus* as a pathogen in farmed and wild fish. *Bulletin. Office international des épizooties* **87**, 517–519.

McVicar, A. H. (1981). An assessment of *Ichthyophonus* disease as a component of natural mortality in plaice populations in Scottish waters. *International Council for the Exploration of the Sea. Demersal Fish Committee G49*, 1–7.

McVicar, A. H. (in press). The effects of *Ichthyophonus* infection in haddock *Melanogrammus aeglefinus* and plaice *Pleuronectes platessa* in Scottish waters. *In* "Proceedings of ICES Special Meeting on Diseases of Commercially Important Marine Fish and Shellfish 1–3 October, 1980, Copenhagen. (Ed. J. E. Stewart). Rapports et Proces — verbaux.

McVicar, A. H. and MacKenzie, K. (1972). A fungus disease of fish. *Scottish Fisheries Bulletin No. 37*, 27–28.

Miyazaki, T. and Kubota, S. S. (1977a). Studies on *Ichthyophonus* disease fishes — I. Rainbow trout fry. *Bulletin of the Faculty of Fisheries, Mie University* **4**, 45–56.

Miyazaki, T. and Kubota, S. S. (1977b). Studies on *Ichthyophonus* disease of fishes — III. Life cycle of *Ichthyophonus* affected rainbow trout. *Bulletin of the Faculty of Fisheries, Mie University* **4**, 67–80.

Munday, B. L. (1976). Infectious diseases of farmed trout. *Australian Veterinary Practitioner* **6**, 46, 49–50.

Munro, A. L. S., McVicar, A. H. and Jones, R. (in press). The epidemiology of infectious disease in commercially important wild marine fish. *In* "Proceedings of ICES Special Meeting on Diseases of Commercially Important Marine Fish and Shellfish 1–3 October, 1980, Copenhagen. (Ed. J. E. Stewart). Rapports et Proces — verbaux.

Plehn, M. and Mulsow, K. (1911). Der erreger der "Taumelkrankheit" der salmoniden. *Zentralblatt für Bakteriologie, Parasitenkunde Infektionskrankheiten und Hygiene* **59**, 63–68.

Reichenbach-Klinke, H. (1954–55). Untersuchungen über die bei Fischen durch Parasiten hervorgerufenen Zysten und deren Wirkung auf den Wirtskörper. *Zeitschrift für Fischerei und deren Hilfswissenschaften.*

Reichenbach-Klinke, H. (1973). *Fish Pathology.* TFH Publications, New Jersey.

Reichenbach-Klinke, H. and Elkan, E. (1965). "The Principal Diseases of Lower Vertebrates." Academic Press, London and New York.

Robertson, M. (1909). Notes on an *Ichthyosporidium* causing fatal disease in sea trout. *Proceedings of the Zoological Society of London, 1909,* 399–402.

Ross, A. J. and Parisot, T. J. (1958). Record of the fungus *Ichthyosporidium* Caullery and Mesnil, 1905, in Idaho. *Journal of Parasitology* **44,** 453–454.

Rucker, R. R. and Gustafson, P. V. (1953). An epizootic among rainbow trout. *Progressive Fish Culturist* **15,** 179–181.

Schäperclaus, N. (1953). Fortpflanzung und systematik von *Ichthyophonus. Aquarien — und Terrarien — Zeitschrift* **6,** 177–182.

Sindermann, C. J. (1958). An epizootic in Gulf of St. Lawrence fishes. *Transactions of the Twenty-third North American Wildlife Conference,* 349–360. Wildlife Management Institute, Washington.

Sindermann, C. J. (1963). Disease in marine populations. *Transactions of the Twenty-eighth North American Wildlife Conference,* 336–356. Wildlife Management Institute, Washington.

Sindermann, C. J. (1966). *Diseases of Marine Fishes.* TFH Publications, New Jersey.

Sindermann, C. J. (1970). "Principal Diseases of Marine Fish and Shellfish." Academic Press, New York and London.

Sindermann, C. J. and Scattergood, L. W. (1954). Diseases of fishes of the western North Atlantic. II. *Ichthyosporidium* disease of the sea herring (*Clupea harengus*). *Research Bulletin of the Department of Sea and Shore Fisheries, Maine* **19,** 1–40.

Sprague, V. (1965). *Ichthyosporidium* Caullery and Mesnil 1905, the name of a genus of fungi or a genus of sporozoans? *Systematic Zoology* **14,** 110–114.

Sproston, N. G. (1944). *Ichthyosporidium hoferi* (Plehn & Mulsow, 1911), an internal fungoid parasite of the mackerel. *Journal of the Marine Biological Association of the United Kingdom* **26,** 72–98.

Williamson, H. C. (1913). Report on diseases and abnormalities in fishes. *Fishery Board for Scotland Scientific Investigations, 1911 NoII March 1913.* 1–39.

incidence rates of the disease, with associated infection rates, mortality rates and pathogenicity must be determined in addition to the prevalence levels. Prevalence levels are commonly measured alone, but they only reveal the residue of the disease in the population, which, as was illustrated by results from haddock, can be very high without the disease having a serious effect on the host population (McVicar, in press).

In farmed rainbow trout, the introduction of *Ichthyophonus* has caused heavy mortalities, amounting to almost 50% of the total stock of one farm (Rucker and Gustafson, 1953). Some variability in the effect of the disease was apparent in the study by Dorier and Degrange (1960) when the rainbow trout stocks of some ponds were almost completely wiped out, some trout survived infection but with retardation of growth and others, although heavily infected on microscopic examination, could not be distinguished macroscopically from uninfected individuals. Similarly, no serious mortalities resulted from an outbreak of the disease in a rainbow trout farm in Scotland caused by using infected haddock as food (personal observations) but significant mortalities were associated with two separate incidents in the trial cultivation of plaice in Scotland (McVicar, 1977). Because of the potentially serious effect, fish farms should avoid the disease by not using fresh marine fish as food, or by treating such material before using. Gustafson and Rucker (1956) suggested freezing may be a suitable method of treatment. Inevitably the costs involved in treatment or of using the more expensive compounded diets increase the feeding costs to the farm over that possible from using fresh fish directly. The natural occurrences of *Ichthyophonus* in salmon and the ease of transmission of the fungus from natural infections into rainbow trout and turbot (McVicar, 1977 and unpublished observations) indicated, however, the vulnerability of these species when reared in sea cages to infection from local wild fish stocks, particularly as large numbers of fish are attracted to the vicinity of cages. However, no outbreaks of the disease resulting from such a route of infection have yet been recorded.

In direct economic terms the spoilage effects of *Ichthyophonus* on the muscle of marine fish is probably of greatest significance. Sproston (1944) considered it highly probable that the disease was "to a large measure responsible for the widespread unpopularity of mackerel as a food unless freshly caught" and suggested proteolytic enzymes released during the growth of *Ichthyophonus* after host capture contributed to the rapid decay of the muscle. Similarly, Sindermann (1958) reported that acute infections in herring caused degeneration and necrosis of the body muscles and that such fish were poor for smoking because they fell from the smoke-house racks, and were not suitable for pickling since they were already partly decomposed. The name "greasers" is currently used by fish merchants in

Aberdeen to describe *Ichthyophonus*-infected haddock, the term referring specifically to the texture of the flesh. The fact that this name has persisted in common usage in Aberdeen for at least 70 years (also being referred to by Williamson in 1913), indicates that the disease has remained a common problem during that time. The spoilage of haddock flesh by the disease (white flecking, texture and smell) has resulted in the rejection of a high proportion of some catches, and fishing vessels under contract to some processors have on occasion been requested to avoid heavily infected grounds (McVicar, in press). Although the disease was not often visible in the flesh of freshly caught haddock, the extensive post-mortem germination typical of the fungus greatly increased the problem. Fish considered normal during initial screening by processors became obviously diseased after chilled storage or smoking, making quality control difficult. In addition, as Sandholzer *et al.* (1945, cited by Johnson and Sparrow, 1961) noted, *Ichthyophonus* could be transferred from infected to uninvaded fillets of oceanpout, in storage at 8°C. In plaice the major economic loss directly attributable to *Ichthyophonus* was due to the severe emaciation and jelly-like texture in muscles of infected fish. In heavily infected areas, fish were commonly rejected at sea or after landing during processing.

Comments made by Reichenbach-Klinke and Elkan (1965), Amlacher (1970) and Reichenbach-Klinke (1973) suggest that *Ichthyophonus* was an incurable disease of fish, particularly in advanced stages of infection. Van Duijn (1956), however, suggested that fungicidal drugs such as phenoxethol could be effective against early stages of the fungus and some success was claimed from using antibiotics such as penicillin injected intra-muscularly or chloromycetin mixed with food. However, the balance of experience suggests that whether in aquarium or farmed fish culture, strict prophylactic measures particularly with regard to treatment of food, are the only rational means of securing freedom from this serious condition.

References

Alderman, D. J. (1976). Fungal diseases of marine animals. *In* "Recent Advances in Aquatic Mycology" (Ed. E. B. G. Jones), pp.223–260. Elek Science, London.

Amlacher, E. (1970). "Textbook of Fish Diseases." TFH Publications, New Jersey.

Caullery, M. J. G. C. and Mesnil, F. (1905). Recherches sur les haplosporidies. *Archives de Zoologie, expérimental et générale* **4**, 101–181.

Chien, C., Miyazaki, T. and Kubota, S. S. (1979a). Studies on *Ichthyophonus* disease of fishes — IV. Comparative study on naturally infected fishes. *Bulletin of the Faculty of Fisheries, Mie University* **6**, 129–146.

Chien, C., Miyazaki, T. and Kubota, S. S. (1979b). Studies on *Ichthyophonus* disease of fishes — V. Culture. *Bulletin of the Faculty of Fisheries, Mie University* **6**, 147–151.

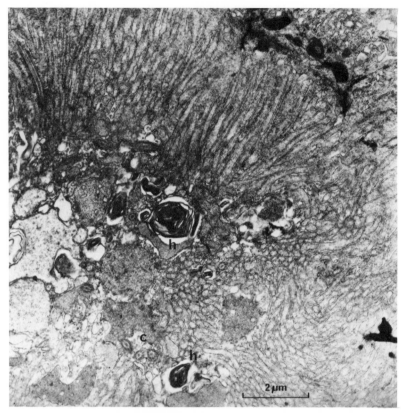

Fig. 17. Ultrastructure of plaice kidney tubule showing *Ichthyophonus* hyphae (h) in the lumen. c = cilium.

individual plaice, and provided the basis for an estimate of the mortality rate due to the disease in natural infections (McVicar, 1981). Indirect fluorescent antibody tests using *Ichthyophonus* from culture and antiserum produced against plaice antibody in rabbits showed antigenicity on the surface of spores and hyphae, but particularly strongly in the vicinity of growing hyphal tips. However, there was no indication that the production of antibody by plaice conferred any protection against *Ichthyophonus*. Similar levels of antibody production were found in turbot (*Scophthalmus maximus*) and some rainbow trout experimentally infected with the fungus but double precipitation lines were produced by turbot.

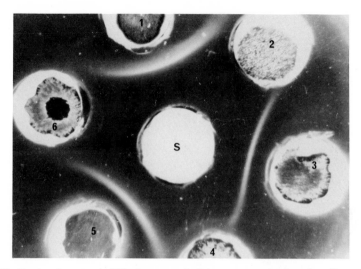

Fig. 18. Ouchterloney gel diffusion test of plaice serum tested against live spore(s). Three infected fish (1, 3, 5) show strong precipitating antibody reactions. One infected plaice (4) shows a weak reaction while one infected plaice (2) and an uninfected control plaice (6) showed no reaction.

Economic Significance

Extensive mortalities of herring in the Gulf of St. Lawrence were attributed by Sindermann (1958) to *Ichthyophonus* infection. During the period 1954–56 dead fish were observed floating in shoals at the surface, the nets of trawlers were frequently fouled with dead and decomposing herring raised from the bottom and dead fish were washed up on the shores of the Gulf. There was evidence for six major epidemics of the disease since the end of the last century (Sindermann, 1963), and Sindermann (1970) considered that the associated drastic reduction in herring abundance made the disease possibly the most important single factor limiting population growth of herring in the western North Atlantic. Loss to the fishery in economic terms must have been considerable. No other records of mass fish kills due to *Ichthyophonus* have been reported in natural populations but significant annual mortalities (>55%) due to the fungus have been estimated by McVicar (1981) in plaice off northern Scotland. Plaice catches from the area have not significantly changed since 1974 (Scottish Fishery Statistics), but the disease was common in that region even before 1960. Data on natural mortality due to disease is also important for assessment and management of fish stocks, and as pointed out by Munro *et al.* (in press)

12

Saprolegnia Infections of Salmonid Fish

A. D. PICKERING and L. G. WILLOUGHBY

Freshwater Biological Association, Ferry House,
Far Sawrey, Nr. Ambleside, Cumbria, U.K.

Introduction

Mycotic infections of fish by freshwater Oomycetes can develop at all stages of the fish's life cycle and as such are of considerable economic significance to the intensive fish cultivation industry. Unless treated, such fungal infections are usually lethal to the fish and extensive zoospore production ensures that infections spread rapidly through a population. The purpose of this review is to examine the nature of such infections, with particular emphasis being given to those of salmonid fish, and to identify those conditions that promote the outbreak of fungal diseases. Not unnaturally, we will draw heavily on our own work at the Freshwater Biological Association but will attempt to present this in the broader framework of the international scientific literature on the subject.

A major problem associated with the study of fungal infections of fish is the tendency for uncritical observers to refer to any fungal growth as saprolegniasis without any formal identification of the fungus or fungi involved. As we have shown in our studies on the perch (*Perca fluviatilis* L.) (Pickering and Willoughby, 1977) fungal-infected epidermal lesions may contain as many as four different aquatic fungi growing together as a mixed colony. A total of six genera of freshwater Oomycetes (*Achlya, Aphanomyces, Leptolegnia, Leptomitus, Pythiopsis, Saprolegnia*) have been isolated from a population of fungal-infected perch in Windermere (Willoughby, 1970; Pickering and Willoughby, 1977; Bucke *et al.*, 1979). Thus, indiscriminate use of the term 'saprolegniasis' for any cotton wool-like growth on a teleost fish may include some fungi (for example *Leptomitus lacteus*) which are not even members of the order Saprolegniales (for a summary of the different Oomycetes that have been isolated from infected fish the reader is referred to Scott and O'Bier (1962), Wolke (1975), Wilson (1976) and Neish and Hughes (1980)).

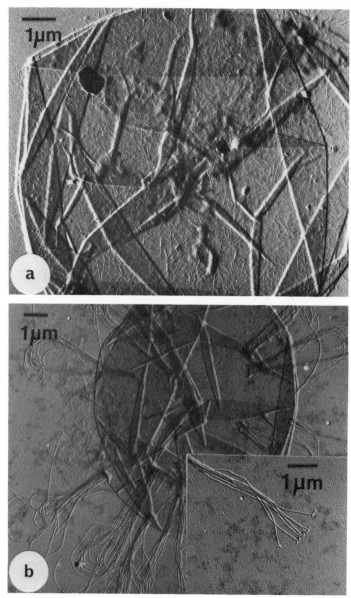

Fig. 1. (a) Empty cyst case from a primary zoospore cyst of *Saprolegnia diclina* Type 1. The cyst case is covered by short, single, unbranched hairs. Preparation shadowed for transmission electron microscopy with gold/palladium. (b) Empty cyst case from a secondary zoospore cyst of *Saprolegnia diclina* Type 1. Note the numerous bundles of long, unbranched hairs. *Enlarged inset:* Each of the hairs ends in a pair of recurved hooks. Preparations shadowed for transmission electron microscopy with platinum/palladium.

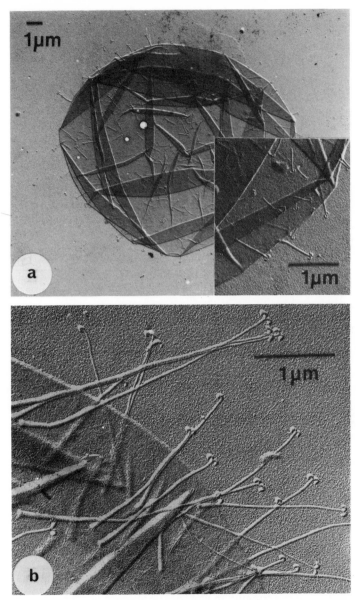

Fig. 2. (a) Empty cyst case from a secondary cyst of *Saprolegnia diclina* Type 3. The cyst case bears many single, short hooked hairs. *Enlarged inset:* shows details of the pair of recurved hooks at the end of each hair. Preparation shadowed for transmission electron microscopy with platinum/palladium. (b) Hooked-hairs on the secondary cyst case of *Saprolegnia hypogyna.* The hairs are significantly longer than those on *Saprolegnia diclina* Type 3 (see inset, Fig. 2a). Preparation shadowed for transmission electron microscopy with platinum/palladium.

Table 2. *Characteristics used by Willoughby (1978) to type* Saprolegnia diclina *isolates.*

Characteristic	Type 1 (salmonid pathogens)	Type 2 (perch pathogens)	Type 3 (saprophytic)
Antheridia	Diclinous	Diclinous	Diclinous
Oogonium production 7°C	Moderate	Prolific	Prolific
20°C	None	None	Prolific
Oogonium shape	Oval-elongate	Round-oval	Round-oval
Oogonium investment	Often intensive → 'birdsnest' appearance	Not intensive	Not intensive
Oospores	Centric or sub-centric often aborting	Centric or sub-centric sometimes aborting	Centric or sub-centric never aborting
Oogonium pitting	Normally absent	Normally present	Normally absent

working with fungal-infected sockeye salmon *Oncorhynchus nerka* (Walbaum) in British Columbia, Canada. Of 20 isolates taken from infected salmon, Neish concluded that 12 belonged to the *Saprolegnia diclina–parasitica* complex, the other isolates being *Saprolegnia* sp. (sexually sterile under laboratory conditions). In view of the taxonomic problems, we have tabulated the main characteristics used by Willoughby (1978) to type *Saprolegnia diclina* isolates (Table 2).

Characteristics of *Saprolegnia diclina* Type 1 and *Saprolegnia* sp. Strains which may Influence their Pathogenicity to Fish

As far as the authors are aware, there is no published work which unequivocally relates specific characteristics of fungal isolates to their pathogenicity. However, we have examined several aspects of the biology of salmonid fungal pathogens and it seems possible that these may reflect the parasitic nature of the fungus. In view of the absence of such information in the literature we think it would be useful to summarize, in the following sections, those characteristics of *S. diclina* Type 1 and the sterile *Saprolegnia* isolates which may be at least partly responsible for their undoubted pathogenicity. It is intended that this should act as a stimulus for further work in this area.

Zoospore encystment

All Oomycetes produce motile spores with two flagella, one of the whiplash type and the other of the tinsel type. In *S. diclina* Type 1 and *Saprolegnia* sp. the zoosporangium releases pyriform primary zoospores with the two flagella inserted at the apex. The primary zoospore swims for a short period of time only, in a weak and erratic manner, before encysting. Electron microscope studies of the primary zoospore cyst case indicate that *S. diclina* Type 1 and *Saprolegnia* sp. isolates are structurally similar in this respect to other *Saprolegnia* species (*S. diclina* Types 2 and 3, *S. australis*, *S. ferax*, *S. hypogyna*). The primary zoospore cyst is normally covered with single, unbranched hairs approximately 1.5μm in length (Fig. 1a) although on one occasion we found primary zoospore cysts of a *S. diclina* Type 3 isolate which were apparently devoid of these hairs (Pickering *et al.*, 1979). Each primary cyst normally releases a secondary zoospore although under certain circumstances the primary cyst may germinate directly (L. G. Willoughby, unpublished observations). Secondary zoospores are reniform, biflagellate spores capable of prolonged, active swimming. This active phase prior to a second encystment is, presumably, an important dispersive factor in the life cycle. It is possible that chemotropism might play a significant role in the movement of zoospores to a potential host fish but as far as we are aware there is no available information on this phenomenon in fungal pathogens of fish. Little is known about the stimuli that trigger encystment of the secondary zoospore but recent work at our laboratory has shown that there may be important differences between pathogenic and non-pathogenic strains with regard to this process. The secondary zoospores of eight out of nine isolates of *S. diclina* Type 1 and two out of five *Saprolegnia* sp. isolates encysted readily in sterilized lake water whereas under similar conditions other *Saprolegnia* isolates (*S. diclina* Type 3, *S. australis*, *S. ferax*, *S. hypogyna*) all continued to show zoospore motility after 18–27 hours (Willoughby *et al.*, 1982). From subsequent germination studies, it seems reasonable to consider sterilized lake water as a dilute nutrient solution and it is possible, therefore, that pathogenic isolates may have the ability to encyst and then grow under conditions of low levels of nutrients, conditions too dilute to trigger encystment in non-pathogenic strains. The external mucus of fish has water-soluble components and at the water/mucus interface low concentrations of nutrients may be available. Mucus removed from the surface of the fish triggers encystment of zoospores of the pathogenic strains and mycelial growth ensues rapidly.

Ultrastructural studies of the secondary cyst reveal interesting similarities between *S. diclina* Type 1 and *Saprolegnia* sp. and differences between these isolates and all other *Saprolegnia* isolates so far examined (Pickering *et al.*,

A second problem related to the identification of fungi involved in infections of freshwater fish is the reluctance of many of the *Saprolegnia* isolates to produce sexual structures under laboratory conditions. Most genera of the family Saprolegniaceae can be identified from hyphal characteristics, the nature of the zoosporangium and subsequent spore release but identification of the different *Saprolegnia* species has traditionally depended on characteristics of the oogonia and antheridia. However, the absence of sexual structures did not deter Coker (1923), in his monograph on the Saprolegniaceae, from ascribing apparently sterile *Saprolegnia* isolates from fish to the species *Saprolegnia parasitica*. Subsequently, Kanouse (1932) gave an account of the complete life history of *Saprolegnia parasitica* in which the sexual organs were described for the first time. As a result of this emendation, non-sexual strains of *Saprolegnia* ought not to be ascribed to any particular species. Willoughby (1978), in a critical analysis of the relationships between *Saprolegnia parasitica* and *Saprolegnia diclina* concluded that, at the present state of knowledge, the binomial *Saprolegnia diclina* Humphrey was appropriate for all isolates in the *S. parasitica–diclina* complex although three distinct types were apparent within this group. We have adopted Willoughby's system of classification for the purpose of this paper and will use *Saprolegnia diclina* Type 1 as synonymous with *S. parasitica* (Kanouse, 1932) and *Saprolegnia* Type 1 (Willoughby, 1968, 1969, 1971, 1972; Pickering and Willoughby, 1977). Sexually sterile strains of *Saprolegnia* isolated from living fish will be referred to as *Saprolegnia* sp. A more complete account of the history of these taxonomic problems is given by Neish and Hughes (1980).

In addition to problems of identification, studies of fungal infections of freshwater fish are complicated by the prolific growth of saprophytic fungi once the fish is dead (Willoughby, 1971). It is most important that isolates are made from living or freshly killed fish if a reliable diagnosis is to be made. Even with living fish it is difficult to prove beyond doubt that a fungal colonist exists as a parasite on the fish and not as a saprophyte on necrotic tissue. The pathogenic potential of several isolates has been clearly demonstrated in experimental inoculation studies (Table 1) although the test fish have not always been of the same species as the host from which the fungus was originally isolated. Thus several members of the family Saprolegniaceae can, under certain circumstances, act as primary pathogens by parasitizing living fish.

Despite the difficulties outlined above, there is little doubt that fungal infections of freshwater fish are serious problems of both natural fisheries and intensive cultivation units. A deeper understanding of the biology of these pathogens, of their interactions with the host fish and of the influence of fisheries management practices on both the parasite and host is

Table 1. *Potential fish pathogens of the family Saprolegniaceae.* (These isolates have been demonstrated to be primary pathogens of fish under controlled experimental circumstances. The studies of Tiffney (1939a) fulfilled all four of Koch's postulates, those of Vishniac and Nigrelli (1957) and Scott and O'Bier (1962) fulfilled the first three postulates but these workers did not re-isolate the fungus in pure form from the experimentally infected fish.)

Pathogenic fungus	Reference
Achlya bisexualis	Scott and O'Bier (1962)
Achlya flagellata	Tiffney (1939a)
Achlya sp.	Tiffney (1939a), Vishniac and Nigrelli (1957)
Dictyuchus sp.	Tiffney (1939a)
Saprolegnia delica (syn. *S. diclina*)	Scott and O'Bier (1962)
Saprolegnia diclina Type 1 (syn. *S. parasitica* Coker emend. Kanouse)	Vishniac and Nigrelli (1957), Scott and O'Bier (1962)
Saprolegnia ferax	Tiffney (1939a), Scott and O'Bier (1962)
Saprolegnia monoica	Scott and O'Bier (1962)
Saprolegnia sp.	Tiffney (1939a), Scott and O'Bier (1962)

essential if we are to combat successfully mycotic infections of freshwater fish.

Identification of the Salmonid *Saprolegnia*

In our experience, fungal infections of the integument of salmonid fish are always associated with a group of closely related strains of *Saprolegnia*. We have isolated fungi from infected salmonids representative of a limited geographical range comprising the English Lake District, the River Lune, Lancashire, and Loch Leven, Scotland. Of 48 isolates in pure culture 36 have been identified as *Saprolegnia diclina* Type 1, the remaining 12 proving to be sexually sterile under our laboratory conditions (*Saprolegnia* sp.). Ultrastructural studies of the secondary zoospore cyst (Pickering *et al.*, 1979; see also below) indicate that these apparently sterile strains are closely related to *Saprolegnia diclina* Type 1. We have never isolated any other species of the Saprolegniaceae from infected salmonids despite the fact that fungal-infected non-salmonids taken from the same water body at the same time often yielded a wide range of aquatic fungi (Pickering and Willoughby, 1977).

Further evidence for this association between salmonid fish and a closely related group of *Saprolegnia* fungi has been obtained by Neish (1977)

1979). Typically, secondary cysts of *S. diclina* Type 1 and *Saprolegnia* sp. bear bundles of long hooked-hairs (Fig. 1b) whereas *S. diclina* Types 2 and 3, *S. australis* and *S. ferax* produce secondary cysts with short, single hooked-hairs (Fig. 2a). This observation is taken as evidence of a close taxonomic relationship between *S. diclina* Type 1 and the particular *Saprolegnia* sp. isolated from salmonid fish. *S. hypogyna* also produces secondary cysts with single hooked-hairs but in this case the hairs are significantly longer than those of the other non-pathogenic species (Fig. 2b). Even within the group of pathogenic strains, however, there is some evidence of significant variation in this character with a direct relationship between the length of the hooked-hairs and the number of hooked-hairs comprising each bundle (Pickering *et al.*, 1979). At one extreme are isolates with long ($<10\mu$m) hooked-hairs aggregated in large bundles ($<$ 12 hairs/bundle) and at the other extreme are isolates with short (2μm) hooked-hairs aggregated in smaller bundles ($\approx$ 4 hairs/bundle). The hooked-hairs are preformed in the so-called bar bodies of the primary cyst and secondary zoospore stages (Fig. 3) and are integrated into the cyst wall during the process of encystment. There is good evidence from the study of primary zoospore encystment that the lining of the capsule-shaped bar bodies forms the outer coat around the settling zoospores and stabilizes them for subsequent secretion of the microfibrillar wall (Heath and Greenwood, 1970). Attachment of the hairs to the cyst wall appears to be firmer in pathogenic strains than in saprophytic isolates (G. M. Beakes, personal communication). It is tempting to conclude, like Manton *et al.* (1951) and Meier and Webster (1954), that the bifurcate hooks on the secondary cysts are concerned with attachment of the cyst to fish. In this connection, it might be expected that the greater development of such structures in isolates from salmonid fish would enhance their pathogenicity although it should be pointed out that little is known about the nature of the infective stage of the fungus under natural conditions. An alternative role for the hooked-hairs, other than directly in attachment to fish, has been suggested by Dr M. W. Dick (personal communication). He is of the opinion that they might be concerned with floatation or even with attachment to the underside of the water meniscus, thus ensuring a high position in the water column and a more favourable situation for encountering a potential fish host.

Some of the pathogenic isolates exhibit marked polyplanetism, the repeated emergence of zoospores from the secondary cyst case. This is indicated by the abundance of empty, secondary cyst cases in preparations for transmission electron microscopy. No systematic study has been made of this phenomenon but it may be of adaptive significance by preserving zoospore motility under conditions which are favourable for encystment but not for subsequent germination and growth. Thus, it seems likely

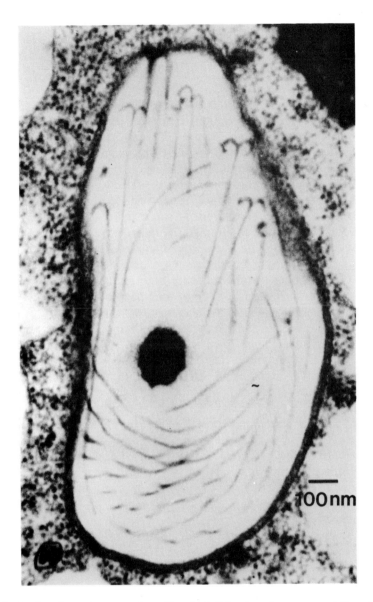

Fig. 3. Section through a secondary "bar-body" in the primary cyst of *Saprolegnia diclina* Type 1. Note the long hooked hairs which would be released during encystment of the subsequent secondary zoospore. Micrograph kindly provided by Dr G. M. Beakes (Newcastle University) — glutaraldehyde fixation with post-osmification.

that the triggers for encystment and for subsequent germination are not identical.

Germination and Growth

In marked contrast to typical freshwater saprophytes of the genus *Saprolegnia*, the majority of isolates from diseased salmonid fish (*S. diclina* Type 1 and *Saprolegnia* sp.) exhibited encystment, germination and growth during the first day of incubation at 10°C in natural lake water, or in a dilute nutrient medium such as sterilized lake water. Furthermore, in an enriched water supply (the effluent from a trout hatchery) linear growth of most salmonid *Saprolegnia* isolates was stimulated further, up to a factor of 2–5 times that achieved in natural lake water whereas under identical conditions, secondary zoospores of saprophytic isolates (*S. australis*, *S. diclina* Type 3, *S. hypogyna*) still failed to encyst and germinate (Willoughby *et al.*, 1982). During these studies it was observed that the germination of pathogenic isolates was frequently of a partially evacuated (indirect) type, a phenomenon originally reported by Willoughby (1972) for *Saprolegnia diclina* Type 1 isolates growing in trout mucus. This has been described in more detail by Willoughby (1977) for isolates growing in sterilized lake water. Partially evacuated germination is characterized by an attached zoospore and very fine initial germ tube (with several cross walls) both devoid of cytoplasmic contents (Fig. 4). It is thought that the first phase of such a germination pattern occurs through the successive production of new cross walls behind the advancing hyphal tip containing the cytoplasm. Using different concentrations of a synthetic fungal growth medium (glucose–yeast extract broth), Willoughby *et al.* (1982) have shown that the occurrence of partially evacuated germination in the pathogenic isolate LIC10 (*S. diclina* Type 1) is strongly dependent on the concentration of the nutrient solution. Cytoplasm-filled (direct) germination occurred in the most concentrated and in the most dilute nutrient solutions used in this investigation but partially evacuated germination predominated at intermediate concentrations.

The biological significance of this response in pathogenic isolates has not been established although it is possible that the 'partially evacuated germling' may act as the infective agent. Under these circumstances the increased length of the germling may increase the efficiency of attachment to the host. It is interesting to record that we have repeatedly observed firm attachment of partially evacuated germlings to the base of plastic petri dishes and in all cases attachment was by means of the empty cyst case and the empty portions of the initial germ tube but not by the cytoplasmic region of the hypha (L. G. Willoughby, unpublished observations).

Alternatively, the increase in length of the germling by means of partially evacuated germination may be a means of extending the area of search for new nutrient sources with a minimal use of the cytoplasmic reserves. Further work is needed to clarify these issues.

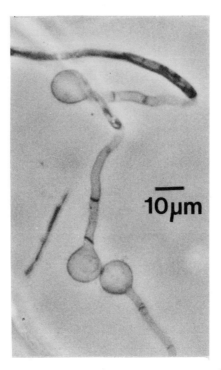

Fig. 4. Indirect germination of secondary zoospores cysts of *Saprolegnia diclina* Type 1. The attached zoospore cyst and initial germ tube (with several cross walls) are both devoid of cytoplasmic contents. Living preparation under phase contrast.

Temperature Considerations

An examination of fungal-infected elvers *Anguilla anguilla* L. from a fish farm utilizing the heated effluent from a power station prompted a wider study of the growth of *Saprolegnia diclina* and *Saprolegnia* sp. isolates from teleost fish under different temperature regimes (Willoughby and Copland, 1982). Marked differences in the tolerance of isolates to both high and low temperatures were found and these seemed to be indicative of ecological adaptation. Some strains (Group A) were able to grow and release zoospores over a wide range of temperatures (3–33°C). Included in this group were all six isolates (*Saprolegnia* sp.) from elvers from the heated effluent together with a *Saprolegnia* sp. isolated from an infected perch. A second group of strains (Group B) were able to grow, produce zoospores and also form resistant chlamydospores at high temperatures (31.5°C) but were much less competent in zoospore production at lower temperatures (3°C). This group includes *S. diclina* Type 1 isolate (isolate C17) from a salmonid fish, the char *Salvelinus alpinus* L., and *Saprolegnia* sp. isolates from non-salmonid fish (the tench *Tinca tinca* L., the carp *Cyprinus carpio* L., the orfe *Leuciscus idus* L.). The third group of fungal strains (Group C) were able to grow and produce zoospores at low temperatures but were less competent in this respect at high temperature. Of 15 isolates from salmonid fish, 14 belonged to Group C. (The exception, isolate C17, was also atypical in other aspects of its biology.) Thus, the temperature–response characteristics of pathogenic fungi isolated from teleosts seem to reflect, to a considerable degree, the thermal preferences of the host fish. Fungal isolates capable of survival and reproduction at high temperatures were derived from fish with an ability to withstand high temperatures (for

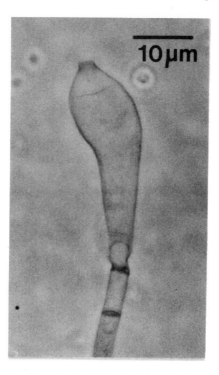

Fig. 5. 'Minisporangium' at the hyphal tip of a germling of *Saprolegnia diclina* Type 1. Its zoospore(s) has been released from the apical pore. Living preparation under phase contrast.

example eels and cyprinids) whereas isolates from stenothermal, cold water salmonids grew more successfully at low temperatures. The mechanisms by which the thermal tolerance of host and pathogen are aligned should be a rewarding subject for further investigation.

Abbreviated Life Cycle

It has already been suggested that polyplanetism may serve to ensure zoospore motility under conditions which trigger encystment but may not be favourable for subsequent germination and growth. Even when germination occurs, if the levels of nutrients in the surrounding water are not sufficiently high, the 'starved germling' may abbreviate the normal life cycle to produce a further zoospore stage (Willoughby, 1977). This abbreviated life cycle may occur in both direct and indirect germlings and features the development of a single sporangium on each thallus (Fig. 5). The sporangium normally releases just one secondary zoospore (reniform, biflagellate). If this spore then encysts and grows, germination is almost always of the direct type. Upon releasing the single zoospore from its sporangium, the germling then autolyses. It seems possible that this abbreviated life cycle is a mechanism whereby zoospore motility (and hence fungal dispersion) is maintained under conditions which stimulate encystment and germination but are not suitable for the normal growth and development of the colony.

Pathology of *Saprolegnia* Infections

Gross Pathology

Saprolegnia infections of salmonid fish are characterized by conspicuous fungal colonies growing on the body surface of the fish (Fig. 6). These cotton wool-like lesions are normally white in colour but may be discoloured by the accumulation of debris between the fungal hyphae or as a result of a simultaneous bacterial infection. The fungus can colonize almost any area of the external surface of the fish although evidence now suggests that the pattern of infection on the body of the fish may not be quite as random as was previously thought. Two independent studies on the mature brown trout have both demonstrated a clear sexual dimorphism in the pattern of *Saprolegnia* infection (White, 1975; Richards and Pickering, 1978). Moreover, there appear to be differences in the patterns of infection of hatchery-reared brown trout when compared with wild fish (Richards and Pickering, 1978). Hatchery-reared fish of both sexes are significantly more frequently infected on all fins than on the rest of the body, whereas in wild fish the male fish are more vulnerable along the dorsal surfaces (particularly around the base of the dorsal and adipose fins) and the females are more vulnerable on the tail region. A statistical comparison of the patterns of infection of male and female fish from both natural and hatchery conditions indicates that there are large areas on the body of the male fish that are more frequently infected than on the female fish and, conversely, there are areas on the caudal and anal fins of the female fish that are significantly more frequently infected than the corresponding areas on the male fish (Richards and Pickering, 1978; for a discussion of this phenomenon see the section on predisposing factors).

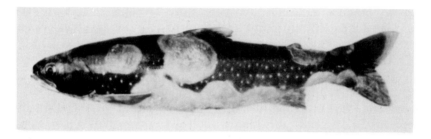

Fig. 6. Windermere char severely infected with the fungus *Saprolegnia diclina* Type 1.

One unexplained feature of the gross pathology of *Saprolegnia* infections of salmonid fish is the frequent occurrence of lesions in the form of a delicate ring of fungus enclosing an apparently uninfected area of the body surface (Willoughby, 1971). It is possible that this represents some form of temporary inhibition or restriction of fungal growth during the early stages of infection (presumably from a point source). In this connection it is interesting that branched hyphae, much (but not all) of which was autolysed and empty of cytoplasmic contents, have been observed in the mucus removed from ostensibly healthy char (Willoughby, 1972). The factors influencing this apparent destruction of fungal hyphae have not been elucidated (see section on defence mechanisms).

Histopathology

Detailed descriptions of the histopathological processes associated with *Saprolegnia* infections of salmonid fish have been provided by Neish (1977) and Pickering and Richards (1980). In general, the penetration of fungal hyphae is restricted to the epidermis and dermis. Muscular lesions are uncommon but occasionally develop when fungal and bacterial penetration to the muscle surface occurs. With small fish, however, hyphae may invade the deeper tissues of the fish and penetrate vital organs, even the central nervous system (Bootsma, 1973; Nolard-Tintigner, 1973). Degenerative changes in the epidermis and dermis include focal areas of cellular necrosis, spongiosis or intercellular oedema and an ultimate sloughing of the epidermis. The local acantholysis that occurs around fungal hyphae in the early stages of infection may be mediated by the chymotrypsin-like enzymic activity of the fungus (Peduzzi *et al.*, 1976; Peduzzi and Bizzozero, 1977). Clumping of melanin granules in the dermal melanophores accentuates the pale appearance of fungal infected lesions. Inflammatory responses are normally absent or weakly developed (Wolke, 1975; Pickering and Richards, 1980) unless bacteria infections also develop. As far as we are aware, there is no evidence that pathogenic *Saprolegnia* strains produce any toxins that might be transmitted systematically.

Osmoregulatory Failure

Once infected, salmonid fish do not normally recover from saprolegniasis unless treated (hatchery conditions) or unless they migrate naturally to estuarine or seawater environments. Death of the fish is undoubtedly due to the massive osmoregulatory problems caused by destruction of the superficial tissues over large areas of the body surface although the survival time is influenced by the precise location of damaged tissue. Gardner (1974), working with UDN-affected salmon with secondary *Saprolegnia* infections, found that infected fish had significantly lower plasma osmotic pressure, sodium and protein concentrations than uninfected fish. Primary *Saprolegnia* infection influences the salt and water balance of the brown trout (Richards and Pickering, 1979) and a significant inverse relationship has been demonstrated between the serum osmotic pressure (or Na^+) concentration) and the degree of severity of the infection. Decreases in the concentrations of K^+, Ca^{2+}, Mg^{2+} and total protein were also evident in infected fish and electrophoretic analysis of the serum proteins indicated a significant decrease in the albumin/globulin ratio (Richards and Pickering, 1979). The *Saprolegnia*-associated drop in serum Na^+ concentration was similar in magnitude to that associated with the fatal exposure of brown trout to acid water (Leivestad *et al.*, 1976). The net rates of loss of electrolytes and proteins together with the increased osmotic influx of water are functions of the extent of fungal colonization over the body surface and will determine the survival time of the fish in fresh water. From our own experience with hatchery-reared brown trout, survival time may be less than 3 days from the first visible signs of infection.

Defence Mechanisms and the Predisposition of Fish to Fungal Infections

The interrelationships between a pathogen, its host and environmental conditions are complex and overt infectious diseases only occur when a susceptible host is exposed to a virulent pathogen under certain environmental conditions (Snieszko, 1974). Thus, it is necessary to consider all three components (pathogen, host and environment) if we are to understand the nature of and the reasons for outbreaks of fungal infection in salmonid fish. The influence of the host and of the environment will be considered in the following sections on defence mechanisms and predisposing factors and some of the aspects of pathogen virulence have already been discussed in the preceding sections. However, one subject that has not yet been considered is the relative abundance of pathogenic *Saprolegnia* spores or propagules in the environment. Reliable methods for quantitative estimation of propagules in fresh water are usually labour-intensive and tedious to operate. This, together with the fact that fungal identification (particularly with *S. diclina* Type 1) may take several weeks, or even months (Neish, 1977), is responsible for the paucity of information on the abundance of pathogenic *Saprolegnia* propagules in natural water bodies. It is hoped that, if confirmed by other workers, the relatively rapid identification of potentially pathogenic isolates by means of the secondary zoospore cyst ultrastructure will do much to remedy this situation. Until the whole genus is surveyed it will not be known how specific this character is; however, the situation appears promising because groups of hooked-hairs have not so far been reported for any member of the Saprolegniaceae other than *S. diclina*.

An estimation of the concentration of total Saprolegniales in Windermere gave values ranging from below 25 to 5,200 litre^{-1} at the lake margin compared with a mean of 11 propagules litre^{-1} in the centre of the lake, with some evidence of a peak during the Autumn period (Willoughby, 1962). It was not possible to distinguish pathogenic from non-pathogenic fungi in this work. In a later study (Willoughby, 1969), it was shown that *Saprolegnia diclina* Type 1 accounted for approximately half the total Saprolegniaceae in water samples from the River Leven (the Windermere outflow). The species of *Saprolegnia* implicated in fish pathology are probably best considered as facultative necrotrophs (Lewis, 1973), forms which are normally saprophytic but which can also exist as parasites. It follows, therefore, that their natural distribution in fresh water need have no correlation with the presence of fish and in this connection we note their ready cultivation on hemp seeds and other vegetable material. It has even been suggested (Dick, 1970) that decaying cast insect exuviae may harbour them and produce zoospore reservoirs for new fish infections. However, there is very little detailed work on the distribution of *Saprolegnia* in fresh water and it will be as well, for the time being at least, to retain the option of obligate necrotrophy (Lewis, 1973) for *S. diclina* Type 1 and the related *Saprolegnia* sp., where the living fish might be the major substratum for growth. It would seem likely that pathogenic *Saprolegnia* spores or propagules are ubiquitous components of the microbial flora of most natural water bodies and that potential hosts are constantly challenged by the pathogen. Under these circumstances, changes in the host and in the environment may be at least as important as changes in the pathogen load of the water in determining the outbreak of fungal infections. Once an outbreak occurs, the presence of infected fish ensures that the spore count in the water rises dramatically (Willoughby and Pickering, 1977).

Defence Mechanisms

Secretion of Mucus. The epidermis and its associated layer of mucus forms an immediate interface between the internal tissues of the fish and its environment. It is generally assumed that the mucous layer somehow acts as a physical barrier to the colonization of the skin by potential pathogens although convincing evidence is not normally forthcoming. However, Willoughby and Pickering (1977) have shown that *Saprolegnia diclina* Type 1 spores can readily adhere to the surface of the brown trout and the char and that the vast majority of these spores are removed or inactivated during the first 24 hours of subsequent quarantine in clean water. Using a more refined experimental approach to produce a pulse of zoospores around the fish for a short period of time only, A. D. Pickering and L. G. Willoughby (unpublished results) monitored the rate of loss of viable *S. diclina* Type 1 spores from the body surface of unhandled, acclimated brown trout. Spore counts were made from a series of fish sampled at different times by plating out skin samples (six skin samples from each fish) on to nutrient agar (see Willoughby and Pickering (1977) for techniques) and counting the resultant colonies. It can be seen (Fig. 7) that the rate of loss of fungal spores from the body surface of the fish was much slower than the rate of loss from the environment during the period of flushing with spore-free water. The loss of spores from the fish did not conform to a true exponential decay, but it is clear that over 95% of the viable fungal spores were removed from mucous layer within 2 hours. In view of the lack of evidence for inactivation of the spores in brown trout mucus (see below) and the fact that the rate of the removal of inert particles (experimentally applied starch grains) from the body of the fish were similar (A. D. Pickering, unpublished results), it would appear that the continuous secretion of mucus by the goblet cells of the salmonid epidermis acts as an extremely effective, physical, cleansing mechanism thereby removing small particles (including potentially pathogenic fungal spores) from the surface of the fish.

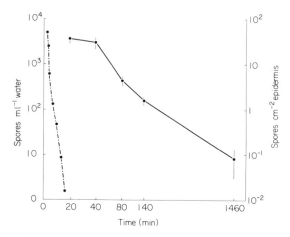

Fig. 7. The loss of viable spores of *Saprolegnia diclina* Type 1 from the surface of the brown trout. At the start of the experiment a high concentration of secondary zoospores ($\approx 7 \times 10^3$ spores ml^{-1}) was introduced into the water and then flushed away with spore-free water. $- - - -$, indicates the loss of spores from the water surrounding the fish; ———, depicts the change in concentration of viable spores on the epidermis of the fish during the subsequent 24 hours. Vertical bars, indicate $\pm$ standard error of the mean and the number of determinations for each point was not less than 20.

Epidermal Antibiotic Activity. The antibiotic properties of certain teleost mucous secretions have been known for a considerable period of time (see, for example, Nigrelli, 1935) and more recently, evidence of a range of potential antibiotic molecules in the mucous layers of fish has been presented. For example, Fletcher and Grant (1968) and Fletcher and White (1973a) identified lysozyme in the mucous secretions of the plaice *Pleuronectes platessa* and in another study (Fletcher and Grant, 1969), they induced specific haemagglutinins in skin mucus following parental administration of human erythrocytes. Antibodies have also been found in the mucus of the gar *Lepisosteus platyrhincus* (Bradshaw *et al.*, 1971) and the catfish *Tachysurus australis* (Di Conza, 1970) although no antibodies to fungi have yet been detected in the epidermal secretions of fish (Wilson, 1976). Specific agglutinin formation in the body mucus has been demonstrated following parental immunization with *Vibrio anguillarum* in the plaice (Fletcher and White, 1973b) and in the rainbow trout *Salmo gairdneri* (Harrell *et al.*, 1976).

In our experience, epidermal mucus taken from salmonid fish acts as an effective growth medium for *S. diclina* Type 1 spores (Willoughby, 1971; Willoughby and Pickering, 1977; Willoughby *et al.*, 1982). Nevertheless, it is possible that salmonid mucus has labile antibiotic properties which are lost once the secretion is removed from the epidermis. Some evidence against this has been obtained from experiments in which char were challenged with a high concentration of *S. diclina* Type 1 secondary zoospores (14,000 spores ml^{-1}). Ten minutes after challenge a mucus sample was taken from the fish and immediately examined by phase contrast microscopy. The mucus sample contained 4,000 spores ml^{-1}, many of which had already germinated (A. D. Pickering, unpublished observations). On the other hand, it has already been pointed out that Willoughby (1972) observed lysed fungal hyphae from the epidermal mucus of an ostensibly healthy char. In view of the marked plasticity of epidermal structure and function in salmonids (Pickering and Richards, 1980) one cannot discount the possiblity of temporal changes in antibiotic properties of their mucous secretions. Furthermore, the nature of the infective agent (cyst or zoospore) may markedly influence its sensitivity to antibiotic factors in the epidermal mucous secretions.

Natural and Acquired Immunity. Little of the extensive literature on teleost immunology concerns the responses of fish to fungal antigens. Early infiltration of lymphocyte-like cells to the sites of *Saprolegnia* infection in the epidermis of the brown trout may indicate a direct immune response (Pickering and Richards, 1980) although such an infiltration is not invariably found and a positive identification of the cell-type involved is still required. Precipitating antibodies against *Saprolegnia* antigens have been detected in the serum of the Atlantic salmon *Salmo salar* L. (Hodkinson and Hunter, 1970) but the likelihood of cross-reactivity (as shown by Peduzzi and Bizzozero (1977) using rabbit antisera raised against four different *Saprolegnia* isolates), and the widespread occurrence of 'natural antibodies' which may react with a variety of microbial extracts (Ingram, 1980) makes the interpretation of such observations difficult. In the field of fish immunology it is apparent that a shift in emphasis from bacteria to fungi is required if we are to elucidate the relative roles of specifically-induced and 'natural' antibodies in the defences of fish against *Saprolegnia* infection.

Predisposing Factors

Traditionally, saprolegniasis has been considered to be a secondary condition with fungal hyphae normally colonizing existing lesions on the fish. Whilst it is undoubtedly true that fungal infections are often secondary to other diseases and to physical damage (see below), there is evidence that *Saprolegnia diclina* Type 1 can also act as a primary pathogen on undamaged, healthy fish (Tiffney, 1939b; Pickering and Christie, 1980). The following sections identify those conditions that increase the susceptibility of salmonid fish to infection (both primary and secondary) by *S. diclina* Type 1 and *Saprolegnia* sp.

Integumental Damage. Epidermal integrity is essential if the secretion of mucus is to act as an efficient, physical protection against fungal invasion. Small breaches in the epidermis can be quickly covered by mucous secretion and by the migration of epidermal cells over the injured area (Bullock *et al.*, 1978) but large wounds are potential sites for *Saprolegnia* colonization. Increased susceptibility of teleost fish to fungal infection as a result of physical damage has been demonstrated by Tiffney (1939b), Hoshina and Ookubo (1956), Vishniac and Nigrelli (1957) and Egusa (1963). It is likely that the increased susceptibility of the fins of hatchery-reared brown trout to *Saprolegnia* infection (Richards and Pickering, 1978) is partly the result of mechanical damage under conditions of unnaturally high stocking density. This association between damage and infection is further borne out by the pattern of infection on the sexually mature, female brown trout in which the tail and anal fins are particularly vulnerable (Richards and Pickering, 1978). It is precisely these areas that are used by the fish to excavate the gravel of the spawning redds and, consequently, one might expect substantial physical damage. Any environmental conditions that are likely to result in physical damage to the fish will also increase the probability of subsequent fungal infection.

Sexual Maturation. The association of *Saprolegnia* infections with sexual maturation in salmonid fish is well documented (Neish, 1977; Richards and Pickering, 1978). This appears to be an expression of a more general decrease in resistance because sexually mature salmonid fish are also more prone to other skin parasites (Pickering and Christie, 1980). Sexual maturation in the male brown trout is associated with a marked epidermal demucification (Pickering, 1977) which may partly account for the fact that mature male fish are more prone to fungal infections than are mature female fish (Richards and Pickering, 1978). However, this cannot be the complete explanation because Pickering and Christie (1980) have demonstrated sexual differences in susceptibility to ectoparasitic infestation even before the sex-linked changes in epidermal mucification occur. It is also unlikely that the increased vulnerability to skin ectoparasites can be explained simply in terms of physical damage to the skin of the spawning fish because Paling (1965) observed that the incidence and severity of infection of the *gills* of brown trout in Windermere by the monogenean *Discocotyle sagittata* Leuckart was significantly greater in mature male fish during the spawning season. Thus, it is reasonable to conclude that physical damage (in both males and females) and epidermal demucification (in the males) probably exacerbate *existing* problems of vulnerability to skin parasites in sexually maturing salmonid fish. Further research is now needed to resolve the nature of this underlying increase in vulnerability during the spawning season.

Other Infections. In addition to their role as primary pathogens, *Saprolegnia diclina* Type 1 and *Saprolegnia* sp. strains may also occur as secondary infections. Secondary fungal infection is associated, in particular, with those conditions that cause ulceration of, or damage to, the superficial tissues of the fish. Three examples have been selected to illustrate this phenomenon, but it should be appreciated that these represent only a small proportion of the body of information concerning secondary fungal infections.

The causative agent of ulcerative dermal necrosis (UDN—a condition of salmonid fish characterized by superficial lesions on the head and opercula (Roberts *et al.*, 1970)) has yet to be identified although recent attention has been given to the possibility of ultraviolet radiation damage (Bullock and Roberts, 1979). Whatever its etiology, one frequent consequence of UDN is secondary infection by *Saprolegnia diclina* Type 1 or *Saprolegnia* sp. (Stuart and Fuller, 1968; Willoughby, 1968, 1969). From our own experience with hatchery-reared brown trout it is clear that bacterial fin rot also often results in secondary *Saprolegnia* infections. A similar association between bacteria and fungi has been found in a so-called fungal disease of cultivated Japanese eels. Critical investigations have shown that the primary pathogens are bacteria and that the fungus *Saprolegnia* sp. is a secondary colonist (Hoshina and Ookubo, 1956; Egusa, 1965; Egusa and Nishikawa, 1965). In all the above cases there can be little doubt that the debilitating effect of the fungus is sufficient to increase significantly the mortality rate of infected fish.

Responses to Stress. Based on his work with Pacific salmon, Neish (1977) emphasized the role of stress in initiating *Saprolegnia* infections. This hypothesis has been further developed by Neish and Hughes (1980) and should act as a stimulus for future work. They postulate that there is a direct link between stress-mediated increases in plasma corticosteroid levels and a fish's susceptibility to saprolegniasis. The mechanisms involved have not been elucidated although immunosuppression, decreased inflammatory responses and impaired wound healing all seem worthy of further investigation. Activation of the pituitary–interrenal axis may occur in response to a variety of different stresses (Donaldson, 1981) and evidence for the modulation of the fish's defence mechanisms by stressful stimuli is now accumulating (see Ellis, 1981). However, from a practical point of view evidence of corticosteroid-mediated increases in susceptibility of fish to fungal infections is more limited. Roth (1972) demonstrated that a variety of hormones, including corticosteroids, had a facilitating effect upon fungus growth on the freshwater teleost *Catostomus commersoni* Lacepede and Robertson *et al.* (1963) found that cortisol-treated rainbow trout developed fungal infections and ichthyophthiriasis. For a more detailed consideration of the responses of fish to stress the reader is referred to Pickering (1981).

Elevated corticosteroid levels occur in certain spawning salmonid fish (Hane and Robertson, 1959; Idler *et al.*, 1959; Phillips *et al.*, 1959) and it seems possible that these may predispose the fish to fungal infections. However, Pickering and Christie (1981) failed to find any marked elevation of blood cortisol levels in maturing, male brown trout even though fish at this stage had previously been shown to be particularly prone to infestations by skin parasites (Pickering and Christie, 1980). A slight elevation of blood cortisol levels was evident in male fish during the later stages of the spawning period. By comparison, a five-fold elevation of cortisol levels in the female fish was coincident with the onset of ovulation (Pickering and Christie, 1981). Thus, in hatchery-reared brown trout the increased susceptibility to skin parasites during sexual maturation is not particularly well correlated with elevated blood cortisol levels. *Saprolegnia* infection itself can act as a stress, with infected fish developing markedly elevated blood cortisol levels (Pickering and Christie, 1981). This aspect of the stress response could not be demonstrated with other ectoparasitic infestations.

Conclusions

Fungal infections of salmonid fish are almost invariably associated with a group of closely related strains identified as *Saprolegnia diclina* Type 1 or *Saprolegnia* sp. Ultrastructural evidence indicates that the sexually sterile isolates (*Saprolegnia* sp.) are closely related to *S. diclina* Type 1. These pathogenic isolates are able to encyst and grow under environmental conditions (with a low nutrient status) that would not promote encystment and growth of closely related saprophytic *Saprolegnia* species. Moreover, there are mechanisms in the pathogenic isolates for reverting to zoospore motility under conditions which are unsuitable for the subsequent growth of the colony. The temperature tolerances of isolates from a range of teleost fish reflect, to a considerable degree, the tolerances of the host fish.

Saprolegnia diclina Type 1 and *Saprolegnia* sp. frequently occur as secondary infections although they can also act as primary pathogens. Infections are normally restricted to the superficial tissues, resulting in a breakdown of the fish's osmoregulatory mechanisms. Much of the defence system of salmonid fish to *Saprolegnia* infections appears to depend upon the removal of infective spores and cysts by means of the continual secretion of mucus by the epidermis. Once an infection is established, it is unusual for a fish to recover naturally. Integumental damage (by physical means or as a result of other primary infections) frequently results in fungal infections and an increase in susceptibility is also associated with sexual maturation in salmonid fish. Some evidence suggests that activation of the pituitary–interrenal axis as part of the stress response in teleost fish predisposes the fish to saprolegniasis.

One of the purposes of this review it to indicate those areas which we believe would benefit from further study. From the mycological point of view, there is almost nothing known of the occurrence, nature and mode of attachment of the infective propagules in nature. However, detailed pure-culture studies on the comparative morphology and physiology of both pathogenic and purely saprophytic strains are providing clues which may prove to be helpful in this connection. With respect to the host fish, the influence of stress responses on the fish's defence systems is a subject that is awaiting thorough investigation. If this review has placed the available information in context and has stimulated interest in the practical research problems still to be tackled, its basic aim will have been realized.

Acknowledgements

The authors would like to thank Dr G. M. Beakes (Newcastle University) for permission to reproduce Fig. 3 and for his critical comments on the manuscript and Mr T. Furnass (FBA) for assistance with the photography.

References

Bootsma, R. (1973). Infections with *Saprolegnia* in pike culture. *Aquaculture* **2**, 385–394.
Bradshaw, C. M., Richard, A. S. and Sigel, M. M. (1971). IgM antibodies in fish mucus. *Proceedings of the Society for Experimental Biology and Medicine* **136**, 1122–1124.

Bucke, D., Cawley, G. D., Craig, J. F., Pickering, A. D. and Willoughby, L. G. (1979). Further studies of an epizootic of perch *Perca fluviatilis* L., of uncertain aetiology. *Journal of Fish Diseases* 2, 297–311.

Bullock, A. M. and Roberts, R. J. (1979). Induction of UDN-like lesions in salmonid fish by exposure to ultraviolet light in the presence of phototoxic agents. *Journal of Fish Diseases* 2, 439–441.

Bullock, A. M., Marks, R. and Roberts, R. J. (1978). The cell kinetics of teleost fish epidermis: mitotic activity of the normal epidermis at varying temperatures in plaice (*Pleuronectes platessa*). *Journal of Zoology* 184, 423–428.

Coker, W. C. (1923). "The Saprolegniaceae". The University of North Carolina Press, Chapel Hill, NC, U.S.A.

Dick, M. W. (1970). Saprolegniaceae on insect exuviae. *Transactions of the British Mycological Society* 55, 449–458.

Di Conza, J. J. (1970). Some characteristics of natural haemagglutinins found in serum and mucus of the catfish (*Tachysurus australis*). *Australian Journal of Experimental Biology and Medical Science* 48, 515–523.

Donaldson, E. M. (1981). The pituitary–interrenal axis as an indicator of stress in fish. *In* "Stress and Fish" (Ed. A. D. Pickering), pp.11–48. Academic Press, London and New York.

Egusa, S. (1965). The existence of a primary infectious disease in the so-called "fungus disease" in pond-reared eels. *Bulletin of the Japanese Society of Scientific Fisheries* 31, 517–526.

Egusa, S. and Nishikawa, T. (1965). Studies of a primary infectious disease in the so-called fungus disease of eels. *Bulletin of the Japanese Society of Scientific Fisheries* 31, 804–813.

Ellis, A. E. (1981). Stress and the modulation of defence mechanisms in fish. *In* "Stress and Fish" (Ed. A. D. Pickering), pp.147–170. Academic Press, London and New York.

Fletcher, T. C. and Grant, P. T. (1968). Glycoproteins in the external mucous secretions of the plaice, *Pleuronectes platessa*, and other fishes. *Biochemical Journal* 106, 12P.

Fletcher, T. C. and Grant, P. T. (1969). Immunoglobulins in the serum and mucus of the plaice (*Pleuronectes platessa*). *Biochemical Journal* 115, 65P.

Fletcher, T. C. and White, A. (1973a). Lysozyme activity in the plaice (*Pleuronectes platessa* L.). *Experientia* 29, 1283–1285.

Fletcher, T. C. and White, A. (1973b). Antibody production in the plaice (*Pleuronectes platessa* L.) after oral and parenteral immunization with *Vibrio anguillarum* antigens. *Aquaculture* 1, 417–428.

Gardner, M. L. G. (1974). Impaired osmoregulation in infected salmon, *Salmo salar* L. *Journal of the Marine Biological Association of the United Kingdom* 54, 635–639.

Hane, S. and Robertson, O. H. (1959). Changes in plasma 17-hydroxycortico-steroids accompanying sexual maturation and spawning of the Pacific salmon (*Oncorhynchus tshawytscha*) and rainbow trout (*Salmo gairdneri*). *Proceedings of the National Academy of Sciences of the United States of America* 45, 886–893.

Harrell, L. W., Etlinger, H. M. and Hodgins, H. O. (1976). Humoral factors important in resistance of salmonid fish to bacterial disease. II. Anti-*Vibrio anguillarum* activity in mucus and observations on complement. *Aquaculture* 7, 363–370.

Heath, I. B. and Greenwood, A. D. (1970). Wall formation in the Saprolegniales II. Formation of cysts by the zoospores of *Saprolegnia* and *Dictyuchus*. *Archiv fur Microbiologie* **75**, 67–79.

Hodkinson, M. and Hunter, A. (1970). Immune response of UDN-infected salmon to *Saprolegnia*. *Journal of Fish Biology* **2**, 305–311.

Hoshina, T. and Ookubo, M. (1956). On a fungi-disease of eel. *Journal of the Tokyo University of Fisheries* **42**, 1–13.

Idler, D. R., Ronald, A. P. and Schmidt, P. J. (1959). Biochemical studies on sockeye salmon during spawning migration. VII. Steroid hormones in plasma. *Canadian Journal of Biochemistry and Physiology* **37**, 1227–1238.

Ingram, G. A. (1980). Substances involved in the natural resistance of fish to infection — a review. *Journal of Fish Biology* **15**, 23–61.

Kanouse, B. B. (1932). A physiological and morphological study of *Saprolegnia parasitica*. *Mycologia* **24**, 431–452.

Leivestad, H., Hendrey, G., Muniz, I. P. and Snekvik, E. (1976). Effects of acid precipitation on freshwater organisms. *Fagrapporter sur Nedors Virkning pa Skog og Fisk* **6**, 87–111.

Lewis, D. H. (1973). Concepts in fungal nutrition and the origin of biotrophy. *Biological Reviews* **48**, 261–278.

Manton, I., Clarke, B. and Greenwood, A. D. (1951). Observations with the electron microscope on a species of *Saprolegnia*. *Journal of Experimental Botany* **2**, 321–331.

Meier, H. and Webster, J. (1954). An electron microscope study of cysts in the Saprolegniaceae. *Journal of Experimental Botany* **5**, 401–409.

Neish, G. A. (1977). Observations on saprolegniasis of adult sockeye salmon, *Oncorhynchus nerka* (Walbaum). *Journal of Fish Biology* **10**, 513–522.

Neish, G. A. and Hughes, G. C. (1980). "Fungal Diseases in Fish". T. F. H. Publications, Inc., Ltd., New Jersey.

Nigrelli, R. F. (1935). On the effect of fish mucus on *Epibdella melleni* a monogenetic trematode of marine fishes. *Journal of Parasitology* **21**, 438.

Nolard-Tintigner, N. (1973). Etude experimentale sur l'epidemiologie et la pathogenie de la Saprolegniose chez *Lebistes reticulatus* Peters et *Xiphophorus helleri* Heckel. *Acta Zoologica et Pathologica Antverpiensia* **57**, 1–127.

Paling, J. E. (1965). The population dynamics of the monogenean gill parasite *Discocotyle sagittata* Leuckart on Windermere trout, *Salmo trutta* L. *Parasitology* **55**, 667–694.

Peduzzi, R. and Bizzozero, S. (1977). Immunochemical investigation of four *Saprolegnia* species with parasitic activity in fish: Serological and kinetic characterization of a chymotrypsin-like activity. *Microbial Ecology* **3**, 107–119.

Peduzzi, R., Nolard-Tintigner, N. and Bizzozero, S. (1976). Recherches sur la Saprolegniose. II. Etude du processus de penetration, mise en evidence d'une enzyme proteolytique et aspect histopathologique. *Revista Italiana di Piscicoltura e Ittiopatologia* **11**, 109–117.

Phillips, J. G., Holmes, W. N. and Bondy, P. K. (1959). Adrenocorticosteroids in salmon plasma (*Oncorhynchus nerka*). *Endocrinology* **65**, 811–818.

Pickering, A. D. (1977). Seasonal changes in the epidermis of the brown trout *Salmo trutta* (L.). *Journal of Fish Biology* **10**, 561–566.

Pickering, A. D. (Ed.) (1981). "Stress and Fish". Academic Press, London and New York.

Pickering, A. D. and Christie, P. (1980). Sexual differences in the incidence and severity of ectoparasitic infestation of the brown trout, *Salmo trutta* L. *Journal of Fish Biology* **16**, 669–683.

Pickering, A. D. and Christie, P. (1981). Changes in the concentrations of plasma cortisol and thyroxine during sexual maturation of the hatchery-reared brown trout, *Salmo trutta* L. *General and Comparative Endocrinology* **44**, 487–496.

Pickering, A. D. and Richards, R. H. (1980). Factors influencing the structure, function and biota of the salmonid epidermis. *Proceedings of the Royal Society of Edinburgh* **79B**, 93–104.

Pickering, A. D. and Willoughby, L. G. (1977). Epidermal lesions and fungal infection on the perch, *Perca fluviatilis* L., in Windermere. *Journal of Fish Biology* **11**, 349–354.

Pickering, A. D., Willoughby, L. G. and McGrory, C. B. (1979). Fine structure of secondary zoospore cyst cases of *Saprolegnia* isolates from infected fish. *Transactions of the British Mycological Society* **72**, 427–436.

Richards, R. H. and Pickering, A. D. (1978). Frequency and distribution patterns of *Saprolegnia* infection in wild and hatchery-reared brown trout *Salmo trutta* L. and char *Salvelinus alpinus* (L.). *Journal of Fish Diseases* **1**, 69–82.

Richards, R. H. and Pickering, A. D. (1979). Changes in serum parameters of *Saprolegnia*-infected brown trout, *Salmo trutta* L. *Journal of Fish Diseases* **2**, 197–206.

Roberts, R. J., Shearer, W. M., Munro, A. L. S. and Elson, K. G. R. (1970). Studies on ulcerative dermal necrosis of salmonids. II. The sequential pathology of the lesions. *Journal of Fish Biology* **2**, 373–378.

Robertson, O. H., Hane, S., Wexler, B. C. and Rinfret, A. P. (1963). The effect of hydrocortisone on immature rainbow trout (*Salmo gairdneri*). *General and Comparative Endocrinology* **3**, 422–436.

Roth, R. R. (1972). Some factors contributing to the development of fungus infection in freshwater fish. *Journal of Wildlife Diseases* **8**, 24–28.

Scott, W. W. and O'Bier, A. H. (1962). Aquatic fungi associated with diseased fish and fish eggs. *Progressive Fish-Culturist* **24**, 3–15.

Snieszko, S. F. (1974). The effects of environmental stress on outbreaks of infectious diseases of fish. *Journal of Fish Biology* **6**, 197–209.

Stuart, M. R. and Fuller, H. T. (1968). Mycological aspects of diseased Atlantic salmon. *Nature, London* **217**, 90–92.

Tiffney, W. N. (1939a). The identity of certain species of the Saprolegniaceae parasitic to fish. *Journal of the Elisha Mitchell Scientific Society* **55**, 134–151.

Tiffney, W. N. (1939b). The host range of *Saprolegnia parasitica*. *Mycologia* **31**, 310–321.

Vishniac, H. S. and Nigrelli, R. F. (1957). The ability of the Saprolegniaceae to parasitize platyfish. *Zoologica* **42**, 131–135.

White, D. A. (1975). Ecology of an annual *Saprolegnia* sp. (Phycomycete) outbreak in wild brown trout. *Verhandlungen der Internationalen Vereinigung fur Theoretische und Angewandte Limnologie, Stuttgart* **19**, 2456–2460.

Willoughby, L. G. (1962). The occurrence and distribution of reproductive spores of Saprolegniales in fresh water. *Journal of Ecology* **50**, 733–759.

Willoughby, L. G. (1968). Atlantic salmon disease fungus. *Nature, London* **217**, 872–873.

Willoughby, L. G. (1969). Salmon disease in Windermere and the River Leven; the fungal aspect. *Salmon and Trout Magazine* **186**, 124–130.

Willoughby, L. G. (1970). Mycological aspects of a disease of young perch in Windermere. *Journal of Fish Biology* **2**, 113–116.

Willoughby, L. G. (1971). Observations on fungal parasites of Lake District Salmonids. *Salmon and Trout Magazine* **192**, 152–158.

Willoughby, L. G. (1972). U.D.N. of Lake District trout and char: outward signs of infection and defence barriers examined further. *Salmon and Trout Magazine* **195**, 149–158.

Willoughby, L. G. (1977). An abbreviated life cycle in the salmonid fish *Saprolegnia*. *Transactions of the British Mycological Society* **69**, 133–135.

Willoughby, L. G. (1978). Saprolegnias of salmonid fish in Windermere: a critical analysis. *Journal of Fish Diseases* **1**, 51–67.

Willoughby, L. G. and Copland, J. W. (1982). Temperature-growth relationships in *Saprolegnia* pathogens of fish, especially eels grown in warm water. *Transactions of the British Mycological Society* (in press).

Willoughby, L. G. and Pickering, A. D. (1977). Viable Saprolegniaceae spores on the epidermis of the salmonid fish *Salmo trutta* and *Salvelinus alpinus*. *Transactions of the British Mycological Society* **68**, 91–95.

Willoughby, L. G., McGrory, C. B. and Pickering, A. D. (1982). Zoospore germination in *Saprolegnia* pathogens of fish. *Transactions of the British Mycological Society* (in press).

Wilson, J. G. M. (1976). Immunological aspects of fungal disease in fish. *In* "Recent Advances in Aquatic Mycology" (Ed. E. B. G. Jones), pp.573–601. Elek Science, London.

Wolke, R. E. (1975). Pathology of bacterial and fungal diseases affecting fish. *In* "The Pathology of Fishes" (Eds W. E. Ribelin and G. Migaki), pp.33–116. The University of Wisconsin Press, Madison, Wisconsin.

Index

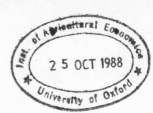